Color Atlas and Synopsis of Pigmented Lesions

Notice

Medicine is an ever-changing science. As new research and clinical experience broaden our knowledge, changes in treatment and drug therapy are required. The authors and the publisher of this work have checked with sources believed to be reliable in their efforts to provide information that is complete and generally in accord with the standards accepted at the time of publication. However, in view of the possibility of human error or changes in medical sciences, neither the authors nor the publisher nor any other party who has been involved in the preparation or publication of this work warrants that the information contained herein is in every respect accurate or complete, and they are not responsible for any errors or omissions or for the results obtained from use of such information. Readers are encouraged to confirm the information contained herein with other sources. For example and in particular, readers are advised to check the product information sheet included in the package of each drug they plan to administer to be certain that the information contained in this book is accurate and that changes have not been made in the recommended dose or in the contraindications for administration. This recommendation is of particular importance in connection with new or infrequently used drugs.

Color Atlas and Synopsis of Pigmented Lesions

The Pigmented Lesion Clinic,
Massachusetts General Hospital:
A Perspective of Three Decades, 1965 – 1995

Raymond L. Barnhill, M.D.
Associate Professor of Pathology
Harvard Medical School
Director of Dermatopathology
Brigham and Women's Hospital
Boston, Massachusetts

Thomas B. Fitzpatrick, M.D., Ph.D., D.Sc. (Hon)
Edward C. Wigglesworth Professor of Dermatology, Emeritus
Chairman Emeritus, Department of Dermatology
Harvard Medical School
Chief Emeritus, Dermatology Service
Massachusetts General Hospital
Boston, Massachusetts

Katrin Fandrey, M.D.
Staedtische Dermatology Clinic
Dortmund, Germany

Robert O. Kenet, M.D., Ph.D.
Department of Medicine
Cornell University Medical College
The American Melanoma Foundation
New York, New York

Martin C. Mihm, Jr., M.D.
Chief of Dermatology and Dermatopathology
Albany Medical College, Albany, New York

Arthur J. Sober, M.D.
Associate Professor of Dermatology
Harvard Medical School, Boston, Massachusetts

McGraw-Hill, Inc.
Health Professions Division

New York • St. Louis • San Francisco • Auckland • Bogotá • Caracas • Lisbon
London • Madrid • Mexico City • Milan • Montreal • New Delhi
San Juan • Singapore • Sydney • Tokyo • Toronto

ISBN 0070051100

Copyright © 1995 by McGraw-Hill, Inc. All rights reserved. Printed in the United States of America. Except as permitted under the United States Copyright Act of 1976, no part of this publication may be reproduced or distributed in any form or by any means, or stored in a data base or retrieval system, without the prior written permission of the publisher.

1 2 3 4 5 6 7 8 9 0 KGP KGP 9 8 7 6 5

ISBN 0-07-005110-0

This book was set in Times Roman by York Graphic Services, Inc. The editors were Dereck Jeffers and Peter McCurdy; the cover designer was Michele Cooper. Phil James prepared the index. Quebecor/Kingsport was printer and binder.

This book is printed on acid-free paper.

*This atlas is dedicated
to our patients,
past, present, future.*

Contents

Preface   ix

Introduction   xi

  Introduction   1
  Chapter 1.   Approach to Clinical Diagnosis   3
  Chapter 2.   Risk-Stratification of Pigmented Lesions Using Clinical Histomorphology (Epiluminescence Microscopy)   15

Section I. Benign Pigmented Lesions   28
  Chapter 3.   Ephelides   29
  Chapter 4.   Café-au-lait Macules   33
  Chapter 5.   Becker's Melanosis   39
  Chapter 6.   Solar Lentigo   43
  Chapter 7.   Lentigo Simplex and Mucosal Melanotic Lesions   53
  Chapter 8.   Mongolian Spot   65
  Chapter 9.   Nevus of Ota and Related Conditions   69
  Chapter 10.   Blue Nevus and its Variants   75
  Chapter 11.   Common Acquired Melanocytic Nevi   83
  Chapter 12.   Halo Nevus   95
  Chapter 13.   Nevus Spilus   100
  Chapter 14.   Segmental Lentiginosis   105

Section II. Difficult Diagnostic Lesions   107
  Chapter 15.   Recurrent Melanocytic Nevus   109
  Chapter 16.   Spindle and Epithelioid Cell Nevus   113
  Chapter 17.   Pigmented Spindle Cell Nevus   117

Section III. Precursors to Primary Melanoma of the Skin
  Chapter 18.   Dysplastic Melanocytic Nevus   123
  Chapter 19.   Congenital Melanocytic Nevus   135

Section IV. Cutaneous Malignant Melanoma   145
  Chapter 20.   Lentigo Maligna and Lentigo Maligna/Melanoma   153

Chapter 21.	Superficial Spreading Melanoma	163
Chapter 22.	Nodular Melanoma	177
Chapter 23.	Acral Lentiginous Melanoma	187
Chapter 24.	Desmoplastic Melanoma	199
Chapter 25.	Mucocutaneous Melanoma	205
Chapter 26.	Unusual Presentations of Melanoma Including Metastatic Melanoma	211

Section V. Nonmelanocytic Pigmented Lesions Entering into the Differential Diagnosis of Melanoma   223

Chapter 27.	Seborrheic Keratosis	225
Chapter 28.	Pyogenic Granuloma	231
Chapter 29.	Sclerosing Hemangioma Variant of Fibrous Histiocytoma	233
Chapter 30.	Angiokeratoma	235
Chapter 31.	Pigmented Basal Cell Carcinoma	241

Index   245

Preface

Several trends make the publication of this atlas timely. The incidence of melanoma has been increasing progressively and dramatically since 1940. It is now one of the most common cancers diagnosed in late adolescence and in young adults. Because of the visual nature of the tumor, it is accessible to the trained eye for diagnosis. Early intervention leads to cure. Since the individuals involved are younger than cancer patients in general, the number of useful years saved is impressive.

Under the new managed health care systems, more health care professionals need to be aware of the clinical features of melanoma and its precursors in order to recognize them early in their course. Not only does the dermatologist well versed in diagnosis need to be capable of recognizing melanoma, so also does the primary care practitioner, such as the general physician, nurse practitioner, and physician assistant.

A newer diagnostic technique covered in this monograph, epiluminescence microscopy, is an addition to the classical techniques for the recognition of suspicious pigmented lesions, and may prove of value in assisting practitioners to distinguish suspicious from non-suspicious lesions. This may translate into a reduction of unnecessary biopsies, which in turn leads to an improvement in the cost effective delivery of care. It is our hope that this atlas will assist the practitioner in the recognition of potential melanomas and thereby save lives.

Introduction

In the early 1960s, one of us (TBF) became interested in the clinical aspects of cutaneous melanoma and began to examine primary melanomas with the Zeiss binocular dermatoscope. Two principal features were noted in early melanoma: variegation of color and irregular borders and especially the gray-blue hue, which was recognized as a distinctive marker for early melanoma. Dr. Wallace Clark, a dermatopathologist, subsequently came to Boston in 1967, and joined TBF, a dermatologist, and the late Dr. John Raker, a surgeon, in establishing the Pigmented Lesion Clinic (PLC) at the Massachusetts General Hospital. It was the first in the world of its kind. Dr. Martin C. Mihm, Jr., at that time a fellow in dermatopathology, joined the new PLC group. Soon after the PLC was started, a "new" tumor type was identified. This melanoma had the clinical features of lentigo maligna melanoma (LMM)—variegation of color and areas of regression—yet this newly discovered lesion was smaller. Although it contained nodules, as did LMM, it was not a macule overall but was instead distinctly raised throughout, i.e., it was a plaque. Clark studied the histologic features of this plaque (or the "surround" portion if a nodule was present) and noted an unusual feature: the abnormal melanocytes invaded the epidermis throughout, in the manner of Paget's disease, and were not confined to the basal cell layer as is typical of LMM. The identification of this "new" cutaneous melanoma by Wallace H. Clark, Jr. was a milestone in the development of our knowledge of the biology of melanoma. Almost simultaneously the late Dr. Vincent McGovern of Australia described the same lesion, calling it *precancerous melanosis*. Clark then later devised a new classification of melanoma, calling the newly described lesion *superficial spreading melanoma*.

The description of early primary melanoma of the skin has been the major factor responsible for the striking improvement in survival of patients with cutaneous melanoma, inasmuch as the prognosis is related to the thickness of the primary tumor. Earlier detection has also resulted in less radical surgery being needed for cure. Our strategy over the past two decades has been to spread the gospel of early detection of melanoma, first to our colleagues and more recently by education of the general public: melanoma is a potentially dangerous, relatively common cancer that can be cured if detected early.

In the spring of 1991, a patient whom we had followed on a regular basis for management of basal cell carcinomas on the back, who had not been seen for three years, was urged by his wife to seek medical attention for a new pigmented lesion on his upper back. This was in fact a primary superficial spreading melanoma, 0.9 mm in thickness. This gentleman was distraught about the lesion. He telephoned every day until the tumor was reviewed by one of our dermatopathologists with expertise in the pathology of melanocytic lesions. But we were able to give him some encouraging news based on our knowledge of prognostic factors for melanoma, such as the large series of melanoma cases followed for eight years recently reported by Wallace Clark and his colleagues; the data were analyzed not only for thickness of the lesion but also for the number of mitoses, the site of the tumor, the extent of tumor infiltrating lymphocytes, the presence or absence of regression, and the patient's gender. We could reassure this patient that the eight-year survival rate was over 80 percent.

This patient illustrates the benefits of early detection of melanoma and application of new knowledge about prognosis developed over the past two decades. Prior to the description of early melanoma, this patient's lesion would not have been suspected until it had become large or ulcerated. Furthermore and most importantly, his wife would not have been aware of suspicious pigmented spots if not for the extensive educational programs that are now in place.

Until very recently, a large fraction of physicians did not carefully examine the skin in a general physical examination—they listened to the heart, recorded blood pressure, palpated lymph nodes and abdomen, inspected the mouth and ears, and examined the rectum for rectal and prostatic carcinomas, but the skin was simply not considered of great importance in the general physical examination. Most general physicians now scrutinize the skin for suspicious pigmented lesions because they have learned that primary melanoma of the skin is a serious malignancy whose prognosis they may influence by early detection. It is then in a curable stage of its evolution.

This atlas and synopsis is an attempt to convey what we have learned about the clinical features of pigmented lesions over the past three decades. The single most significant accomplishment of the PLC has been the description of the early stages of cutaneous melanoma. This alerted health professionals that melanoma of the skin can be cured if it is detected early and that this now common cancer is one serious malignancy that can be diagnosed by a single noninvasive technique—examination of the skin with the naked eye by informed and experienced observers, this is to say, by all health professionals.

Color Atlas and Synopsis of Pigmented Lesions

Introduction

1. Approach to Clinical Diagnosis

As with other areas of medicine, the evaluation and management of melanocytic lesions of the skin are essentially an exercise in obtaining a directed clinical history and careful clinical examination, with a few additional techniques contributing to diagnosis. In this section the essential steps in clinical diagnosis of melanocytic lesions will be outlined (Table 1-1).

CLINICAL HISTORY

One of the immediate goals of the clinical history should be to establish whether and to what extent the patient is at risk for malignant melanoma (Tables 1-2 to 1-4). A knowledge of risk factors for melanoma and success in obtaining such relevant information from patients are critical for a thorough assessment of the patient (Table 1-2). Thus the clinical history should include inquiries as to personal or family history of melanoma and/or atypical moles, a new or recently changing pigmented lesion, immunosuppression as from organ transplantation or lymphoma, and history of severe sunburns, sun sensitivity, or excessive sun exposure.

Perhaps the most common clinical problem associated with pigmented lesions is a new or changing lesion (see Table 1-1). The physician's clinical history should attempt to establish how long the lesion has

Table 1-1 Guidelines for Clinical Diagnosis of Cutaneous Melanoma

Clinical history directed toward risk factors for melanoma
    Duration of lesion in question
    Duration of changes, if any
    Specific changes
Family history of melanoma or dysplastic nevi
Total-body skin examination
    Assessment of pigmentary characteristics and nevus phenotype
    Hair color
    Skin phototype
    Freckling tendency
    Estimation of number of nevi on skin surface
    Estimation of presence and number of clinically atypical nevi
    Assessment of individual gross morphologic features of individual nevi for presence of atypical features
    Use of sidelighting, as needed
    Use of Wood's lamp, as needed

Table 1-2 Risk Factors for Cutaneous Melanoma

FACTOR	ESTIMATED RELATIVE RISK*
Changing pigmented lesion	Very high
Xeroderma pigmentosum	500
FAMM† kindred: prior melanoma	500
FAMM kindred: atypical nevi but no prior melanoma	150
Numerous common nevi	5–65
Atypical nevi	7–20
Giant congenital nevus	5–15
Previous melanoma	9
Lentigo maligna	5–10
Immunosuppression	4–7
Red or blond hair	2–7
Tendency to freckle	2–4
Sun sensitivity	2–3
Excessive sun exposures	2–4
Melanoma in first-degree relative	2–12
Few or no common nevi	0.3
Asian, Hispanic, or African-American persons	0.08–0.15
Age <15 years	0.01

*Average = risk 1. Estimates derived from bibliography

†FAMM = familial atypical mole melanoma

SOURCE: Adapted from Williams ML, Sagebiel RW: Melanoma risk factors and atypical moles. *West J Med* 160:343, 1994.

Table 1-3 Five Steps in Assessing the Risk of Melanoma

CHECKLIST FOR DETECTING HIGH-RISK PERSONS

1. Carefully question the patient for family history of melanoma or atypical nevi.
2. Question the patient regarding personal history of sun exposure.
   (a) Does he or she burn easily, never tan, or tan poorly (skin phototypes I and II)?
   (b) Did he or she ever have a severe sunburn in childhood or adolescence?
3. Assess the total number of all types of moles.
4. Search for dysplastic melanocytic nevi.
5. Search for congenital melanocytic nevi.

Table 1-4 Stratification of Risk for Development of Cutaneous Melanoma

Greatly elevated risk:
  Changing mole
  Dysplastic nevi in familial melanoma
  >50 nevi ≥2 mm
Moderately elevated risk:
  One family member with melanoma
  History of prior melanoma
  Sporadic dysplastic nevi
  Congenital nevus
Slightly elevated risk:
  Immunosuppression
  Sun sensitivity
  Severe sunburns
  Freckling
Lower than average risk:
  Children <10 years
  African-Americans, Asians, Native Americans, dark-complexioned
    Caucasians

SOURCE: Adapted from Rhodes AR et al: Risk factors for cutaneous melanoma: A practical method of recognizing predisposed individuals. *JAMA* 258:3146, 1987.

been present, over what interval of time the lesion has been changing, and the specifics of how the lesion has changed. The development of a new melanocytic lesion, particularly one greater than 5 to 6 mm in diameter in a patient beyond the age of 30 to 40 years, is of concern and is a valid indication for consideration of biopsy. In general, changes in melanocytic lesions that are of significance take place over weeks or usually months. Change occurring over a matter of days and then stopping is usually secondary to trauma or inflammation. A persistently changing lesion has been established as one of the principal signs suggesting development of melanoma. Also, the nature of the change should be documented. Changes in size, i.e., increase in area or elevation, development of an irregular border, changes in color (either darkening or lightening), crusting, bleeding, and the presence of tenderness, pain, or itching are signs and symptoms associated with melanoma (Table 1-5). It should be emphasized that not all changing lesions can be ascribed to trauma, inflammation, or malignant transformation. Gradual enlargement or change in color may occur with an individual's growth or puberty. Enlargement and darkening of moles (melanocytic nevi) may occur normally in pregnancy. Finally, sun exposure may produce darkening or occasional development of new moles.

The physician should attempt to verify whether moles usually greater than 1 to 1.5 cm in greatest diameter are congenital (present at birth) and thus possibly associated with somewhat greater risk for development of melanoma compared with ordinary acquired nevi. Congenital onset of nevi can sometimes be corroborated by perinatal photographs, if available.

FAMILY HISTORY

Individuals who are being evaluated for cutaneous melanocytic lesions should be questioned regarding history of melanoma, atypical moles, or congenital nevi in blood relatives. The presence of a family history of melanoma confers on blood relatives an increased risk for melanoma (see Table 1-2).

EXAMINATION OF SKIN

In general, all individuals should be offered a total-body skin examination, including scalp, genitalia, intertriginous areas, and interdigital spaces. The examination should be conducted in a brightly lit room. Natural light or a halogen light source is optimal for assessment of color. A mobile or hand-held light source is also useful for sidelighting individual lesions to assess surface topography (see below).

A Wood's lamp (black light, source of long-wave ultraviolet light) may be employed to accentuate epidermal hyper- or hypopigmentation, as, for example, in lentigo maligna, halo nevus, or regression of a melanocytic lesion. Other useful instruments include a hand-held magnifying lens or loupe and a ruler for recording sizes of pigmented lesions. (See also Chap. 2.)

ASSESSMENT OF GROSS MORPHOLOGIC FEATURES

General Assessment of Risk Factors for Melanoma: Pigmentary Characteristics and Nevus Pattern

One of the most important aspects of the skin examination is an initial global appraisal of the individual's risk factors for melanoma, i.e., pigmentary characteristics and nevus phenotype. This general assessment enables one to gauge the individual's general risk for melanoma as low, intermediate, or high. Of particular significance is a general assessment of nevus phenotype, i.e., overall number of nevi on

Table 1-5 Percentage of Patients Presenting with Particular Signs and Symptoms by Primary Tumor Thickness*

Thickness (mm)	<0.85	0.85–1.69	1.70–3.64	≥3.65
Size change	55	49	51	72
Color change	49	47	45	58
Elevation	36	51	59	82
Bleeding	13	25	48	63
Ulcer	5	15	33	50
Tenderness	8	7	14	19
Itching	20	30	29	46

*Values represent percentage manifesting the presence of symptom or increase in sign.

SOURCE: From Sober AJ et al: Detection of "thin" primary melanomas. CA 33:160, 1983.

the skin surface and whether they are "normal" or clinically unusual or atypical. Such an assessment is probably best accomplished by observing the undressed patient from across the room. The reason that the latter evaluation is so important is that both quantitative and qualitative abnormalities of nevi have been established as among the most important risk factors for melanoma (Tables 1-6 and 1-7). Although absolute figures are not available, melanoma risk is probably directly related to total number of ordinary nevi on the skin surface. As detailed in Table 1-8, as general guidelines, most individuals have fewer than 25 normal moles. More than 50 nevi is considered excessive and is associated with elevated melanoma risk.

Independent of number of nevi, clinically abnormal ("dysplastic") nevi are also associated with increased melanoma risk (see Table 1-7). Although at present there are no minimum criteria for what constitutes an abnormal or clinically atypical nevus, such nevi, in general, are characterized by larger size (>6 mm, but not always), irregular and ill-defined borders, and increasingly complex patterns of pigmentation/color. In reality, there is a continuum that encompasses "normal" nevi, clinically "atypical" nevi, and melanoma, with progressively abnormal attributes as outlined in Table 1-9.

In addition to appraising numbers and features of nevi, the examiner should make note of other pigmentary characteristics as-

Table 1-6 Relative Risk of Melanoma in Relation to Numbers of Benign Nevi

STUDY	COUNTRY	NEVUS DEFINITION	NEVUS COUNTS	RELATIVE RISK
Holly et al.	U.S.	≥2 mm, whole body "nondysplastic"	11–25	1.6
			26–50	4.4
			51–100	5.4
			>100	9.8
Weiss et al.	Germany	"Benign" nevi	10–50	4.3
			>50	15
Krüger et al.	Germany	≥2 mm, trunk (males)	5–10	2.9
			11–20	5.5
			>20	33
			>40	133
Swerdlow and Green	Scotland	≥2 mm, whole body	10–24	4.4
			25–49	8.7
			≥50	64
Green et al.	Australia	≥2 mm, left arm	2–4	16
			5–10	15
			>10	20

SOURCE: Adapted from Williams ML, Sagebiel RW: Melanoma risk factors and atypical moles. *West J Med* 160:343, 1994.

Table 1-7 Melanoma Risk Associated with Clinically Atypical (Dysplastic) Nevi: Comparison of Occurrence in Melanoma Patients vs Controls

STUDY	COUNTRY	DEFINITION	1 OR MORE DYSPLASTIC NEVI (%)		RELATIVE RISK
			MELANOMA PATIENTS	CONTROLS	
Roush et al. and Nordlund et al.	Australia	>5 mm, irregular border, and haphazard pigmentation	34%	7%	7.7
MacKie et al.	Scotland	>5 mm and either irregular borders, irregular pigmentation, or inflammation	38%	20%	2.1–4.5*
Holly et al.	U.S.	At least 3 of 6 criteria: ill-defined border, irregular border, irregular pigmentation, >5 mm, erythema, accentuated skin markings	55%	17%	3.8–6.3†
Halpern et al.	U.S.	>4 mm, macular component, variegation of color, and irregular or indistinct border	39%	7%	8.8
Garbe et al.	West Germany	At least 3 of 5 criteria: >5 mm, irregular margins, ill-defined border, color variation, macular and papular components	45%	5%	7

*Relative risks for one or two atypical nevi, 2.1; for three or more atypical nevi, 4.5.
†Relative risks for one to five atypical nevi, 3.8; for six or more atypical nevi, 6.3.

SOURCE: Adapted from Williams ML, Sagebiel RW: Melanoma risk factors and atypical moles. *West J Med* 160:343, 1994.

sociated with elevated (generally low relative risk) melanoma risk (see Table 1-2): red or blond hair, blue or green eyes, very fair skin (skin phototype I or II, "Celtic" skin type) (Table 1-10), and freckling tendency.

For purposes of risk assessment, the general impression of nevus phenotype should be recorded, e.g., 0 to 25, 25 to 50, >50, >100 normal nevi and presence and number of clinically atypical nevi (size >6 mm, irregular borders, haphazard color).

Table 1-8 Nevus Phenotypes

	NORMAL NEVUS PATTERN	ABNORMAL NEVUS PHENOTYPE
Number	None to few (<25) nevi	Many (>50) nevi
Size	<5 mm	Variable: small to large, often several >5 mm
Color/borders	Uniform or homogeneous color, well-circumscribed	Some to many nevi with irregular or haphazard color, erythema, irregular or ill-defined borders

SOURCE: Adapted from Williams ML, Sagebiel RW: Melanoma risk factors and atypical moles. *West J Med* 160:343, 1994.

Table 1-9 Clinical Characteristics of Common Acquired Nevi, Dysplastic Nevi, and Malignant Melanoma

CHARACTERISTIC	COMMON ACQUIRED NEVI	DYSPLASTIC NEVI	MALIGNANT MELANOMA
Size	<5–6 mm	4–12 mm	Usually >10 mm
Border	Regular Well defined	Irregular Ill defined	More irregular Ill defined
Symmetry	Symmetry	Asymmetry	Greater asymmetry
Coloration	Homogeneous Regular	Haphazard	Haphazard (More complexity)
Colors	Tan, brown, dark brown, flesh	Tan, brown, dark brown, black, pink	Tan, brown, dark brown, black, pink, red, gray, blue, white
Surface	Usually papular	Macular component	Macular, raised, nodular
Skin markings	Accentuated	Accentuated, "pebbling"	Accentuation, obliteration, ulceration

Table 1-10 Classification of Various Human Skin Phototypes

RESPONSE TO SHORT SUN EXPOSURE IN RELATION TO SKIN COLOR
OF THE UNEXPOSED SKIN (BUTTOCKS)

A. Pure white, white, and beige skin color
Skin phototype I	Pure white	Tender sunburn, no tan
Skin phototype II	Pure white	Tender sunburn, light tan
Skin phototype III	White	Nontender sunburn, dark tan
Skin phototype IV	Beige	No sunburn, dark tan

B. Brown skin color
Skin phototype V		No sunburn, dark tan

C. Black skin color
Skin phototype VI		No sunburn, dark tan

NOTE: The original scientific paper in which this classification was first introduced was Fitzpatrick TB: Soleil et peau. *J Med Esthet* 2(7):33, 1975.

Assessment of Gross Morphologic Features of Individual Pigmented Lesions (Table 1-11)

SYMMETRY The overall symmetry of a melanocytic lesion is one of its most important attributes. Benign melanocytic lesions such as lentigines or benign nevi tend to have an overall orderliness, whereas increasingly atypical lesions such as dysplastic nevi and melanoma are progressively more asymmetric (see Table 1-9). However, there are exceptions, such as some nodular melanomas, which may be symmetric in appearance.

SIZE The dimensions of a melanocytic proliferation provide one of the best correlates with atypicality. The size of a lesion should be recorded along two axes: greatest diameter (length) and width. In general, benign lesions are relatively small, usually 6 mm or less in diameter, while increasing size is generally associated with a greater likelihood of atypia (see Table 1-9). Simple lentigines (as contrasted with solar lentigines) usually measure about 2 to 3 mm, junctional nevi approximately 3 to 5 mm, and compound and dermal nevi 3 to 6 mm. Dysplastic nevi range from 4 to 12 mm or larger. Melanonychia striata (pigmented bands in finger- or toenails) generally should not exceed 6 mm in breadth. Exceptions to these generalizations may be observed.

Melanomas are usually greater than 10 mm in longest diameter. The dimensions vary among the different subtypes of melanoma. Lentigo maligna melanomas may be as large as 10 cm, while nodular melanomas average about 1 cm but may be as small as 4 to 5 mm.

BORDER CHARACTERISTICS Benign melanocytic lesions are characterized by regular and well-defined borders. Perifollicular hypopigmentation in melanocytic nevi may occasionally result in some irregularity of borders. Dysplastic nevi may exhibit some degree of irregularity of borders and may have ill-defined or "hazy" margins. Melanomas are likely to have more irregular, notched, or scalloped borders. Paradoxically, under epiluminescence microscopic examination, the pigment pattern of melanomas ends abruptly (see Chap. 2).

SURFACE PROFILE The degree to which a melanocytic lesion is completely flat (macular) or raised (papular) may be evaluated by gentle palpation or by side (tangential) lighting. Freckles, café au lait spots, lentigines, and junctional nevi are macular, while compound and dermal nevi are papular (see below). The ill-defined peripheral zones of some dysplastic nevi, however, may be macular. Lentigo maligna is usually completely flat, whereas virtually all melanomas have surface elevation. In general, advanced melanomas are characterized by dome-shaped, polypoid, or ulcerated nodules.

SURFACE TOPOGRAPHY The technique of directing a stream of light tangentially across a pigmented lesion is used to assess surface markings. The lentigo simplex is associated with no distortion of skin cleavage lines, while nevi with junctional components generally have accentuated skin markings. Dysplastic nevi may have a "cobblestone" or pebbled appearance when studied with tangential lighting. Obliteration or loss of skin markings may occur with melanoma. Scaling, crusting, and ulceration also may be associated with development of melanoma. Congenital nevi may exhibit a pebbled, "pigskin," or rugose surface. Finger- or toenail deformity associated with nail pigmentation should alert one to the possibility of early subungual melanoma.

COLORATION Evaluation of color is one of the most important aspects of clinical diagnosis of melanocytic lesions. Attention should be given to the overall symmetry or regularity of color and to the number of colors present. In general, the color pattern in melanocytic lesions encompasses a large spectrum from a uniform one-color appearance typical of benign nevi to a complex, chaotic admixture of several colors as found in most melanomas. Lentigines and junctional or compound nevi are frequently characterized by a homogeneous shade of tan, brown, or dark

---

Table 1-11 Gross Morphologic Features Assessed in Melanocytic Lesions*

Symmetry
Size, in mm (length and width)
Border characteristics
    Regular or irregular
    Well-defined or ill-defined
Macular, papular, or both
Surface topography
    Accentuation or obliteration of skin cleavage lines, pebbling, ulceration, crusting
Coloration

---

*The ABCDE system for recognizing early melanoma utilizes these characteristics in the mnemonic Asymmetry, Border irregularity, Color (haphazard or variegated), Diameter (greater than 6 mm), and Enlargement (history of increase in size).

brown. Perifollicular hypopigmentation in nevi with an otherwise uniform color may produce a somewhat variegate pattern. Dysplastic nevi frequently have two or more colors in regular or irregular distribution. Melanomas demonstrate complexity and disorder of coloration. In addition to various shades of brown, there may be an admixture of red, gray, white, blue, pink, and black. Foci of gray and white usually correlate with regression. The presence of blue-black is particularly suggestive of melanoma. It should be emphasized that the development of a black area, particularly an asymmetric one, within any melanocytic lesion is suspicious for melanoma.

As would be expected, there are exceptions to these guidelines concerning color pattern. Some nodular melanomas are amelanotic, or flesh-colored, whereas others have a uniform color. Occasionally, lentigo maligna melanoma may be amelanotic. The biopsy of these lesions often carries a "rule out basal cell carcinoma" diagnosis.

In general, color correlates with location (or absence) of melanin in the skin. The color black generally indicates melanin in the stratum corneum (upper epidermis). Brown correlates with lower epidermal or papillary dermal pigment, whereas shades of blue correspond to melanin in the deeper (reticular) dermis. Gray to white indicates loss or absence of melanin. Pink and red are related to prominent vascularity and inflammation.

The ABCDE System for Recognizing Early Melanoma This mnemonic was introduced in the United States in an effort to familiarize primary care physicians and the lay public with the cardinal features of early melanoma. The various characteristics outlined in Table 1-11 were discussed above.

Other Ancillary Techniques for Evaluating Melanocytic Lesions

SIDELIGHTING This technique entails directing a beam of light obliquely across the lesion being examined, as already mentioned. The procedure is useful for several reasons. First of all, the examiner is able to determine the degree to which the lesion is macular, papular, or both. This may be helpful because certain lesions are characteristically macular, such as lentigines and junctional nevi, while others are papular, such as compound nevi. This technique can reveal not only surface flatness or elevation but also the extent to which the skin markings of a melanocytic lesion are altered, distorted, or perhaps obliterated. Sidelighting of flat lesions can distinguish melanocytic nevi from lentigines and other lesions such as café au lait macules: nevi have accentuated skin markings versus no alteration in these other lesions. Furthermore, dysplastic nevi may have an even more exaggerated surface, resulting in a so-called cobblestone or pebbled appearance. Congenital nevi also may have a pebbled, "pigskin," or rugose surface texture. Papillomatous nevi and, occasionally, melanomas can exhibit keratinous excrescences or a verrucoid appearance, mimicking seborrheic keratoses.

A feature suggestive of melanoma is loss of surface markings. Scaling, ulceration, and crusts also may be present in melanoma. Dermal nevi also may demonstrate diminished surface markings.

EXAMINATION WITH WOOD'S LAMP The Wood's lamp (black-ray) is a mercury vapor lamp that has an emission spectrum in the long-wave ultraviolet region (340 to 450 nm with a peak at 365 nm). Examination of the skin with a Wood's lamp can be helpful in accentuating differences in epidermal but not dermal pigmentation. Thus use of the lamp may better define the extent of hypermelanotic lesions such as lentigo maligna and the radial growth of other subtypes of melanoma. Such evaluation can be useful for determining the configuration and dimensions of a lesion. Evaluating the loss of pigmentation with the Wood's lamp is equally valuable. This instrument may enhance areas of hypopigmentation indicative of regression or reveal a surrounding band (or "halo") of diminished pigmentation. One circumstance in which use of the Wood's lamp is almost essential is examination of a patient with metastatic melanoma from an unknown primary lesion. In this instance, the patient undergoes total-body Wood's lamp evaluation for evidence of a residual or regressed primary melanoma, which may manifest as a circumscribed lesion with hypopigmentation in the appropriate area of lymphatic drainage in the case of nodal metastases.

ADDITIONAL READINGS

Barnhill RL, Roush GC: Correlation of clinical and histopathologic features in clinically atypical melanocytic nevi. *Cancer* **67**:3157, 1991

Bolognia JL, Shapiro PE: Perifollicular hypopigmentation: A cause of variegate pigmentation and irregular border in melanocytic nevi. *Arch Dermatol* **128**:514, 1992

Evans RD et al: Risk factors for the development of malignant melanoma: I. Review of case-control studies. *J Dermatol Surg Oncol* **14**:393, 1988

Fitzpatrick TB: Soleil et peau. *J Med Esthet* **2**(7):33, 1975

Fitzpatrick TB, Clark WH Jr: Problems in the diagnosis of malignant melanoma, in *Tumors of the Skin* (The University of Texas M.D. Anderson Hospital and Tumor Institute, Seventh Annual Clinical Conference on Cancer, 1962). Chicago, Year Book Medical Publishers, 1963, pp. 169–183

Fitzpatrick TB et al: Clinical characteristics, in *Cutaneous Melanoma,* edited by CM Balch et al. Philadelphia, Lippincott, 1992, pp. 223–233

Friedman RJ et al: Early detection of malignant melanoma: The role of physician examination and self-examination of the skin. *CA* **35**:130, 1985

Garbe C et al: Markers and relative risk in a German population for developing malignant melanoma. *Int J Dermatol* **28**:517, 1989

Green A et al: Common acquired naevi and the risk of malignant melanoma. *Int J Cancer* **35**:297, 1985

Greene MH et al: High risk of malignant melanoma in melanoma-prone families with dysplastic nevi. *Ann Intern Med* **102**:458, 1985

Greene MH et al: Malignant melanoma in renal-transplant recipients. *Lancet* **1**:1196, 1981

Halpern AC et al: Dysplastic nevi as risk markers of sporadic (nonfamilial) melanoma. *Arch Dermatol* **127**:995, 1991

Holly EA et al: Number of melanocytic nevi as a major risk factor for malignant melanoma. *J Am Acad Dermatol* **17**:459, 1987

Kaplan EN: The risk of malignancy in large congenital nevi. *Plast Reconstr Surg* **53**:421, 1974

Keefe M et al: A study of the value of the seven-point checklist in distinguishing benign pigmented lesions from melanoma. *Clin Exp. Dermatol* **15**:167, 1990

Koh HK: Cutaneous melanoma. *N Engl J Med* **325**:171, 1992

Kraemer KH et al: Xeroderma pigmentosum—Cutaneous, ocular, and neurologic abnormalities in 830 published cases. *Arch Dermatol* **123**:241, 1987

Krüger S et al: Epidemiologic evidence for the role of melanocytic nevi as risk markers and direct precursors of cutaneous malignant melanoma. *J Am Acad Dermatol* **26**:920, 1992

MacKie RM et al: The number and distribution of benign pigmented moles (melanocytic naevi) in a healthy British population. *Br J Dermatol* **113**:167, 1985

Mihm MC Jr et al: Early detection of primary cutaneous malignant melanoma: A color atlas. *N Engl J Med* **289**:989, 1973

Nordlund JJ et al: Demographic study of clinically atypical (dysplastic) nevi in patients with melanoma and comparison subjects. *Cancer Res* **45**:1855, 1985

Quaba AA, Wallace AF: The incidence of malignant melanoma (0 to 15 years of age) arising in "large" congenital nevocellular naevi. *Plast Reconstr Surg* **78**:174, 1986

Rhodes AR et al: Case report: Nonepidermal origin of malignant melanoma associated with a giant congenital nevocellular nevus. *Plast Reconstr Surg* **67**:782, 1981

Rhodes AR et al: Risk factors for cutaneous melanoma—A practical method of recognizing predisposed individuals. *JAMA* **258**:3146, 1987

Roush, GC et al: Diagnosis of the dysplastic nevus in different populations. *J Am Acad Dermatol* **14**:419, 1986

Saida T et al: Clinical guidelines for the early detection of plantar malignant melanoma. *J Am Acad Dermatol* **23**:37, 1990

Saida T, Ohshima Y: Clinical and histopathologic characteristics of early lesions of subungual malignant melanoma. *Cancer* **63**:556, 1989

Sober AJ et al: Detection of "thin" primary melanomas. *CA* **33**:160, 1983

Sober AJ et al: Early recognition of cutaneous melanoma. *JAMA* **242**:2795, 1979

Swerdlow AJ, Green A. Melanocytic naevi and melanoma: An epidemiological perspective. *Br J Dermatol* **117**:137, 1987

Weinstock MA, Sober AJ: Risk of progression of lentigo maligna to lentigo maligna melanoma. *Br J Dermatol* **16**:303, 1987

Weiss J et al: Malignant melanoma in southern Germany—different predictive value of risk factors for melanoma subtypes. *Dermatologica* **183**:109, 1991

Wick MM et al: Clinical characteristics of early cutaneous melanoma. *Cancer* **45**:2684, 1980

Williams ML, Sagebiel RW: Melanoma risk factors and atypical moles: *West J Med* 160:343, 1994.

2. An Introduction to the Living Gross Tissue Pathology of Pigmented Lesions Using in Vivo Oil-Immersion Cutaneous Microscopy (Epiluminescence Microscopy)

During the past several decades, the clinical diagnosis of melanoma has evolved from recognition of the clinical signs of advanced cutaneous melanoma, such as bleeding or ulceration, to identification of the more subtle clinical features of early melanoma, such as asymmetry, border irregularity, color variability, diameter, and enlargement (the ABCDE's). More recently, clinicians have begun to look at the *subsurface* tissue morphology of pigmented structures of the epidermis, dermal-epidermal junction, and papillary dermis, providing a more accurate method of predicting histopathologic diagnoses, including melanoma in situ. Pigmented cutaneous lesions that are at high risk, low risk, or almost no risk of being melanoma or potential melanoma precursors can be identified by inspecting their *clinical histomorphology*—that is, their in vivo gross tissue morphology—using oil-immersion microscopy of living skin.

DEFINITION

To inspect the tissue morphology of pigmented structures situated below the stratum corneum (cornified layer of the epidermis), we use a technique called *epiluminescence microscopy,* or ELM. ELM involves applying oil to the skin surface, illumination, and magnification and is, in fact, oil-immersion cutaneous microscopy. ELM is also known as *skin-surface microscopy, cutaneous microscopy, incident-light microscopy, dermoscopy, dermatoscopy,* and *Auflickmikroskopie.* Mineral oil, applied to the surface of a pigmented lesion, "clears the skin" by minimizing light reflection, scattering, and refraction at the air-skin interface, rendering the stratum corneum transparent and thereby enabling visualization of the morphology of pigmented tissue structures near the dermal-epidermal junction.

A new dimension of the gross morphology of skin becomes visible with ELM. These *clinical histomorphologic* features are some of the same cutaneous structures that are observed in cross section with conventional histopathologic examination; however, with ELM they are generally viewed at lower magnification (typically at 7.5× to 40×, although occasionally at 100× to 400×), without tissue stains, and as intact three-dimensional pigmented structures in vivo. Such clinical histomorphologic features and their spatial pattern across the lesion can provide diagnostic clues suspicious for melanoma. In addition, benign lesions that mimic melanoma frequently can be identified, and potential melanoma precursors, such as clinically atypical nevi [i.e., nevi with architectural disorder and with or without cytologic atypia (dysplastic or Clark's nevi)], often can be recognized by characteristic features.

THE PIGMENT NETWORK

The predominant ELM feature of many melanocytic lesions is a reticular pigment network pattern (Fig. 2-1). The network results from the pattern of rete ridges in

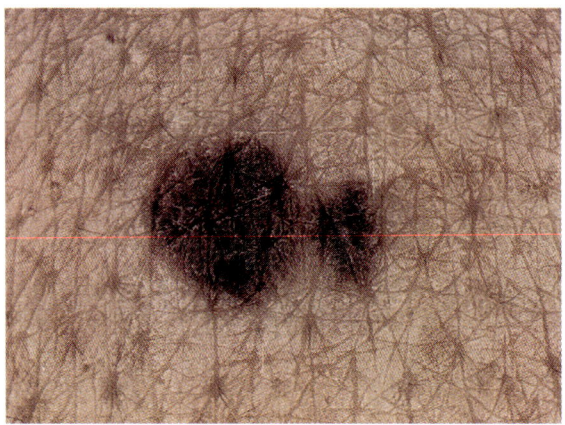

A

Figure 2-1 (a) *(Clinical surface view, without oil): This is a relatively small (6-mm-diameter) flat brown dumbell-shaped lesion. Note that the skin markings are visible in this surface view.* (b) *(Gross subsurface tissue morphology as seen with ELM, with oil): Under ELM with oil, the skin markings can no longer be seen because light reflection from the skin-air interface is eliminated, and a reticular pigment network pattern can be seen. The lines in the network correspond to the pigmented rete ridges at the dermal-epidermal junction. The holes in the network correspond to the dermal papillae. When a network pattern can be seen with ELM, the lesion has a very high probability of being a melanocytic lesion such as a nevus or melanoma (as opposed to a nonmelanocytic lesion that can mimic melanoma). Melanomas of increasing thickness tend to have reticular pigment networks that are progressively more and more distorted or obscured by other ELM features.* (c) *(Digital enhancement of subsurface morphology): With computer enhancement of the ELM subsurface view, this reticular pigment network pattern can be seen clearly. This type of computer-based image enhancement can be used as a teaching tool to help train the eye to recognize subtle ELM features.* (Reprinted with permission from RO Kenet et al: Clinical diagnosis of pigmented lesions using digital epiluminescence microscopy: Grading protocol and atlas. *Arch Dermatol* 129:157, 1993.)

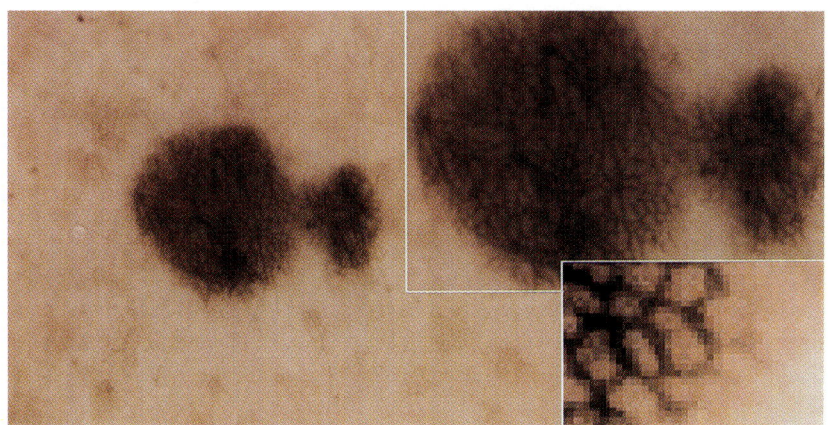

B

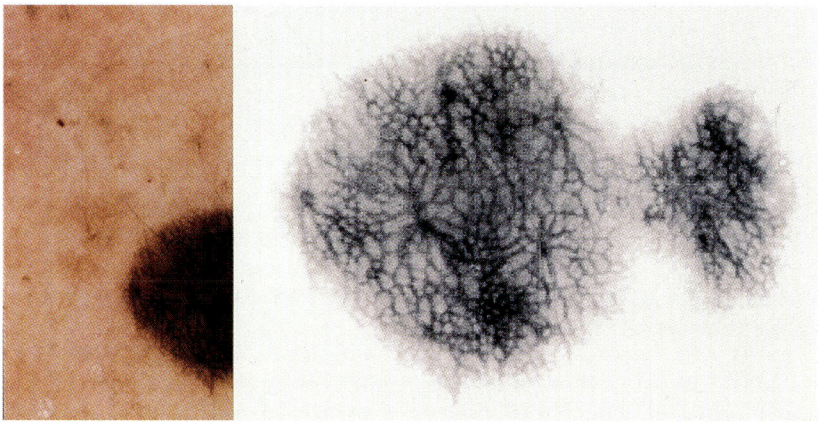

C

the epidermis and the density and distribution of melanin pigment along the rete ridges. The holes in the network correspond to the superficial papillary plate of the dermal papillae. ELM examination of junctional or relatively flat compound melanocytic nevi typically reveals a relatively uniform, regular pigment network that fades at the lesion periphery. The pigment network corresponds to pigmented and elongated epidermal rete ridges usually accompanied by an increased number of melanocytes in the basal cell layer. The first step in ELM interpretation consists of careful inspection of the gross living tissue morphology of a pigmented lesion for the presence of a reticular pigment network. If a pigment network can be seen anywhere in the lesion, the lesion has a high probability of being melanocytic. (There is one main exception to this rule: occasionally, a pigmented seborrheic keratosis may have a small region with a pigment network.)

USE OF ELM TO ENHANCE CLINICAL DIAGNOSIS

There is a body of data that suggests that ELM can improve the accuracy of clinical pigmented lesion examination, especially for clinically equivocal lesions, both for dermatologists and potentially more so for nondermatologists who obtain sufficient training and develop sufficient expertise. Several studies suggest that ELM, when performed by physicians with special training in ELM interpretation, can increase the sensitivity and specificity for the clinical detection of (1) thin melanoma and (2) lesions that mimic melanoma. Physicians can begin to learn ELM by using it in their daily practices to expand the panoply of clinical and gross architectural features of histology that can be seen with routine clinical physical examination. However, there is a rather steep learning curve to master the subtleties of ELM interpretation. It is presently recommended that dermatologists develop sufficient hands-on experience and/or seek specialized training prior to relying on their own interpretation of ELM patterns for difficult cases. This is especially true when screening for thin melanomas that may not have yet developed classic ELM features of melanoma.

Nevertheless, ELM is actually gross histopathology in vivo and therefore can provide a clinician with a better understanding of why certain lesions have particular clinical morphologic features and hence a conceptual basis for clinicopathologic correlation of pigmented lesions. With the latter goal in mind and as an introduction to ELM diagnosis, selected ELM images are presented along with conventional clinical images in this *Atlas*.

STEPS IN ELM ASSESSMENT

ELM evaluation of a pigmented cutaneous lesion consists of six steps: (1) placing a thin layer of mineral oil (or other clear liquid) on the skin, (2) smoothing the oil with a transparent surface, (3) illuminating the lesion with incident light, (4) inspecting pigmented structures below the skin surface with a magnifying instrument, such as a hand-held lens, a hand-held monocular or binocular scope, a stereo microscope, a camera, or an electronic or digital imaging system, (5) recognizing specific ELM diagnostic features that correspond to specific histologic structures, and (6) assigning a likely diagnosis or a level of risk to the lesion based on the set of ELM features present or not present in the lesion. Even if the diagnosis is not obvious based on both the traditional clinical features and the clinical histomorphologic features visible with ELM, a likely risk group nevertheless may be assigned to a lesion via a method known as risk stratification. Assignment of a lesion to a risk group can then be used to help choose the most appropriate management strategy for that lesion.

RISK STRATIFICATION FOR MELANOMA SCREENING

Risk stratification of pigmented lesions is defined as the grouping or assignment of lesions into various risk groups according to their probability of being melanoma, a melanoma precursor, a banal melanocytic lesion, or a nonmelanocytic lesion. The risk group is assigned based on the set of features present and/or absent in a lesion. These features include both traditional clinical features (i.e., ABCDE) and clinical histomorphologic features (i.e., global, local, and network ELM features; see Table 2-1).

Table 2-2 demonstrates how ELM criteria can be used in melanoma screening to stratify pigmented lesions into groups with different relative risks of being melanoma or a melanoma precursor. For example, a lesion with any one of the ELM features most specific for melanoma would, in this strategy, fall into the highest-risk group and would require biopsy (Table 2-2, *upper row*). High-risk lesions would include those with (1) a multicomponent pattern (defined as a lesion with three or more distinct regions with different ELM appearances, including one dark region with markedly thickened and darkened network lines that histologically represent tubular-shaped fascicles of melanocytes running horizontally in the epidermis; (see Fig. 21-6), (2) a nodular pattern (consisting of several raised dark regions with irregular edges that appear to be partially obliterating a pigment network pattern and that histologically correspond to the vertical growth phase of melanoma; (see Fig. 22-4), (3) clinical histomorphologic features of the radial growth phase of melanoma such as pseudopods (see Fig. 21-6), radial streaming (see Fig. 22-4), or sharp network margins (see Fig. 21-6), or (4) other ELM features that can be associated with melanoma, such as a whitish veil (which corresponds to compact orthokeratosis of the stratum corneum, sometimes with hypergranulosis of the epidermis; (see Fig. 21-6) or blue-gray veil (which corresponds to melanin and/or hemosiderin in the mid- to deep dermis either in melanophages, melanocytes, or extracellularly; see Fig. 22-4).

Any lesion with criteria sensitive but not specific for melanoma would fall into the second highest-risk group (see Table 2-2, *center row*). Pilot data suggest that such features may include (1) pigment dots (if black, they correspond to pigment in the stratum corneum), (2) peripheral erythema (which corresponds to dilated capillaries at the periphery of the lesion), (3) marked overall pigment network irregularity (see Fig. 21-6), (4) peripheral dark patches (defined as regions of pigment network at the periphery of the lesion that are relatively darker than the average lesion pigmentation; (see Fig. 21-6), and (5) marked variation in the thickness of pigment network lines.

Any lesion without features of melanoma but with features sensitive for the histologic features of a markedly atypical (or dysplastic) nevus—i.e., architectural dis-

Table 2-1 ELM Grading Protocol

EPILUMINESCENCE MICROSCOPY (ELM) DIAGNOSTIC FEATURES	PRELIMINARY INTERPRETATION GUIDELINES
	Step 1: Global ELM features
Network pattern	Suggests melanocytic lesion
Globular pattern	Suggests compound or dermal nevus
Multicomponent pattern	Suggests melanoma
Nodular pattern	Suggests melanoma
Saccular pattern	Suggests hemangioma or angiokeratoma
Homogeneous pattern	Brown is indeterminate; blue suggests blue nevus if network absent
	Step 2: Local ELM features
Pseudopods	Suggests melanoma, if network present
Radial streaming	Suggests melanoma, if network present
Irregular extensions	Suggests melanoma, if network present
Whitish veil (milky way)	Suggests melanoma, if network present
Blue-gray areas	Suggests melanoma, if network present
Pigment dots	Peripheral dots may help screen for melanoma or severe atypia, but nonspecific
Brown globules	Nonspecific
Depigmentation	Need more data
Erythema (capillary prominence)	May help screen for melanoma or severe atypia, but nonspecific
Telangiectasia	May occur in melanoma or basal cell carcinoma
Comedo-like openings	Suggests seborrheic keratosis
Milia-like cysts	May suggest seborrheic keratosis but can occur in nevi
Red-blue areas	May suggest hemangioma or angiokeratoma if network absent
Maple leaf areas	May suggest pigmented basal cell carcinoma
	Step 3: Network features
Network irregularity	
Mean irregularity	If marked, may help screen for melanoma or severe atypia, but nonspecific
Focal absence of network	May help screen for severe atypia, but nonspecific
Network holes	
Size: mean and variability	
Network lines	
Thickness: mean, variability	
Darkness: mean, variability	Variability may help screen for melanoma, but nonspecific
Markedly thick and dark lines	Suggests melanoma

Table 2-1 ELM Grading Protocol *(continued)*

EPILUMINESCENCE MICROSCOPY (ELM) DIAGNOSTIC FEATURES	PRELIMINARY INTERPRETATION GUIDELINES
Network patches	
Dark network patches: central, peripheral	If peripheral may help screen for melanoma or severe atypia, but nonspecific
Light network patches (relative hypopigmentation): central, peripheral	May help screen for severe atypia, but nonspecific
Network margins	
Sharp network margins	Suggests melanoma
Network branching	
High-order (treelike) branching	Suggests melanoma

Adapted from Kenet RO et al: *Arch Dermatol* 129:157, 1993.

order with severe cytologic atypia—would fall into the third highest-risk group (Table 2-2, *lower row*). For example, central hypopigmentation may be a sensitive but nonspecific feature for atypical (or dysplastic) nevi and is consistent with the observation that such nevi tend to have pigment network patterns with patches of lighter pigmentation (see Fig. 18-3). Other factors, including clinical history and clinical judgment may influence the ultimate decision regarding biopsy in these latter two risk groups.

Further investigation is needed to identify the clinical histomorphologic features of the earliest melanomas that may not yet have developed macroscopic features of radial growth. However, preliminary data suggest that some thin melanomas (particularly those less than 0.5-mm Breslow thickness, including melanomas in situ) often do not manifest classical ELM features of radial growth such as pseudopods or radial streaming. Such very early melanomas may demonstrate more subtle perturbations of a reticular pigment network pattern, such as (1) thickened and darkened network lines (or trabeculae) that appear to correspond histologically to fascicles of melanocytes running horizontally in the epidermis at the level of the dermoepidermal junction (Fig. 2-2), (2) a markedly irregular overall network pattern (see Fig. 21-6), (3) small irregular regions of confluent brown, dark brown, or nearly black pigment in the setting of an overall irregular network pattern (see Figs. 20-1 and 20-2), and/or (4) a network pattern (without other features) in which the darkest part of the lesion is at the periphery or in which there is an abrupt margin of the network rather than a gradual fading of the network into the surrounding skin.

RISK STRATIFICATION FOR SURGICAL COST CONTAINMENT

Perhaps one of the most interesting but overlooked values of ELM comes in serving the goal of cost containment to limit

Table 2-2 ELM Risk Stratification: Melanoma Screening (Pilot Data)

Specific for melanoma	• Multicomponent pattern • Nodular pattern • Pseudopods / radial streaming • Whitish or blue-gray veil • Sharp network margins	Highest-risk: Biopsy
Sensitive (but not specific) for melanoma	• Pigment dots • Peripheral erythema • Marked network irregularity • Peripheral dark patches • Line-thickness variability	2nd highest risk: Probable biopsy
Sensitive for architectural disorder with severe cytologic atypia	• Central hypopigmentation • Regional network loss	3rd highest risk: Consider biopsy

unnecessary surgery for low-risk pigmented lesions. This is especially relevant for patients with many lesions or for lesions on cosmetically sensitive sites. ELM features found to be most specific for certain benign lesions can be used to stratify lesions into one of several low-risk groups as a means of limiting unnecessary surgery for certain types of lesions. Table 2-3 illustrates, based on pilot data, a potential cost-containment protocol for lesions that demonstrate certain ELM features that are relatively specific for low-risk lesions, for which biopsy can be avoided, curtailed, or replaced by serial ELM examinations.

Certain no-risk nonmelanocytic lesions can be identified by characteristic clinical histomorphologic patterns seen with ELM (see Table 2-3). For example, if a lesion has a saccular pattern (consisting of multiple purplish or red smooth-bordered sacs) in the absence of any evidence of a pigment network (see Fig. 22-8), then the lesion is most likely a hemangioma and would fall into the lowest-risk group that does not require biopsy (see Table 2-3, *upper row*). Minimal-risk seborrheic keratoses can be identified by a characteristic pattern of multiple comedo-like openings with multiple milia-like cysts in the absence of a pigment network (see Fig.

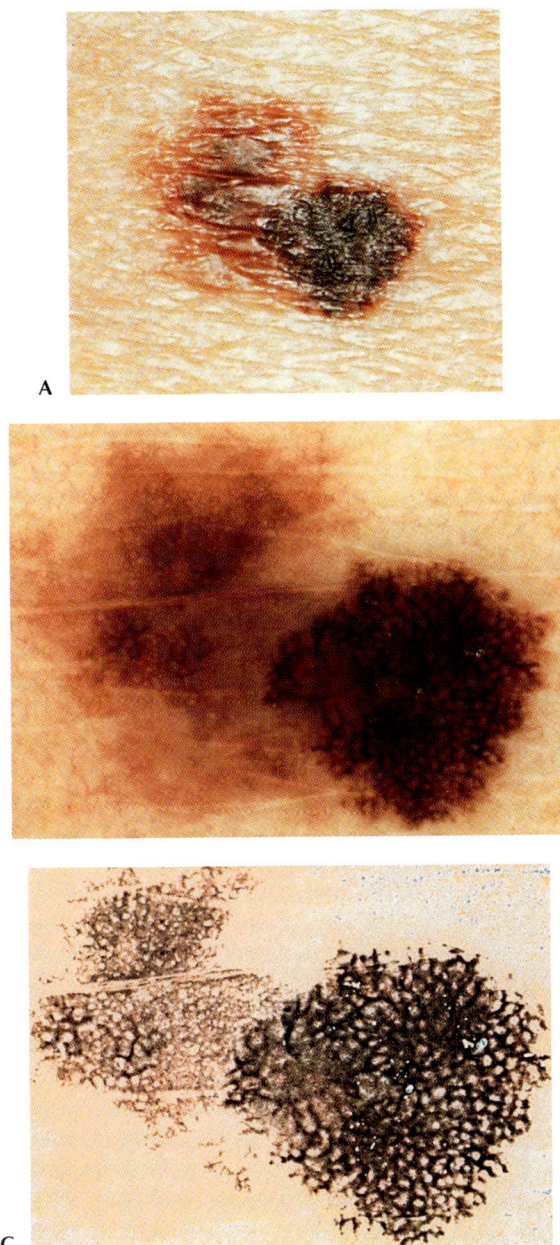

Figure 2-2 *Malignant melanoma in situ.* (a) *(Clinical surface view, without oil):* This is a small dark lesion with irregular borders. (b) *(Gross subsurface tissue morphology as seen with ELM, with oil):* Note the dark region with significantly thickened and darkened network lines. This region also demonstrates a "sharp margin" between the lesion and surrounding skin. These are features that suggest melanoma. (c) *(Digital enhancement of subsurface morphology):* With computer enhancement of the ELM subsurface view, the thickened and darkened network lines that end abruptly in the lower right portion of the lesion can be clearly seen. (Parts a and b courtesy of H. Peter Soyer, M.D., University of Graz, Austria.)

Table 2-3 ELM Risk Stratification: Cost Containment (Pilot Data)

Category	Features	Risk/Action
Benign nonmelanocytic	• Saccular pattern* (hemangioma) • Multiple comedo-like openings* (seborrheic keratosis) *With no network	Lowest risk: No biopsy
Benign melanocytic	• Globular pattern* (compound / dermal) *With no network	2nd lowest risk: Usually no biopsy
Low risk melanocytic	• Regular brown network (darker in center than periphery)	3rd lowest risk: Follow-up exam

27-2). A lesion with a globular pattern (see Fig. 11-3), in the absence of a pigment network, is most likely a papillomatous dermal or compound nevus, which usually requires no biopsy (see Table 2-3, *center row*).

An important frontier of ELM research lies in identifying criteria specific for low-risk melanocytic lesions that are safe to follow clinically (see Table 2-3, *lower row*). Preliminary data suggest that a lesion with a homogeneous brown pigment network that thins and fades at the periphery and that does not have any clinical histomorphologic features suggestive of melanoma may be the type of low-risk lesion that is safe to follow clinically in compliant patients. If such criteria can be confirmed, physicians may less frequently need to biopsy for medicolegal reasons those low-risk pigmented lesions which deviate in minor ways from clinical criteria for benignity. In such circumstances, ELM would enable the physician to employ clinical judgment with greater certainty. Thus stratifying the risk of pigmented lesions using ELM can help determine the most appropriate management strategy for pigmented lesions in both melanoma screening and surgical cost-containment strategies.

TELEMEDICINE AND REMOTE DIAGNOSIS

The rapid advancement of global telecommunications networks that inevitably will unite telephones, televisions, faxes, and computers may soon allow any medical practitioner nearly instant access to any ELM expert to assist in the interpretation of a pigmented lesion. In the future, by interpreting digital images of the living-tissue morphology of pigmented skin lesions, dermatologists may be able to assist primary-care physicians in providing expert and cost-effective skin cancer screening during routine physical examinations.

ADDITIONAL READINGS

Bahmer FA et al: Terminology in surface microscopy. *J Am Acad Dermatol* **23**(6):1159, 1990

Braun-Falco O et al: Das dermatoskop, eine vereinfachung der auflichtmikroskopie von pigmentierten hautveranderungen. *Hautarzt* **41**:131, 1990

Fitzpatrick TB, Kenet RO: Evolution of diagnostic accuracy of primary cutaneous malignant melanoma: I. Clinical criteria (abstract). *Melanoma Res* **3**(suppl 1):4, 1993

Fritsch P, Pechlaner R: Differentiation of benign from malignant melanocytic lesions using incident light microscopy, in *Pathology of Malignant Melanoma*, edited by AB Ackerman. New York, Masson, 1981, pp 301–312

Goldman L: Some investigative studies of pigmented nevi with cutaneous microscopy. *J Invest Dermatol* **16**:407, 1951

Kenet RO: Epiluminescence or surface microscopy, in *Dermatology in General Medicine*, 4th ed, edited by TB Fitzpatrick et al. New York, McGraw-Hill, 1993, pp 1108–1110

Kenet RO: Trends in dermatology: Differential diagnosis of pigmented lesions using epiluminescence microscopy, in *1992 Year Book of Dermatology*, edited by AJ Sober and TB Fitzpatrick. St. Louis, Mosby–Year Book, 1992, pp xxi–xxxii

Kenet RO et al: Clinical diagnosis of pigmented lesions using digital epiluminescence microscopy: Grading protocol and atlas. *Arch Dermatol* **129**:157, 1993

Kenet RO et al: Melanoma screening with digital epiluminescence microscopy (abstract). *Melanoma Res* **3**(suppl 1):4, 1993

Kenet RO et al: Early detection of melanoma by visualizing perturbations of pigment network morphology using digital epiluminescence microscopy (abstract). *J Cutan Pathol* **20**:549, 1993

Kenet RO et al: Grading protocol for clinical diagnosis of pigmented lesions using digital epiluminescence microscopy (abstract). *J Cutan Pathol* **19**(6):530, 1992

Kenet RO et al: Melanoma and melanoma precursors—Pigment pattern characterization in vivo using computer-assisted epiluminescence microscopy (abstract). *J Cutan Pathol* **17**(5):304, 1990

Kreusch J: Incident light microscopy: Reflections on microscopy of the living skin. *Int J Dermatol* **31**:618, 1992

Kreusch J, Rassner G: *Auflichtmikroskopie pigmentierter Hauttumoten: Ein Bildatlas.* Stuttgart, Thieme-Verlag, 1991

Kreusch J, Rassner G: Standardisiette auflichtmikroskopische Unterscheidung melanozytischer und nichtmelanozatischer Pigmentmale. *Hautarzt* **42**(2):77, 1991

Kreusch J, Rassner G: Strukturanalyse melanozytischer Pigmentmale dutch Auflichtmikroskopie: Ubersicht und eigne Erfahtungen. *Hautarzt* **41**(1):27, 1990

MacKie RM: An aid to the preoperative assessment of pigmented lesions of the skin. *Br J Dermatol* **85**:232, 1971

Pehamberger H et al: In vivo epiluminescence microscopy: Improvement of early diagnosis of melanoma. *J Invest Dermatol* **100**:356S, 1993

Pehamberger H et al: In vivo epiluminescence microscopy of pigmented skin lesions: I. Pattern analysis of pigmented skin lesions. *J Am Acad Dermatol* **17**:571, 1987

Saphier J: Die Dermatoskopie: I. Mitteilung. *Arch Dermatol Syphilol* **128**:1, 1921

Saphier J: Die Dermatoskopie: II. *Arch Dermatol Syphilol* **132**:69, 1921

Sober AJ: Digital epiluminescence microscopy in the evaluation of pigmented lesions: A brief review. *Semin Surg Oncol* **9**:198, 1993

Soyer HP, Kerl H: Microscopie de surface des tumeurs cutanées pigmentées. *Ann Dermatol Venereol* **120**:15, 1993

Soyer HP et al: Surface microscopy: A new approach to the diagnosis of cutaneous pigmented tumors. *Am J Dermatopathol* **11**(1):1, 1989

Soyer HP et al: Zur auflichtmikroskopie von pigmenttumoren der haut. *Hautarzt* **39**:223, 1988

Soyer HP et al: Early diagnosis of malignant melanoma by surface microscopy. *Lancet* **2**:803, 1987

Steiner A et al: Statistical evaluation of epiluminescence microscopy criteria for melanocytic pigmented skin lesions. *J Am Acad Dermatol* **29**:581, 1993

Steiner A et al: In vivo epiluminescence microscopy of pigmented skin lesions: II. Diagnosis of small pigmented skin lesions and early detection of malignant melanoma. *J Am Acad Dermatol* **17**:584, 1987

Stolz W et al: Skin surface microscopy. *Lancet* **2**:864, 1989

Yadav S et al: Histopathologic correlates of structures seen on dermoscopy (epiluminescence microscopy). *Am J Dermatopathol* **15**:297, 1993

Section I

Benign Pigmented Lesions

3. Ephelides

Ephelides are small, well-circumscribed pigmented macules found only on sun-exposed skin.

Synonym: freckles

EPIDEMIOLOGY

Ephelides are common in individuals with fair skin color, especially in combination with blond or red hair. They are not present at birth but usually appear in the first 3 years of life. Since freckling can be seen in some families over generations, autosomal dominant inheritance is likely.

ETIOLOGY

Hyperpigmentation in ephelides is the result of increased sun-induced melanogenesis and transport of an increased number of fully melanized melanosomes from melanocytes to keratinocytes. They are thought to be the result of the behavior of clones of mutant melanocytes after exposure to ultraviolet radiation.

CLINICAL FEATURES

Ephelides occur only on sun-exposed areas of the body, mainly on the face, the dorsal aspects of the arms, and the upper part of the chest and the back; they are not found on mucous membranes (Figs. 3-1 and 3-2). Ephelides are well demarcated and round, oval, or irregular in shape; they are usually 1 to 3 mm in diameter, but some may be several millimeters in diameter (Fig 3-3). Depending on the intensity of sun exposure, they vary in color from light to dark brown but almost never become as dark as lentigines or junctional nevi; they may increase in number and distribution and show a tendency to confluency, but they decrease later in life.

HISTOLOGIC FEATURES

The epidermis exhibits a normal configuration. The keratinocytes show an increase in melanin content, predominantly in the basal cell layer. Occasionally, melanophages are seen in the papillary dermis. The number of melanocytes in ephelides does not differ significantly from normal. However, examination of dopa-stained sections has been reported to show both significantly fewer melanocytes and an increased number of melanocytes per unit area in ephelides. The melanocytes in ephelides are larger and have more branching of dendrites and a higher dopa positivity than those in adjacent normal epidermis, apparently indicating greater functional activity.

BIOLOGIC BEHAVIOR AND PROGNOSIS

Ephelides are completely benign and show no propensity for malignant transformation. As mentioned earlier, the tendency to develop ephelides decreases with advanc-

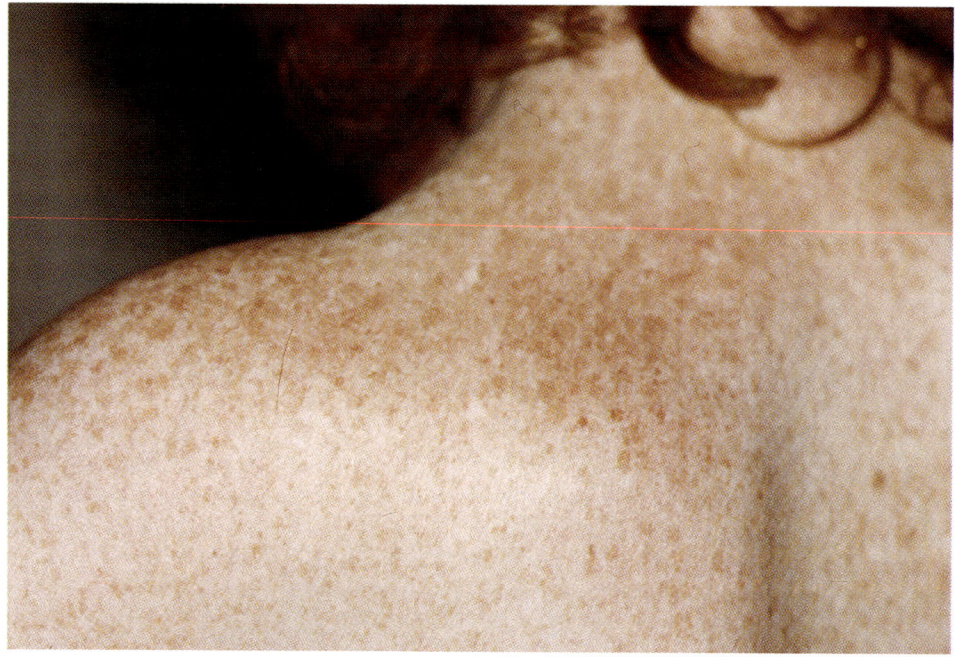

Figure 3-1 *Ephelides. The shoulder of this woman exhibits myriads of small, discrete, tan and brown lesions. Note that the patient has red hair.*

ing age. Recently, Rhodes et al. have suggested that some ephelides may overlap or represent a subtype of solar lentigo. Lesions studied by these authors exhibited melanocytic hyperplasia and occasional cytologic atypia, features shared with solar lentigo. Further studies are needed to clarify the significance of the latter findings. Clinically, ephelides become less prominent with age, but even when they are clinically inapparent in older individuals with ordinary light, they remain visible upon Wood's lamp examination.

DIFFERENTIAL DIAGNOSIS

Ephelides must be distinguished from simple lentigines, solar lentigines, café au lait macules, and junctional nevi.

In general, ephelides are lighter in color than simple lentigines, are located on sun-exposed skin, and are responsive to solar

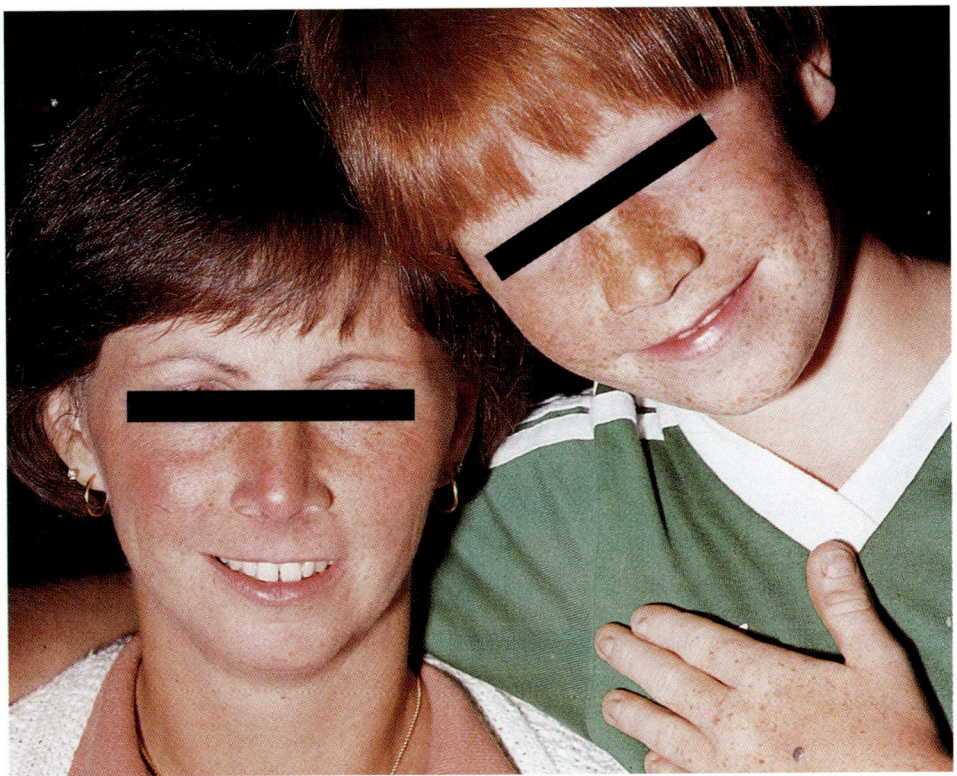

Figure 3-2 *Ephelides. This is a mother and son. Note the striking freckling on the exposed parts, sparing the upper eyelid in the mother, and, again, the red hair.*

exposure. In contrast, simple lentigines may occur on any site and are persistent. Probably the greatest difficulty in differential diagnosis of ephelides is discriminating them from solar lentigines, which are generally, as the name implies, more prevalent with advancing age than are ephelides. Solar lentigines are also persistent and often are larger, darker, and more irregular than ephelides (see Table 6-1). Nonetheless, the two lesions may be impossible to distinguish in some instances. Café au lait macules are usually solitary and larger than ephelides.

MANAGEMENT

Since darkening of ephelides depends on ultraviolet radiation, sun exposure should be minimized and sunscreens with a high sun-protecting factor (SPF) should be used to prevent the appearance of new ephelides.

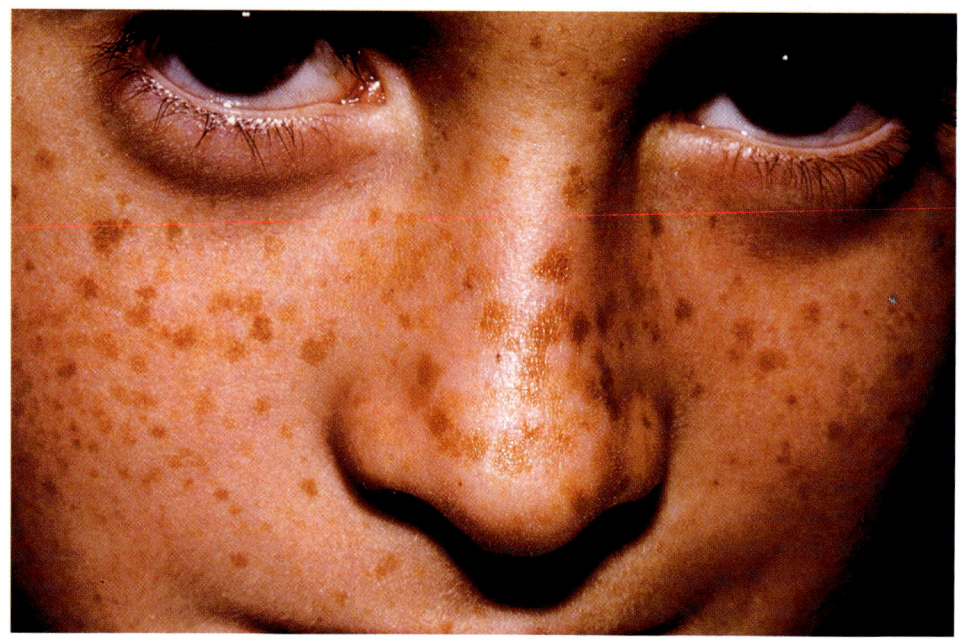

Figure 3-3 *Ephelides. There are discrete macules with slightly variegated color, less than 3 mm in diameter, on the exposed parts. Note the sparing of the lesions under the lower eyelid, which is not such a sun-exposed area.*

ADDITIONAL READINGS

Breathnach AS: Melanocyte distribution in forearm epidermis of freckled human subjects. *J Invest Dermatol* **29**:253, 1957

Breathnach AS, Wyllie LM: Electron microscopy of melanocytes and melanosomes in freckled human epidermis. *J Invest Dermatol* **42**:389, 1964

Brues AM: Linkage of body build with sex, eye color and freckling. *Am J Hum Genet* **2**:215, 1950

Burnet FM: Intrinsic mutagenesis, an interpretation of the pathogenesis of xeroderma pigmentosum. *Lancet* **2**:495, 1974

Gilchrest BA et al: Localization of melanin pigmentation in the skin with Wood's lamp. *Br J Dermatol* **96**:245, 1977

Rhodes AR et al: Sun-induced freckles in children and young adults: A correlation of clinical and histopathologic features. *Cancer* **67**:1990, 1991

4. Café au Lait Macules

Café au lait macules (CALM) are well-circumscribed, uniformly light to dark brown spots.

EPIDEMIOLOGY

CALM can occur as an isolated lesion or as multiple lesions; the latter could be a marker for multisystem disease and occur in various syndromes. Single CALM are found in 10 to 20 percent of the normal population, and about 1 percent of all healthy young adults have up to three CALM. They may be present at birth but usually develop in early childhood and increase in size with age.

ETIOLOGY

The hyperpigmentation observed in CALM is due to increased melanogenesis and an increased melanin content of keratinocytes. However, the basic defect leading to this localized pigmentary disturbance has not yet been elucidated.

CLINICAL FEATURES

The term *café au lait* refers to the lesions' characteristic homogeneous color of coffee with milk, which can be light to dark brown. CALM are completely macular, often have an oval morphology, and the margins are well defined and usually regular (Fig. 4-1). They may be located anywhere on the body, except the mucous membranes. CALM are usually 2.0 to 5.0 cm in diameter in adults but may vary from freckle-like lesions <2.0 mm to macules >20 cm in size.

HISTOLOGIC FEATURES

Light microscopy shows a normally configured epidermis with a slightly increased melanin content in the basilar keratinocytes. The number of melanocytes is normal or slightly increased. The adnexal epithelium is spared of hyperpigmentation, and only rarely does one see melanophages in the upper dermis. In dopa-stained epidermis from most patients with neurofibromatosis, the density of melanocytes is higher in both CALM and normal adjacent skin in comparison with healthy individuals. The melanocytic density in isolated CALM of otherwise normal persons, however, is usually less than in surrounding skin. Melanin macroglobules (large pigment particles) which may be found in CALM are not specific for neurofibromatosis, since they are occasionally found in isolated CALM without underlying disease and occur in several other conditions such as simple lentigines, Becker's nevus, congenital nevi, dysplastic nevi, and sometimes even normal skin.

On electron microscopy, the melanosomes are usually dispersed singly in melanocytes and are usually homogeneous, electron dense, and ellipsoidal when fully melanized.

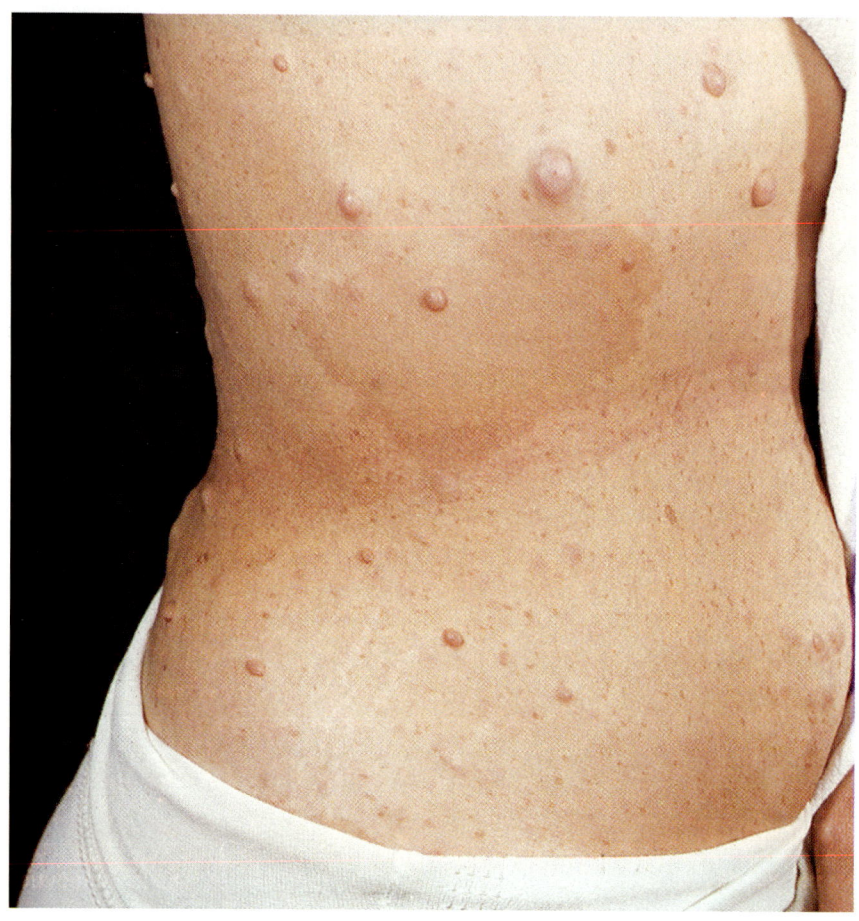

Figure 4-1 *Café au lait macule. Multiple neurofibromas and large CALM.* (From TB Fitzpatrick et al (eds): *Dermatology in General Medicine,* 4th ed. New York, McGraw-Hill, 1993, p 967, with permission.)

BIOLOGIC BEHAVIOR

CALM grow proportionately to body growth and remain stable in size after body growth has ceased. They demonstrate no tendency toward malignancy.

ASSOCIATED DISEASES AND SYNDROMES (See Table 4-1)

Neurofibromatosis (von Recklinghausen's disease) is an autosomal dominant disease of neural crest–derived cells. Its cutaneous manifestations may occur in conjunction with systemic manifestations, which mainly affect the central nervous system. Besides neurofibromata and multiple freckle-like macules in the axillae and other intertriginous areas, multiple CALM are the leading cutaneous features in neurofibromatosis; they are present in more than 99 percent of all patients with neurofibromatosis. Usually they are present at birth, but they can occur months later. The presence of six or more CALM that are >1.5 cm in diameter in adults or five or more such macules that are ≥0.5 cm in diameter in children younger than 5 years has been considered diagnostic, but more reliable are the pigmented hamartomas of the iris called *Tisch nodules*.

Albright's syndrome includes polyostotic fibrous dysplasia of the bones, endocrine dysfunction causing precocious puberty (more often in females than in males), and melanotic macules that are present in nearly two-thirds of patients with this disease. The macules may be present at birth but more commonly develop in the first few years of life. They are usually several centimeters in diameter, few in number, and may be indistinguishable both clinically and histologically from CALM in neurofibromatosis (Fig. 4-2). However, the distribution of the lesions may be somewhat helpful for diagnosis: they favor the forehead, nuchal area, sacrum, and buttocks. They also tend to be unilateral in a linear or segmented arrangement with irregular margins, often involving the

Table 4-1 Diseases and Syndromes Associated with Café au Lait Macules

DISEASE/SYNDROME	PERTINENT FEATURES
Neurofibromatosis	See text
Albright's syndrome	See text
Tuberous sclerosis (epiloa)	Autosomal dominant
	Epilepsy
	Mental retardation
	Adenoma sebaceum
	Shagreen patch
	Periungual fibromas
	"Ash-leaf" (hypopigmented) macules
Silver-Russell syndrome	CALM in 45% of patients
	Short stature
	Skeletal asymmetry
	Shortened, incurved fifth fingers
	Abnormal sexual development
Watson's syndrome	Pulmonary stenosis
	Mental retardation
	Perineal freckling
Westerhof's syndrome	Mental retardation
	Growth retardation
	Hypopigmented macules
Bloom's syndrome	CALM in over 50% of patients
	Growth retardation
	Congenital facial telangiectactic erythema
	Photosensitivity

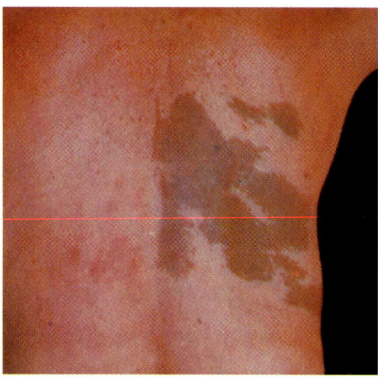

Figure 4-2 *Melanotic macule. This patient has Albright syndrome and polyostotic fibrous dysplasia. These lesions are identical to CALM in neurofibromatosis, but there are no neurofibromas present.* (From TB Fitzpatrick et al (eds): *Dermatology in General Medicine,* 4th ed. New York, McGraw-Hill, 1993, p 967, with permission.)

same side as the bone lesions and situated directly above them. Axillary freckling does not occur in Albright's disease.

DIFFERENTIAL DIAGNOSIS

Hyperpigmented macules that might be confused with CALM include postinflammatory hyperpigmentation, phytophotodermatitis (berloque), melasma, Becker's melanosis, freckles, solar lentigo, flat congenital melanocytic nevi, and epidermal nevi. Postinflammatory hyperpigmentation and phytophotodermatitis are both usually distinguished by the history of an antecedent inflammatory process, have a darker pigmentation than CALM, are often more widely distributed, and differ morphologically from CALM. Phytophotodermatitis often exhibits a bizarre configuration based on external contact of the plant or photosensitizing agent. Melasma is usually easily distinguished from CALM by its mottled appearance and its location on the face of women. Distinction of CALM from Becker's melanosis is discussed in Chap. 5. Freckles (ephelides) are located on sun-exposed skin and fade with lack of sunlight exposure. Solar lentigo is also located on sun-exposed skin and favors individuals over 30 years of age. Solar lentigo exhibits variations in pigment pattern, in contrast to the uniform color of CALM. Relatively flat congenital melanocytic nevi and epidermal nevi also may be confused with CALM on occasion. In contrast to CALM, these lesions are elevated on sidelighting. Both generally have surface alterations as opposed to the normal topography found in CALM. Sometimes a biopsy is necessary for differentiation.

MANAGEMENT

CALM have never been reported to undergo malignant change. Since hyperpigmentation is not sun-related, there is no need to use sun-protective preparations. Furthermore, they cannot be bleached by hydroquinone-containing agents.

ADDITIONAL READINGS

Bell SD, MacDonald DM: The prevalence of café-au-lait patches in tuberous sclerosis. *Clin Exp Dermatol* **10**:562, 1985

Benedict PH et al: Melanotic macules in Albright's syndrome and in neurofibromatosis. *JAMA* **205**:72, 1968

Bloom D: Congenital telangiectatic erythema resembling lupus erythematosus in dwarfs: Probably a syndrome entity. *Am J Dis Child* **88**:754, 1954

Crowe FW, Schull WJ: Diagnostic importance of café-au-lait spot in neurofibromatosis. *Arch Intern Med* **91**:758, 1953

Crowe FW et al: *A Clinical, Pathological and Genetic Study of Multiple Neurofibromatosis.* Springfield, Ill, Charles C. Thomas, 1956

Jimbow K et al: Ultrastructure of giant pigment granules (macromelanosomes) in the cutaneous pigmented macules of neurofibromatosis. *J Invest Dermatol* **61**:300, 1973

Johnson BL, Charneco DR: Café-au-lait spot in neurofibromatosis and in normal individuals. *Arch Dermatol* **102**:442, 1970

Mosher DB et al: Disorders of pigmentation, in *Dermatology in General Medicine,* 4th ed, edited by TB Fitzpatrick et al. New York, McGraw-Hill, 1993, pp 903–995

Nakagawa H et al: The nature and origin of the melanin macroglobule. *J Invest Dermatol* **83**:134, 1983

Riccardi VM: Von Recklinghausen neurofibromatosis. *N Engl J Med* **305**:1617, 1981

Silver HK: Asymmetry, short stature, and variations in sexual development: A syndrome of congenital malformations. *Am J Dis Child* **107**:495, 1964

Silvers DN, Greenwood RS, Helwig EB: Café-au-lait spots without giant pigment granules: Occurrence in suspected neurofibromatosis. *Arch Dermatol* **110**:87, 1974

Watson GH: Pulmonary stenosis, café-au-lait spots, and dull intelligence. *Arch Dis Child* **42**:303, 1967

Westerhof W et al: Hereditary congenital hypopigmented and hyperpigmented macules. *Arch Dermatol* **114**:931, 1978

Whitehouse D: Diagnostic value of the café-au-lait spot in children. *Arch Dis Child* **41**:316, 1966

5. Becker's Melanosis

Becker's melanosis is a unilateral, hyperpigmented, and often hypertrichotic macule or slightly elevated patch.

Synonyms: Becker's nevus, Becker's pigmentary hamartoma, nevoid melanosis, pigmented hairy epidermal nevus

EPIDEMIOLOGY

Becker's melanosis (BM) has been described in all races. Although it is usually acquired, some cases are congenital. The lesions mostly occur in the second and third decades of life and are six times more common in males than in females. Familial occurrence has been reported. The prevalence among 19,302 army recruits aged 17 to 26 was 0.52 percent.

ETIOLOGY

The etiology of BM remains unclear. It is believed to be an organoid harmartoma of ectodermally and mesodermally derived tissues, and a segmented increase in androgen receptors and probable heightened sensitivity to androgens have been postulated. The latter characteristics would explain its onset during or after puberty leadng to its clinical and histologic manifestations, which include hirsutism, acanthosis, dermal thickening, acne, and hypertrophic sebaceous glands. Androgen stimulation also would explain the accentuated smooth-muscle elements often found in the dermis of BM patients. Hyperpigmentation, similar to that found in "sexual skin," is due to increased melanin content in the epidermal keratinocytes and is often preceded by extensive sun exposure that has resulted in sunburns.

CLINICAL FEATURES

The onset of BM is usually noted in the second or third decade of life, often following intense sunbathing. The lesions commonly have a unilateral distribution on the shoulders (Fig. 5-1), the submammary area, and the back, but they also have been described on the forehead, cheeks, eyelids, neck, abdomen, hips, lower leg, and buttocks. Normally, BM appears as a single lesion, but multiple lesions have been reported. The arrangement may be linear or zosteriform. BM ranges in size from a few centimeters in diameter to palm size or larger. There may be slow centrifugal extension of pigmentation. Hyperpigmentation varies from uniformly tan to dark brown. The lesions are well demarcated, but the margins are usually irregular. The center of the lesion may show slight thickening and corrugation of the skin. Hairiness usually develops after pigmentation, and the hairs become coarser and darker with time. Sometimes hypertrichosis is subtle and can only be appreciated by comparison with the contralateral side. The hypertrichosis and pigmentation may not overlap completely. In some cases, perifollicular papules may be a marker for coexistent proliferation of the muscular arrectores pilorum. Acniform lesions strictly limited to the area of hyper-

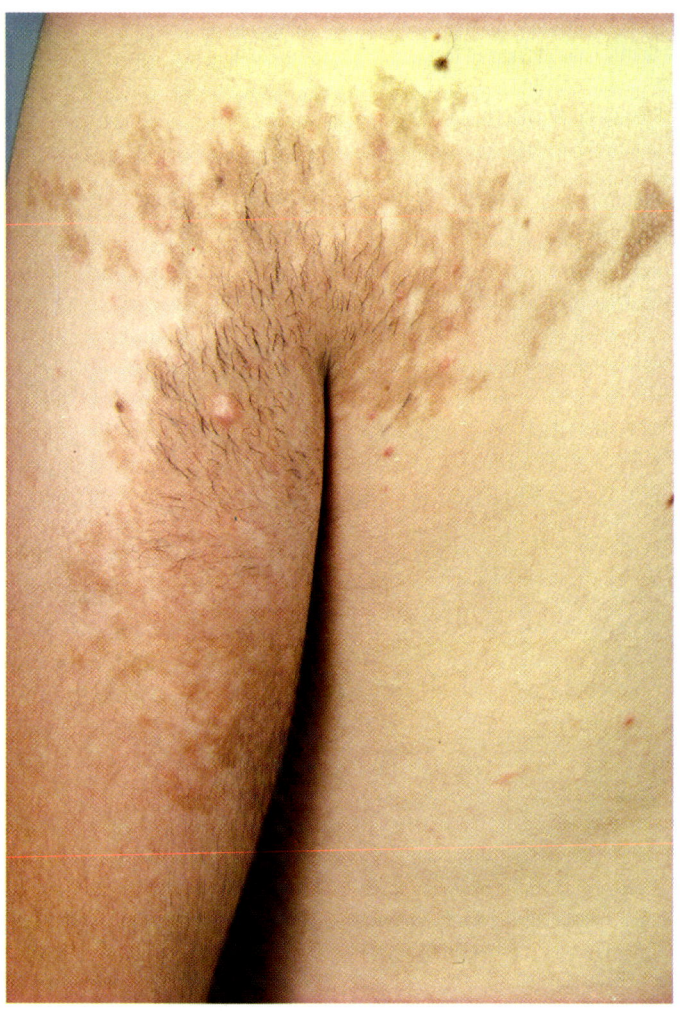

Figure 5-1 *Becker's melanosis over the posterior shoulder showing hyperpigmentation and coarse hairs.* (From TB Fitzpatrick et al (eds): *Dermatology in General Medicine*, 4th ed. New York, McGraw-Hill, 1993, p 863, with permission.)

pigmentation also have been reported. Normally, the lesions are asymptomatic, but some patients report pruritus.

HISTOLOGIC FEATURES

Light microscopy shows variable papillomatosis, acanthosis, and hyperkeratosis. Regular elongation of the rete ridges and hyperplasia of the pilosebaceous units may be observed. The epidermis usually exhibits little, if any, deviation from the normal. The melanin content of the keratinocytes is increased, whereas the number of melanocytes is normal or only slightly increased. Melanophages may be found in the papillary dermis. A concomitant smooth-muscle hamartoma is often but not invariably present in the dermis.

Electron microscopy reveals characteristics consistent with increased melanin synthesis. These changes are similar to those caused by ultraviolet radiation stimulation of normal epidermis.

BIOLOGIC BEHAVIOR AND PROGNOSIS

After development, BM enlarges slowly for a year or two but then remains stable in size. The color may fade with time, but hypertrichosis usually persists. BM is a benign lesion, and malignant transformation has not been reported.

ASSOCIATED ABNORMALITIES

In contrast to the hyperplasia of the ectodermal and mesodermal tissues in BM, occasional developmental abnormalities have been found associated with BM and are generally hypoplastic in nature. These abnormalities include hypoplasia of the ipsilateral breast, areola, nipple, and arm, ipsilateral arm shortening, lumbar spina bifida, thoracic scoliosis, and pectum carinatum, as well as enlargement of the ipsilateral foot. In cases of BM with associated abnormalities, the male-female ratio is reversed 2:5 in comparison with patients with BM without abnormalities.

DIFFERENTIAL DIAGNOSIS

The differential diagnosis primarily includes congenital melanocytic nevus, café au lait macule, and epidermal nevus. A congenital nevus may be confused with BM because of hyperpigmentation, large size, and presence of hypertrichosis. In most instances, however, congenital nevi are distinguished from BM because of the presence of the former at birth, elevation on sidelighting (if not a grossly obvious plaque), and regular borders. Café au lait macules are often present at birth or appear shortly thereafter, are completely macular on sidelighting, and are not hairy. Although epidermal nevi and BM are related because they are hamartomas with epidermal involvement, epidermal nevi are distinguished by the greater tendency to follow lines of cutaneous morphogenesis, e.g., the lines of Blaschko (a linear or whorled pattern). Epidermal nevi are often more extensive, more warty, less pigmented, and not hairy as compared with BM.

MANAGEMENT

Since BM is occasionally mistaken for a hairy congenital nevus, a biopsy may be needed to establish the correct diagnosis.

ADDITIONAL READINGS

Burgreen BL, Ackerman AB: Acneiform lesions in Becker's nevus. *Cutis* **21**:617, 1978

Copeman PM, Wilson Jones E: Pigmented hairy epidermal nevus (Becker). *Arch Dermatol* **92**:249, 1965

Glinick SE et al: Becker's melanosis: Associated abnormalities. *J Am Acad Dermatol* **9**:509, 1983

Person JR, Longcope C: Becker's nevus: An androgen-mediated hyperplasia with increased androgen receptors. *J Am Acad Dermatol* **10**:235, 1984

Tymen R et al: Nevus tardif de Becker. *Ann Dermatol Venereol* **108**:41, 1981

Urbanek RW, Johnson WC: Smooth muscle hamartoma associated with Becker's nevus. *Arch Dermatol* **114**:104, 1978

6. Solar Lentigo

Solar lentigines are sharply demarcated, usually uniformly pigmented macules from 5 to 30 mm in diameter and induced by exposure to sunlight. Their color does not fade when exposure is stopped.

Synonyms: lentigo senilis, liver spot, old age spot, senile freckle

EPIDEMIOLOGY

Solar lentigines are found in 90 percent of the Caucasian population older than 60 years, and incidence increases with advancing age. They also can be found in younger individuals after acute or chronic sun exposure. Lentigines are more common in Caucasians but also occur in Asians.

ETIOLOGY

Solar lentigines result from epidermal hyperplasia with variable proliferation of melanocytes and accumulation of melanin in keratinocytes in response to ultraviolet radiation.

CLINICAL FEATURES

Solar lentigines are well-circumscribed, round, oval, or irregularly bordered macules of yellow, tan, or brown color (Fig. 6-1). More lightly pigmented lesions are usually homogeneous, whereas darker ones tend to have a mottled appearance. Solar lentigines usually appear as multiple lesions; they vary in size from about 1 to 3 cm in diameter, with a tendency to confluency. Solar lentigines occur on sun-exposed areas, predominantly the dorsal aspects of hands and forearms, the face, and the upper chest and back. A particular variant that may be termed *sunburn, hypermelanotic,* or *"ink spot" solar lentigo* is characterized by a striking jet-black color and a stellate outline (Figs. 6-2 and 6-3).

HISTOLOGIC FEATURES

Histologic examination discloses an epidermal proliferation with elongation of the rete ridges with club-shaped or bud-like extensions and branching or fusing of rete ridges forming a reticulated pattern. The epidermis between the rete ridges may appear thinned. There is increased basal-layer pigmentation, especially in the basaloid cells of the rete ridges. In some, but not all, cases, the melanocytes are increased in number. Melanocytes in dopa-stained sections of solar lentigines exhibit increased melanogenesis, and these cells have more numerous as well as longer and thicker dendritic processes than the melanocytes of normal skin. The upper dermis often contains melanophages and occasionally a mild perivascular infiltrate of lymphocytes.

Electron microscopic studies reveal abundant melanosome complexes in keratinocytes which appear to be larger than in normal surrounding skin. As in light mi-

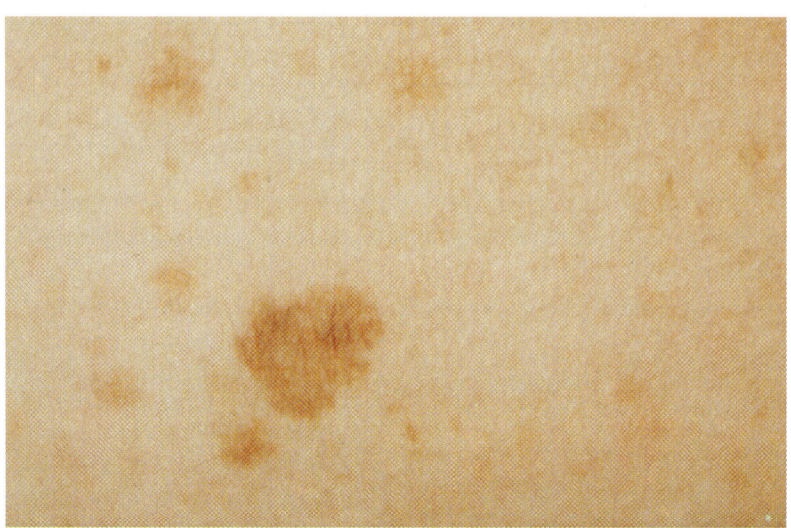

Figure 6-1 *Solar lentigo. This lesion developed on the upper back of a young white male, skin phototype II, following a blistering sunburn.* (From TB Fitzpatrick et al (eds): *Dermatology in General Medicine*, 4th ed. New York, McGraw-Hill, 1993, p 1056, with permission.)

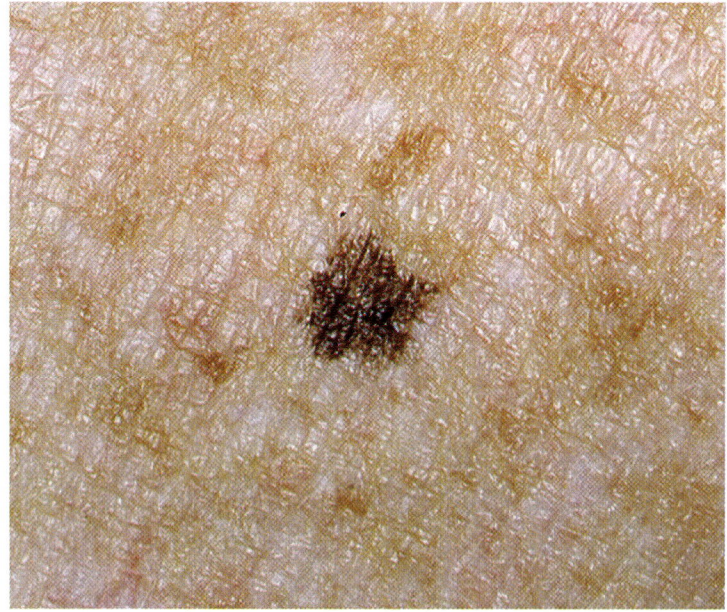

Figure 6-2 *Solar lentigo, hyperpigmented type, which is often seen after a severe sunburn, most often on the upper back.*

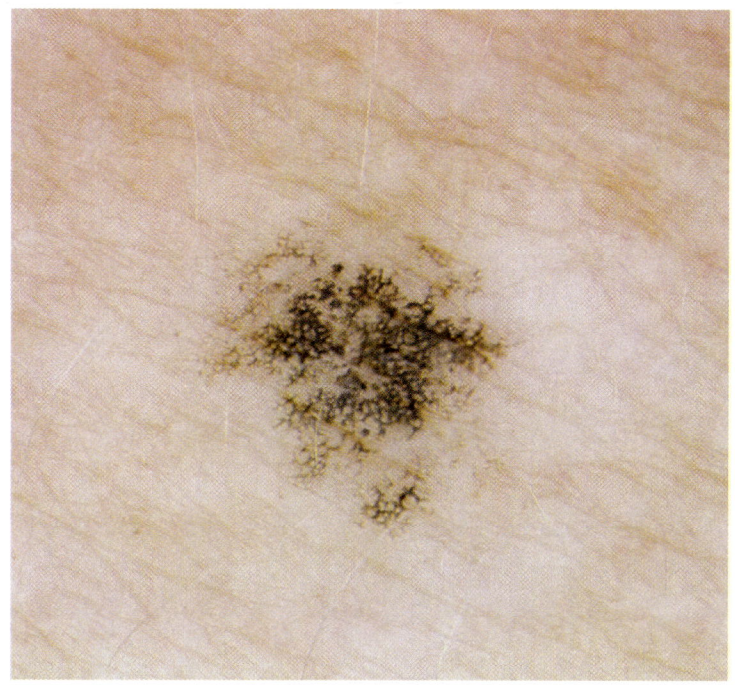

A

Figure 6-3 *Solar lentigo, hyperpigmented type. (a) (Clinical surface view, without oil): This is a relatively small (5-mm-diameter) dark brown lesion with somewhat patchy pigmentation and irregular borders. (b) (Gross subsurface tissue morphology as seen with ELM, with oil): ELM reveals a pigment network pattern with somewhat thicker and darker lines than what is typical of junctional nevi. Note that the network is somewhat "patchy." However, the lesion tends to be darkest in the center and tends to fade out at the periphery. Melanomas may be darkest at the periphery rather than the center of the lesion and may have a "sharp network margin" rather than fading out at the periphery. (c) (Digital enhancement of subsurface morphology): Digital enhancement demonstrates in more detail that the network lines are thicker than typical junctional nevi and that the darkest lines are primarily not at the border of the lesion. (Reprinted with permission from RO Kenet et al: Clinical diagnosis of pigmented lesions using digital epiluminescence microscopy: Grading protocol and atlas. Arch Dermatol 129:157, 1993.)*

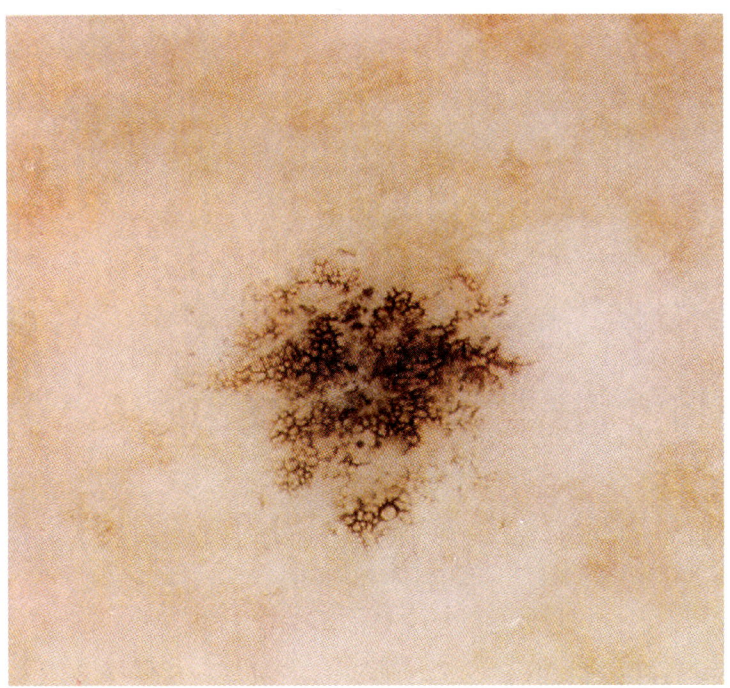

B

Figure 6-3 *(cont.)*

croscopy, the melanocytes show marked dopa reactivity due to increased activity, elongated dendrites, large numbers of melanosomes, enlarged perikarya, and hypertrophic Golgi complexes and mitochondria. Even in the upper layers of the epidermis, numerous large dispersed melanosomes are present, indicating a delay in their lysosomal destruction.

SPECIAL INVESTIGATIONS

Solar lentigines show an irregular border and a reticulated pigment pattern when examined by tangential lighting and hand-lens magnification. Solar lentigines may be visible under Wood's lamp illumination when not apparent in normal light.

BIOLOGIC BEHAVIOR AND PROGNOSIS

Solar lentigines may develop at almost any age and may fade slightly with age or after the cessation of ultraviolet exposure, or they may persist indefinitely. The development of cytologic atypia in solar lentigines on occasion suggests a relationship of solar lentigines to lentigo maligna. The relationship of solar lentigines to freckles (if any) has not been clarified.

Histologic overlap suggests that solitary lichen planus–like keratosis and reticulated seborrheic keratosis evolve from solar lentigo.

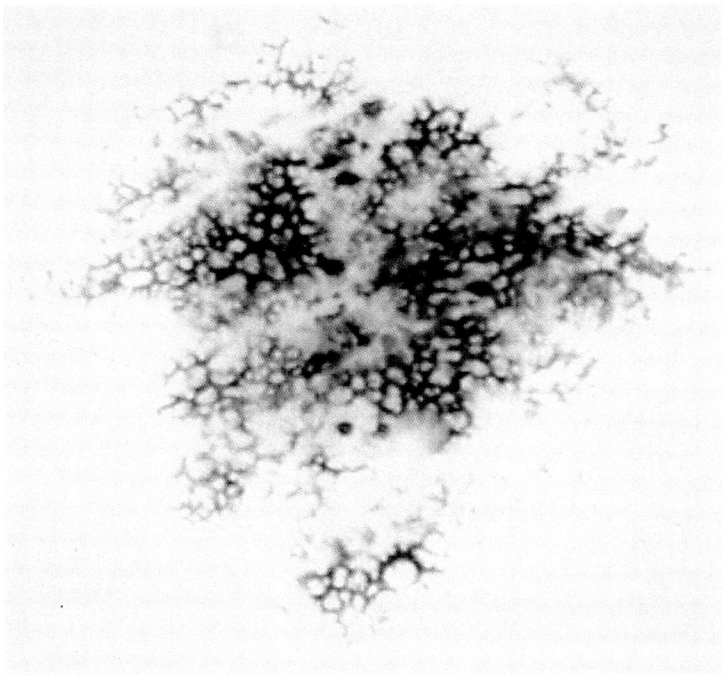

C

Figure 6-3 *(cont.)*

ASSOCIATED DISEASES AND SPECIAL FORMS

PUVA (psoralen + ultraviolet A) lentigo is a well-defined hyperpigmented macule commonly developing in individuals undergoing long-term PUVA chemotherapy (Fig. 6-4). About 50 percent of PUVA-treated persons develop PUVA lentigines after an average of 5 to 7 years of photochemotherapy. The frequency and severity of the lesions are positively correlated with greater numbers of treatments, age of starting therapy, and male sex. There is a negative association with skin phototypes V and VI. In contrast to typical solar lentigines, PUVA lentigines occur on sun-protected skin subjected to PUVA treatment. These lesions usually exhibit darker pigmentation and more of a stellate appearance in contrast to solar lentigines. PUVA lentigines often persist for 2 years or more after the end of PUVA photochemotherapy. Histologically, the PUVA-induced lesions display lentiginous hyperplasia of large melanocytes which often exhibit mild cytologic atypia. On ultrastructural examination, the melanosomes in PUVA lentigines are usually large in comparison with the melanosomes in solar lentigines and single. Because of the frequent presence of cytologic atypia in PUVA lentigines, patients treated with PUVA should be monitored for the development of melanoma.

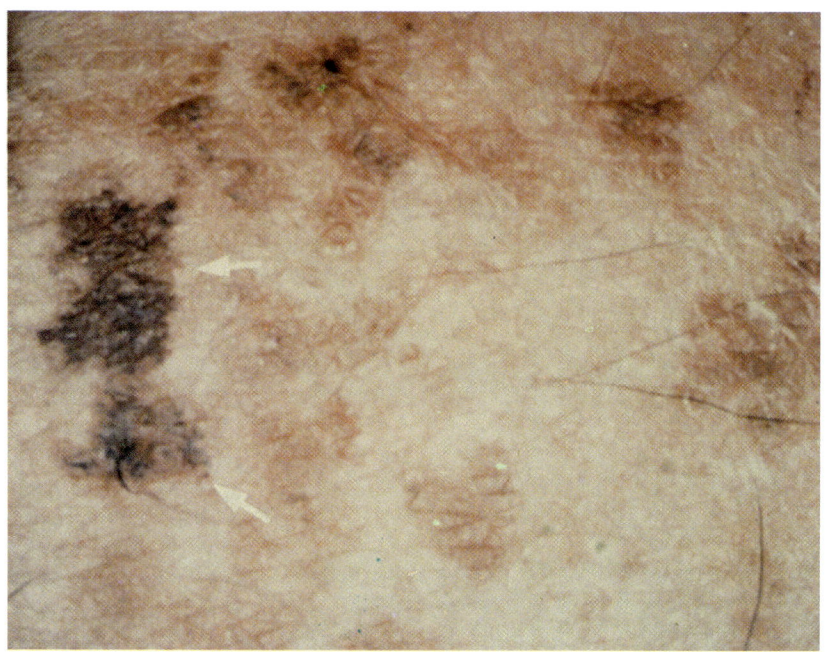

Figure 6-4 *Photochemotherapy (PUVA)-induced lentigines on the buttock of a man who had received PUVA for psoriasis.* (From TB Fitzpatrick et al (eds): *Dermatology in General Medicine,* 4th ed. New York, McGraw-Hill, 1993, p 1057, with permission.)

Solar lentigines are also found in *xeroderma pigmentosum* (Fig. 6-5), a rare genetic disease in which clinical and cellular hypersensitivity to ultraviolet radiation and defective DNA repair are associated with skin malignancies.

DIFFERENTIAL DIAGNOSIS

The differential diagnosis of solar lentigines include freckles, flat varieties of seborrheic keratosis, simple lentigines, pigmented actinic keratosis, lentigo maligna, junctional melanocytic nevi, and large cell acanthomas. Table 6-1 outlines the similarities and differences between solar lentigines and ephelides. There is essentially a continuum extending from solar lentigo to flat varieties of seborrheic keratosis. Demonstration of a keratotic surface with horn cysts is consistent with seborrheic keratosis. Other principal processes that may be confused with solar lentigo are pigmented actinic keratosis (also known as *spreading pigmented actinic keratosis*) and lentigo maligna. Biopsy may be needed for final diagnosis. Pigmented actinic keratosis may exhibit the rough surface and scaling that suggest actinic keratosis rather than solar lentigo. Lentigo maligna has a characteristically macular topography. Furthermore, lentigo maligna often exhibits greater variation in pigmentation and irregularity of borders compared with solar lentigo. Simple lentigines and junctional nevi tend to be well-circumscribed lesions with homogeneous pigmentation. Simple lentigines are often smaller and more heavily pigmented than solar lentigines.

MANAGEMENT

Solar lentigines do not require therapy but may be treated for cosmetic reasons with light applications of liquid nitrogen. Hydroquinone-containing bleaching preparations are not effective. Preventive measures including sunscreens or avoidance of sun exposure may be even more effective than treatment.

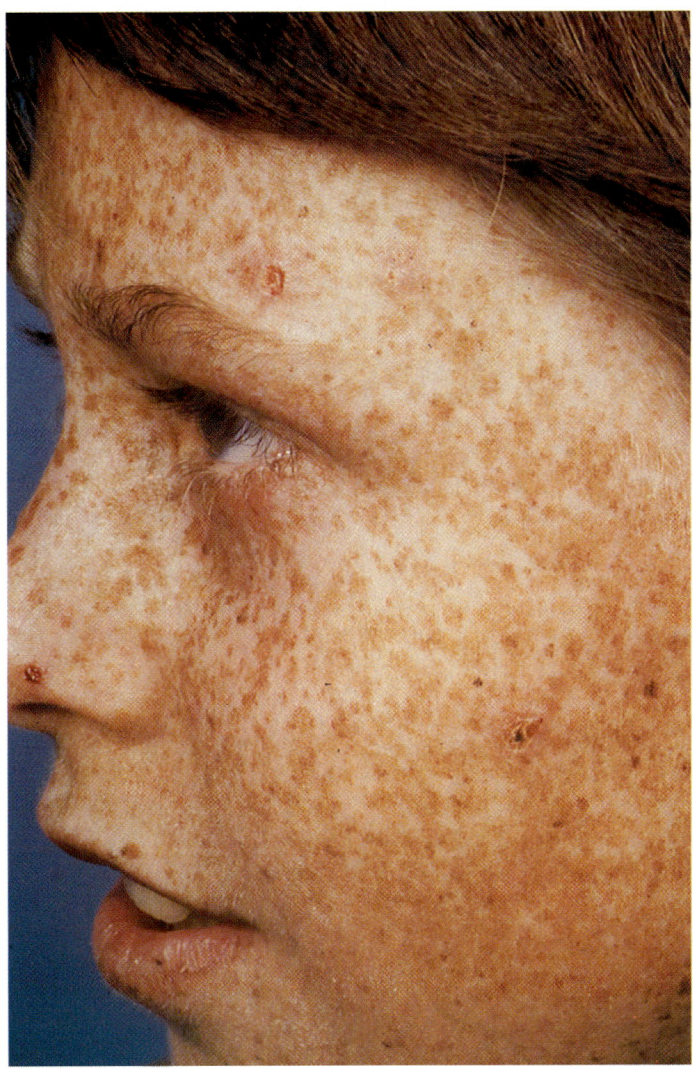

Figure 6-5 *Xeroderma pigmentosum. Mild involvement with a few solar keratoses but marked freckle-like lentigines on the face and lips of a child.* (From TB Fitzpatrick et al: *Color Atlas and Synopsis of Clinical Dermatology,* 2nd ed. New York, McGraw-Hill, 1992, p 625, with permission.)

Table 6-1 Comparative Clinical Features of Freckles and Solar Lentigines

	EPHELIDES (FRECKLES)	SOLAR LENTIGINES
Epidemiology		
Age of appearance	Early childhood	Over age 30
Skin color	White	White, brown, and dark brown
Hair color	"Celtic" types with red or blond hair	Any type
Skin phototype	More common in I, II	More common in I, II, III but also in IV and V
History		
Precipitating factors	Bursts of high-intensity sun exposure convert latent predetermined melanocytes to permanent freckles	Repeated sun exposure over time changes a cluster of melanocytes
Duration of lesions	Fade without sun exposure	Persist for life
Relation to season	Much darker in summer, fade in winter and over time with aging	May darken in summer but do not fade in winter
Heredity	Probably autosomal dominant	No data
Physical examination		
Type of lesion		
Size	Macules, 1–5 mm	Macules 5–15 mm or larger
Color	Light or medium brown	Medium or dark brown
Shape	Round, polycyclic	Round, polycyclic
Border	Jagged	Smooth
Arrangement	Uncountable numbers	Countable, average 3–10
Distribution	On all exposed areas, on the face, forearm, back, rare on dorsa of hands	Principally on the face, neck and common on dorsa of hands
Electron Microscopy	Melanocytes *between* freckle macules contain pheomelanosomes	Large melanosome complexes within keratinocytes

ADDITIONAL READINGS

Braun-Falco O, Schoefinius H-H: Lentigo senilis: Übersicht und eigene Untersuchungen. *Hautarzt* **7**:277, 1971

Breathnach AS: Melanocyte distribution in forearm epidermis of freckled human subjects. *J Invest Dermatol* **29**:253, 1957

Breathnach AS, Wyllie LM: Electron microscopy of melanocytes and melanosomes in freckled human epidermis. *J Invest Dermatol* **42**:389, 1964

Gschnait F et al: Long-term photochemotherapy: Histopathological and immunofluorescence observations in 243 patients. *Br J Dermatol* **103**:11, 1980

Hodgson C: Senile lentigo. *Arch Dermatol* **87**:197, 1963

Jones SK et al: UVA-induced melanocytic lesions. *Br J Dermatol* **117**:111, 1987

Kanerva L et al: A semiquantitative light and electron microscopic analysis of histopathologic changes in photochemotherapy-induced freckles. *Arch Dermatol Res* **276**:2, 1984

Mehregan AH: Lentigo senilis and its evolutions. *J Invest Dermatol* **65**:429, 1975

Miller RA: Psoralens and UVA-induced stellate hyperpigmented freckling. *Arch Dermatol* **118**:619, 1982

Montagna W et al: A reinvestigation of solar lentigines. *Arch Dermatol* **116**:1151, 1980

Nakagawa H et al: Morphologic alterations of epidermal melanocytes and melanosomes in PUVA lentigines: A comparative ultrastructural investigation of lentigines induced by PUVA and sunlight. *J Invest Dermatol* **82**:101, 1984

Rhodes AR et al: Sun-induced freckles in children and young adults. *Cancer* **67**:1990, 1991

Rhodes AR et al: The PUVA-induced pigmented macule: A lentiginous proliferation of large, sometimes cytologically atypical, melanocytes. *J Am Acad Dermatol* **9**:47, 1983

Rhodes AR et al: The PUVA lentigo: An analysis of predisposing factors. *J Invest Dermatol* **81**:459, 1983

Wilson PD, Kligman AM: Experimental induction of freckles by ultraviolet-B. *Br J Dermatol* **106**:401, 1982

7. Lentigo Simplex and Mucosal Melanotic Lesions

Lentigo simplex is a sharply demarcated macule of uniform or variegate hyperpigmentation located anywhere on the body (without predilection for sun-exposed skin) and usually measuring less than 5 mm in diameter. Histologically, this lesion shows lentiginous melanocytic hyperplasia. Lentiginosis is an eruptive form of lentigo simplex which occasionally may be a marker for multisystem disease. The terms *lentiginosis* and *melanosis* also describe lesions with or without melanocytic hyperplasia, respectively, that appear on mucosal sites, such as the conjunctiva, vulva, or penis, and exhibit basal-layer hyperpigmentation. *Melanotic macules* involve labial and oral mucosal sites and are characterized by hyperpigmentation of the basal layer but exhibit little or no lentiginous melanocytic hyperplasia.

Synonyms: simple lentigo, lentiginosis, genital lentiginosis, melanosis, mucosal melanotic macule

EPIDEMIOLOGY

The frequency of lentigo simplex in children and adults is unknown; lentigines are found in all races and seem to occur equally in both sexes. Isolated lesions are often present at birth, more commonly in black than in white newborns. In darkly pigmented races, lentigo simplex is the most common histologic pattern of pigmented lesions on acral cutaneous sites. Lentigines simplex may increase in number during childhood or puberty and sometimes occur in an eruptive form as so-called lentiginosis with or without obvious precipitating factors. Pigmented bands on the nails showing the histology of a lentigo simplex are common in dark-skinned races, especially black individuals. They are found in up to 12 percent of Japanese, whereas they are extremely rare in white individuals.

Oral melanotic macules are found primarily in adults over 40 years of age; approximately 80 percent occur in white individuals. Some authors report a slight female predilection, whereas others describe both sexes affected equally. The most common sites are the vermilion border, followed by the gingiva, the buccal mucosa, and the palate. Up to 30 percent of melanomas in the oral cavity of Caucasians are preceded by melanosis for several months or years. Sixty-six percent of infiltrative oral melanomas in Japanese individuals arise in association with oral melanosis. The labial (lip) melanotic macule occurs mostly between the second and fourth decades of life and has a strong predilection for white females.

The incidence of lentiginosis or melanosis of the female genital area is probably higher than reported. Fifteen percent of 106 females between the ages of 16 and 42 years had genital "nevi." Most lesions are found on the labia minora, but they can occur as well on the labia majora, the vaginal introitus, the cervix, the periurethral area, and the perineum. In a study of 100 random autopsies, 3 cases showed melanosis of the genitalia, and all 3 were elderly women. In general, lentiginosis and melanosis of the female genitalia are benign conditions; atypia is uncommon, and progression to melanoma has not been reported.

In a study of 10,000 men between 17 and 25 years of age, 14.2 percent were noted to have "pigmented nevi" of the genitalia. It is uncertain what proportion was penile lentigo or melanosis, since no clinical descriptions or histologic studies were reported. The ages of patients with penile lentiginosis or melanosis reported in the literature range from 15 to 72 years. The lesions occurred on the glans penis and penile shaft. In a study of pigmented lesions in newborn infants, no lesions were found on the genitalia. Since histologic atypia has been reported in a case of penile lentigo, close follow-up, including biopsies from different sites as judged appropriate, is necessary to rule out atypicality. The incidence of conjunctival melanosis is unknown, but it can be assumed that primary acquired melanosis (PAM) is a precursor lesion of melanoma in this area, since a significant number of melanomas are associated with PAM. Lentigo simplex occasionally develops in scars following excision of malignant melanoma.

ETIOLOGY

An increased number of melanocytes in the basal layer of the epidermis leads to an increased production of melanin, resulting in hyperpigmented macules. The cause of lentigo simplex is unknown, but the appearance of similar macules in disorders affecting other tissues of neuroectodermal origin such as Peutz-Jeghers, LEOPARD, and LAMB syndromes may indicate a generalized defect of neural crest derivatives. Some penile lesions are reported to follow injury, irritation, or PUVA therapy. In women, hormonal factors are thought to play a role. Isolated lentigines may be influenced by genetic factors, since they are frequently found in dark-skinned races.

CLINICAL FEATURES

Lentigines simplex are light brown to black homogeneous pigmented macules occurring anywhere on the body, including mucous membranes and nail beds, without any predilection for sun-exposed areas (Figs. 7-1 to 7-7). They are well circumscribed, round, or oval, have regular borders, and are usually less than 5 mm (often under 3 mm) in diameter (see Fig. 7-1). Lesions on the mucous membranes frequently have irregular, ill-defined borders and mottled, nonhomogeneous pigmentation with areas devoid of pigment; these lesions may be several centimeters in diameter and may resemble early malignant melanoma (see Figs. 7-2 to 7-5). They occur as solitary or multiple lesions. Generalized lentigines may be an isolated phenomenon without underlying disease, either present at birth or appearing during childhood or adulthood. Unilateral lentiginosis and generalized lentiginosis in association with other abnormalities have been described as well (see Fig. 7-6). The latter will be discussed below.

HISTOLOGIC FEATURES

Lentigo simplex exhibits increased numbers of melanocytes in the basal layer of elongated epidermal rete ridges. Increased melanin in the basal layer and sometimes

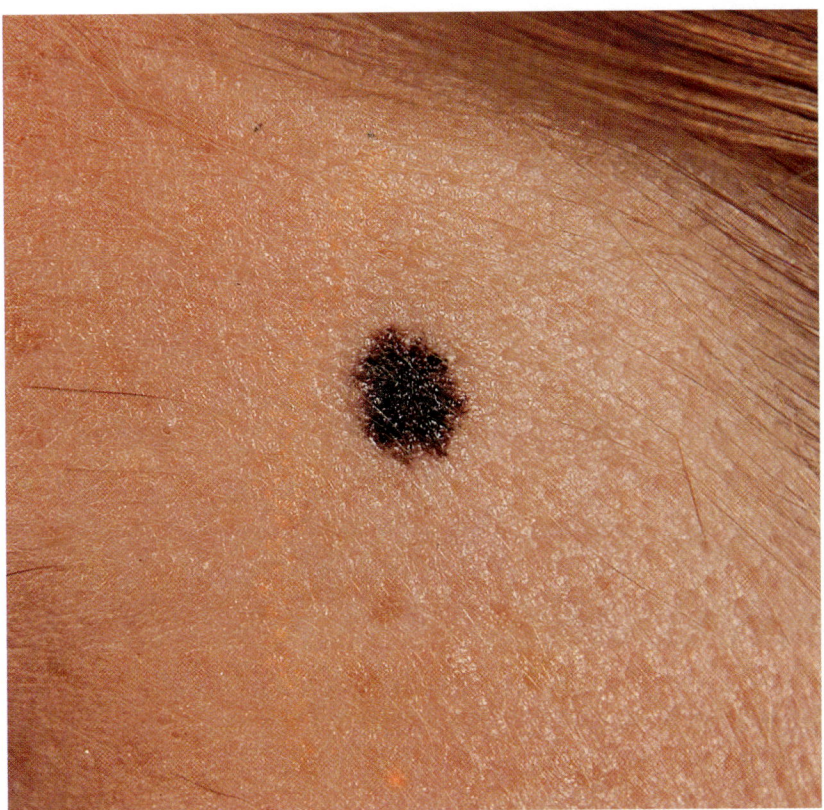

Figure 7-1 *Lentigo simplex. This is a dark brown macule which is almost indistinguishable from a junctional nevus, but histologically, it is distinctively a lentigo.*

even in the upper layers of the epidermis and stratum corneum is commonly observed. Melanophages and a mild inflammatory infiltrate are often present in the upper dermis.

Lesions on mucous membranes, including the lips, show acanthosis with or without elongation of the rete ridges. Slight melanocytic hyperplasia is usually observed but may be absent. Hyperkeratosis, telangiectasia, activated fibroblasts, and large dendritic melanocytes are described in labial melanotic macules. Some acral and mucosal lesions have been reported to exhibit cytologic atypia of the melanocytes.

Melanin macroglobules have been described in lentigo simplex on ultrastructural examination. They are found within melanocytes but also in keratinocytes and melanophages. These are not specific for lentigo simplex, since they have been described in other pigmented lesions (see Chap. 6).

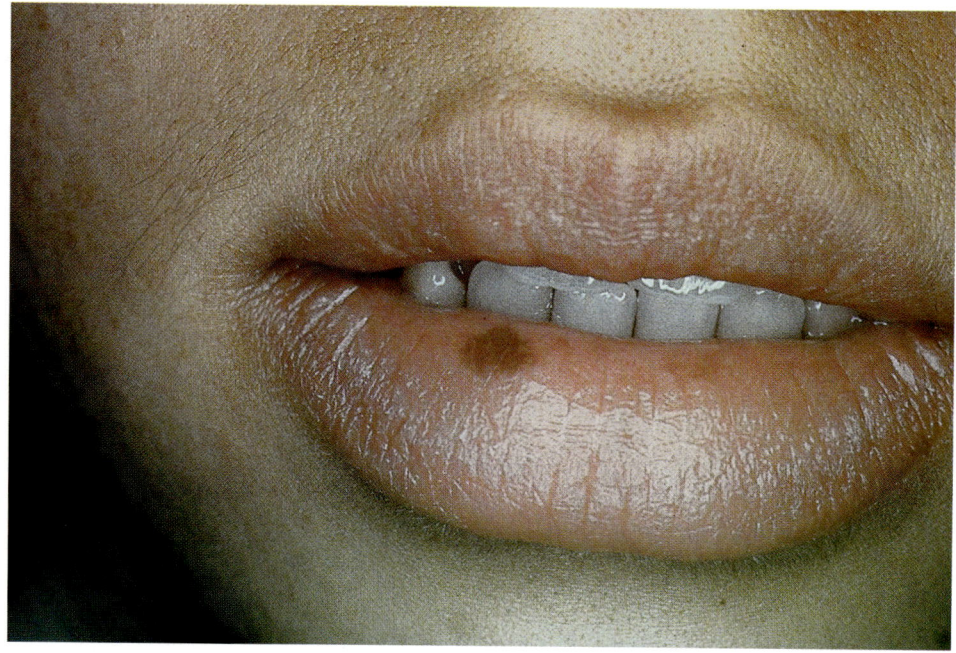

Figure 7-2 *Labial lentigo (lower lip). This lesion, which is not infrequently seen in patients with skin phototypes I and II, has a uniform brown color.*

BIOLOGIC BEHAVIOR AND PROGNOSIS

In contrast to lentigo simplex occurring on the skin, lesions on mucous membranes often slowly increase in size over months to years, with or without changes in the degree of pigmentation; some of them are believed to be precursor lesions for malignant melanoma. Since the presence of preexisting congenital lentigines has been reported in several patients with acral melanoma, such lentigines may be precursor lesions, but more research is needed to establish this relationship to acral lentiginous melanoma.

SPECIAL FORMS AND ASSOCIATED SYNDROMES (SEE TABLE 7-1)

Multiple lentigines syndrome: Synonyms for this condition include *LEOPARD syndrome, lentiginosis syndrome, progressive cardiomyopathic lentiginosis,* and *cardiocutaneous syndrome,* as well as *generalized lentigo and generalized lentiginosis.* Multiple lentigines syndrome is an autosomal dominant disorder with high penetrance and variable expressivity. Multiple lentigines are present at birth or appear during early infancy and may increase in number during childhood. The lesions oc-

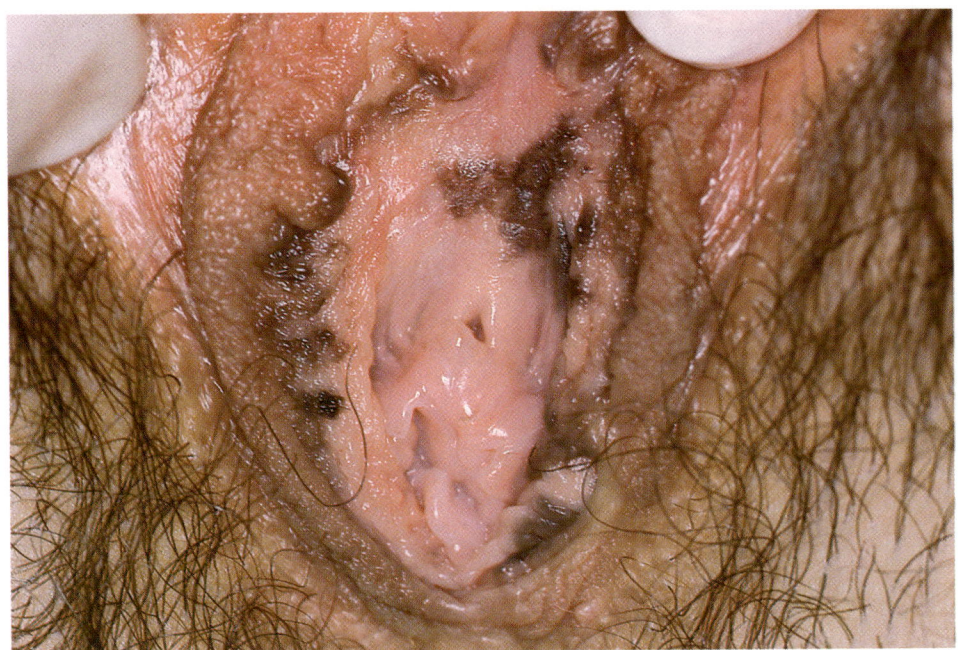

Figure 7-3 *Genital (vulvar) lentiginosis. These asymptomatic lesions on the vulva were present in a 41-year-old woman, appearing 8 years before. The lesions are scattered gray-brown-black macules. Biopsy of the pigmented lesions did not reveal any atypical melanocytes, nor were any nevus cells present. No treatment was attempted, although certain types of laser therapy might be tried in the future.*

cur on both sun-exposed and sun-protected sites, including genitalia, palms, and soles, and are associated with somatic abnormalities. The acronym *LEOPARD* refers to: *l*entigines, *e*lectrocardiographic conduction defects, *o*cular hypertelorism, *p*ulmonary stenosis, *a*bnormalities of genitalia, *r*etardation of growth, and *d*eafness. Variants of this syndrome with incomplete expression have been described.

The *Peutz-Jeghers syndrome* is an autosomal dominant disorder characterized by mucocutaneous lentigines which are present at birth or appear during childhood in combination with intestinal polyposis. The skin lesions are predominantly perioral and periorbital as well as involving the ventral aspects of hands and feet. Mucosal lesions may affect the palate, tongue, buccal mucosa, and conjunctivae. Large lentigines are occasionally noted and resemble café au lait macules. Macules on the oral mucosa may be dark brown or blue-brown in color.

DIFFERENTIAL DIAGNOSIS

The differential diagnosis of the solitary lentigo simplex involves primarily the junctional and relatively flat forms of

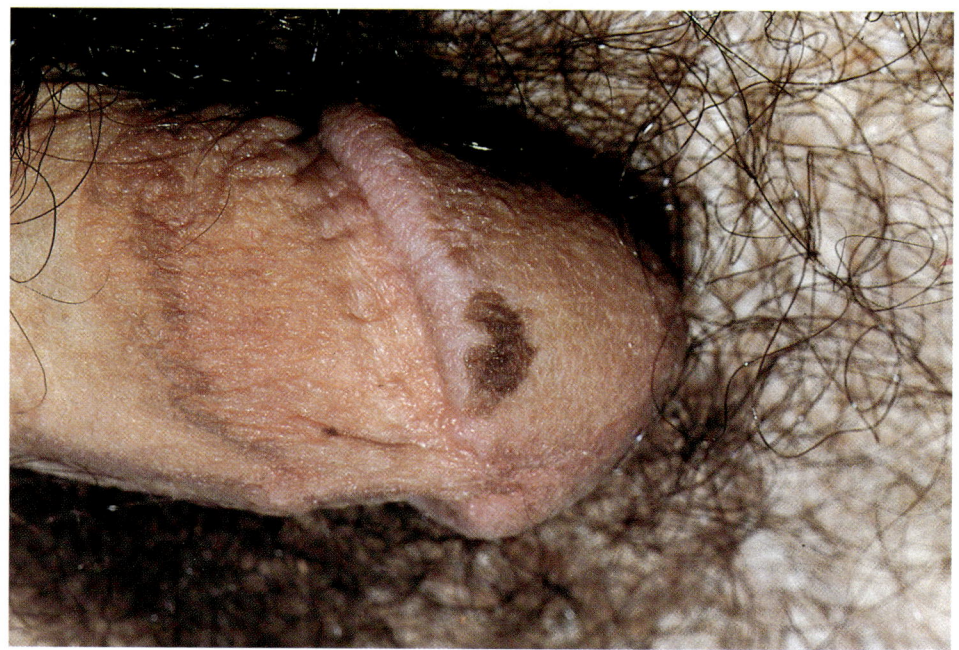

Figure 7-4 *Penile lentigo. This lesion, which looks rather ominous, has variegation of color and irregular borders but is benign and not a premalignant lesion.*

compound melanocytic nevus, solar lentigo, and freckle. In some instances, malignant melanoma, pigmented spindle-cell nevus, café au lait macule, hemangioma, and cutaneous hemorrhage might enter into the differential diagnosis. Although there is a continuum from simple lentigo to junctional melanocytic nevus, the simple lentigo is distinguished from melanocytic nevi by the absence of distorted skin markings when viewed with sidelighting. Lentigo simplex is often smaller (less than 3 to 4 mm) than melanocytic nevi, which are usually 4 to 6 mm in size. However, histopathologic examination may be essential for discrimination of lentigo simplex from a melanocytic nevus. Lentigo simplex is distinguished from a solar lentigo usually by its smaller size, symmetry, uniform pigmentation, and distribution on sites that are not necessarily sun-exposed. However, this distinction may not be possible in some instances without histologic evaluation. The simple lentigo differs from a freckle because of anatomic site, i.e., not being exclusively localized to a sun-exposed area, sharp circumscription, and usually uniform, darker pigmentation. The café au lait macule is usually larger and characterized by lighter color than the simple lentigo. Malignant melanoma, pigmented spindle-cell nevus, and blue nevus are usually distinctive as compared with

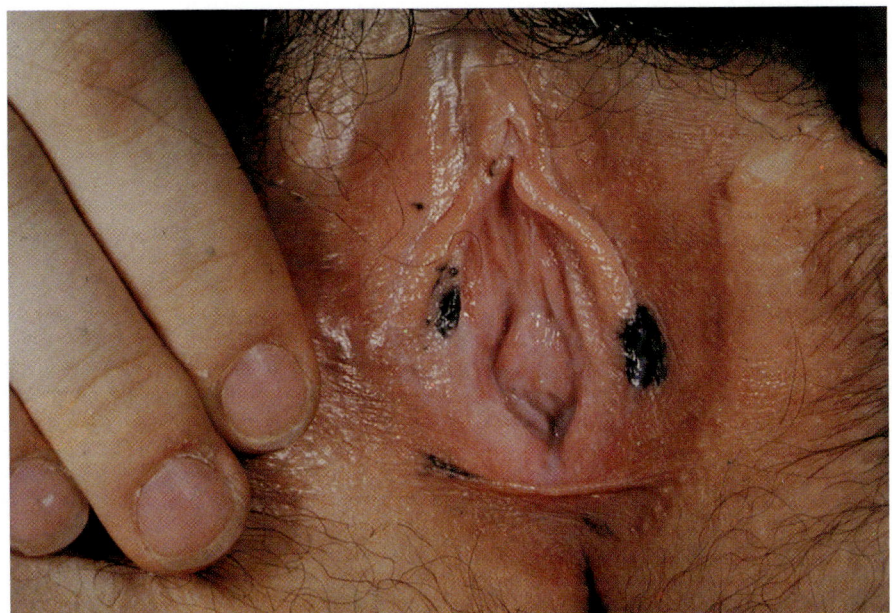

Figure 7-5 *Lentigo simplex. Acquired darkly pigmented lentigines on the vulva of a 13-year-old white girl who has LAMB syndrome.* (From TB Fitzpatrick et al (eds): *Dermatology in General Medicine,* 4th ed. New York, McGraw-Hill, 1993, p 1050, with permission.)

simple lentigo, but on occasion, the latter entities may enter into the differential diagnosis. The latter entities usually are characterized by larger size and show elevation, or at least distortion, of skin cleavage lines. Malignant melanoma usually exhibits asymmetry, irregular borders, and variegation of color. The involvement of mucous membranes by lentigines as single lesions or in a multicentric pattern has been termed *lentiginosis* or *melanosis.* The clinical appearance of such lesions may be strikingly abnormal with irregular borders and considerable variation in the pigment pattern. In most instances, such lesions are stable for many years. However, sampling for histologic evaluation is essential to exclude an atypical proliferation.

MANAGEMENT AND FOLLOW-UP

In general, there is no need to treat benign-appearing lentigo simplex. Lesions on acral or mucous membranes should be evaluated carefully and, if clinically atypical, should be considered for biopsy to assess melanocytic atypia. Lentigines occurring in the patterns of the multiple lentigines syndrome or Peutz-Jeghers syndrome are of practical significance and require further investigation as an indication of systemic disease.

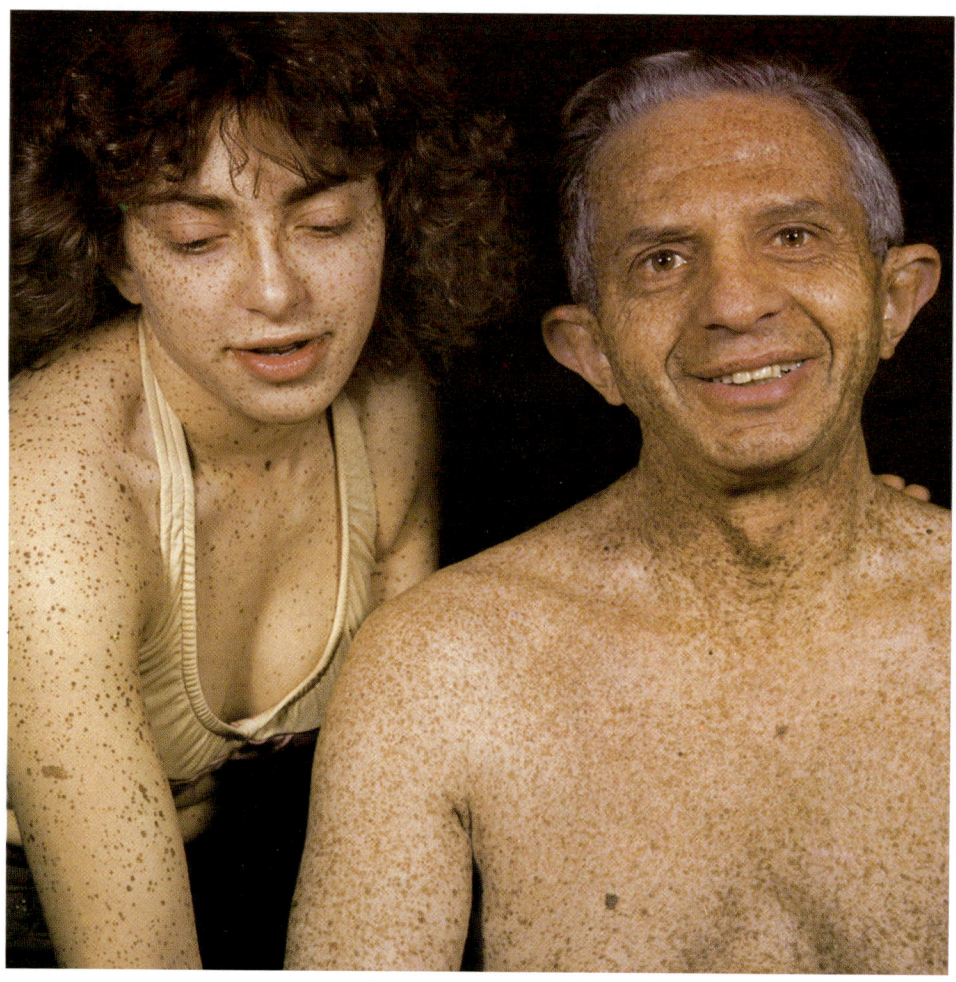

Figure 7-6 *LEOPARD syndrome. Father and daughter both have pulmonic stenosis and extensive freckle-like lentigines in the exposed and unexposed areas. Some lesions are larger than 2.0 to 3.0 mm.* (From TB Fitzpatrick et al: *Color Atlas and Synopsis of Clinical Dermatology,* 2nd ed. New York, McGraw-Hill, 1992, p 645, with permission.)

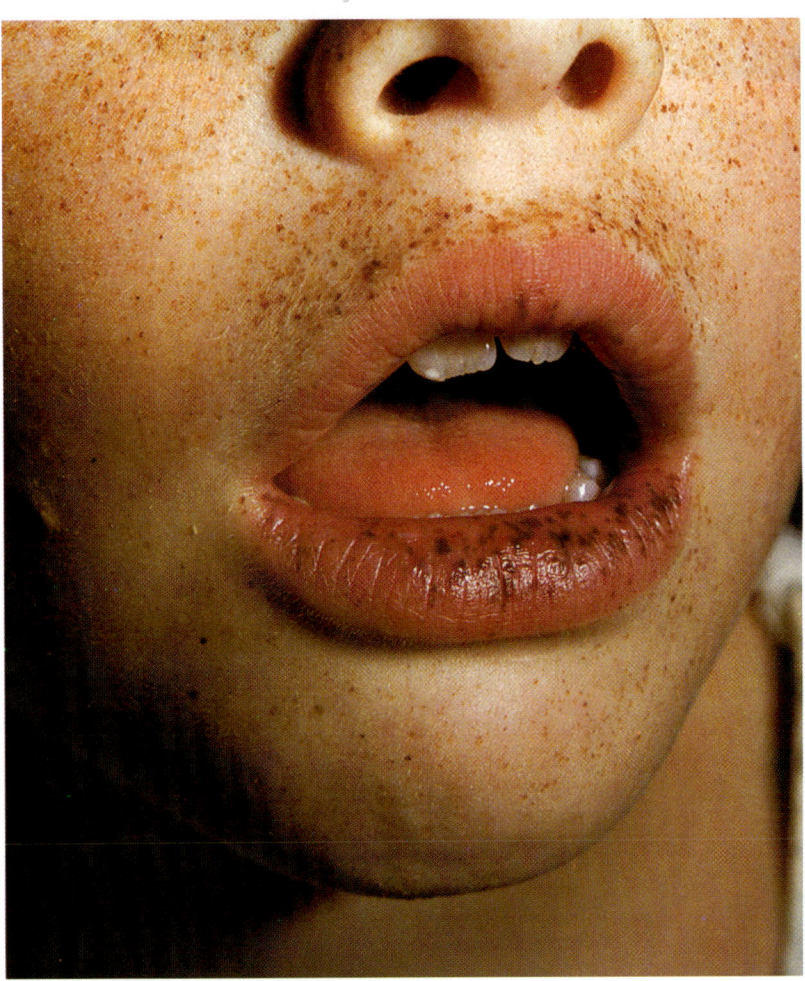

Figure 7-7 *Peutz-Jeghers syndrome. Lentigines, which are dark brown to gray blue, appear on the lips, around the mouth, and on the fingers. Lip macules may, over time, disappear.* (From TB Fitzpatrick et al (eds): *Dermatology in General Medicine*, 4th ed. New York, McGraw-Hill, 1993, p 965, with permission.)

Table 7-1 Special Forms of Lentigo Simplex and Associated Syndromes

DISEASE/SYNDROME	PERTINENT FEATURES
Multiple lentigines (LEOPARD) syndrome	See text
Peutz-Jeghers syndrome	See text
Eruptive lentiginosis	Young adults Development over months to years Disseminated distribution
Localized lentiginosis	
Lentiginosis perigenitoaxillaris	Lentigines limited to axillae and genital area
Partial unilateral lentiginosis	Dermatomal distribution with or without CNS abnormalities
Inherited patterned lentiginosis in blacks (variant of racial pigmentation)	Autosomal dominant Onset in early childhood Centrofacial with involvement of lips, palms, soles, elbows, buttocks Oral mucosal involvement (gingiva, buccal mucosae, soft palate)
Centrofacial lentiginosis	Autosomal dominant Onset in first year of life "Butterfly-like" distribution on nose and cheeks, but occasionally forehead, eyes, upper lip Usually sparing of mucous membranes Bone, endocrine, neurologic abnormalities
LAMB syndrome	*L*entigines (face and genitalia) *A*trial myxomas *M*ucocutaneous myxomas *B*lue nevi
Laugier-Hunziker syndrome	Hyperpigmentation of lips, buccal mucosa, and nails
Carney's syndrome	See "Ephelides" (Chap. 3)
Cronkhite-Canada syndrome	Lentigines of buccal mucosa, hands, feet Hair loss, nail dystrophy, intestinal polyposis

ADDITIONAL READINGS

Alper J, Holmes LB: The incidence and significance of birthmarks in a cohort of 4641 newborns. *Pediatr Dermatol* **1**:58, 1983

Barnhill RL et al: Genital lentiginosis: A clinical and histopathologic study. *J Am Acad Dermatol* **22**:453, 1990

Bhawan J, Cahn TM: Atypical penile lentigo. *J Dermatol Surg Oncol* **10**:99, 1984

Buchner A, Handen LS: Melanotic macule of the oral mucosa. *Oral Surg* **48**:244, 1979

Carney JA et al: The complex of myxomas, spotty pigmentation, and endocrine overactivity. *Medicine* **64**:270, 1985

Coleman WP III et al: Nevi, lentigines, and melanomas in blacks. *Arch Dermatol* **116**:548, 1980

Coskey RJ: Eruptive nevi (letter). *Arch Dermatol* **111**:1658, 1975

Daniel ES et al: The Cronkhite-Canada syndrome: An analysis of clinical and pathologic features and therapy in 55 patients. *Medicine* **61**:293, 1982

Dociu I et al: Centrofacial lentiginosis: A survey of 40 cases. *Br J Dermatol* **94**:39, 1976

Eady RAJ et al: Eruptive nevi: Report of two cases, with enzyme histochemical, light and electron microscopic findings. *Br J Dermatol* **97**:267, 1977

Folberg R, McLean IW: Primary acquired melanosis and melanoma of the conjunctiva: Terminology, classification and biologic behavior. *Hum Pathol* **16**:129, 1985

Jackson R: Melanosis of the vulva. *J Dermatol Surg Oncol* **10**:119, 1984

Jeghers H et al: Generalized intestinal polyposis and melanin spots of the oral mucosa, lips, and digits: A syndrome of diagnostic significance. *N Engl J Med* **241**:993, 1949

Kopf AW, Bart RS: Penile lentigo. *J Dermatol Surg Oncol* **8**:637, 1982

Laugier P, Hunziker N: Pigmentation melanique lentiguilaire, essentielle de la muqueuse jugale et des levres. *Arch Belg Dermatol Syphiligr* **26**:391, 1970

Leicht S et al: Atypical pigmented penile macules. *Arch Dermatol* **124**:1267, 1988

Leyden JJ et al: Diffuse and banded melanin pigmentation in nails. *Arch Dermatol* **105**:548, 1972

Maize JC: Mucosal melanosis. *Dermatol Clin* **6**:283, 1988

O'Neill JF, James WD: Inherited patterned lentiginosis in blacks. *Arch Dermatol* **125**:1231, 1989

Page LR et al: The oral melanotic macule. *Oral Surg Oral Med Oral Pathol* **44**:219, 1977

Rhodes AR et al: Mucocutaneous lentigines, cardiomucocutaneous myxomas, and multiple blue nevi: The "LAMB" syndrome. *J Am Acad Dermatol* **10**:72, 1984

Shapiro L, Zegarelli DJ: The solitary labial lentigo: A clinicopathologic study of 20 cases. *Oral Surg Oral Med Oral Pathol* **31**:87, 1971

Sison-Torre EQ, Ackerman AB: Melanosis of the vulva: A clinical simulator of malignant melanoma. *Am J Dermatopathol* **7**(suppl):51, 1985

Utsunomiya J et al: Peutz-Jeghers syndrome: Its natural course and management. *Johns Hopkins Med J* **136**:71, 1975

Voron DA et al: Multiple lentigines syndrome: Case report and review of the literature. *Am J Med* **60**:447, 1976

Weathers DR et al: The labial melanotic macule. *Oral Surg Oral Med Oral Pathol* **42**:196, 1976

8. Mongolian Spot

A Mongolian spot is an ill-defined macular discoloration with a characteristic uniform gray to steel-blue appearance, varying in its size and intensity, and showing a tendency to disappear in early childhood; the typical site of appearance is the lumbosacral area.

Synonym: congenital dermal melanocytosis

EPIDEMIOLOGY

Mongolian spots are usually present at birth or appear within the first weeks of life; very few cases describe an onset after early childhood. Both sexes seem to be affected equally. The lesions usually regress in early childhood but can persist lifelong and were found in 4.1 percent of 9996 Japanese males between 18 and 22 years of age. They occur in all races, with a frequency of 100 percent in Malaysians, 90 to 100 percent of Mongolians, Japanese, Chinese, and Koreans, 87 percent of Bolivian Indians, 76 percent of mixed races in Bolivia, 65 percent of blacks in Brazil, 52 percent of mixed races in Brazil, 46 to 99 percent of Polynesians, 17 percent of whites in Bolivia, but only 1.5 percent of whites in Brazil, 1.8 percent of Italians, and rarely in other European whites. The racial differences in the frequency of this abnormality suggest that genetic factors influence melanocytic migration.

ETIOLOGY

The hyperpigmentation in Mongolian spots is secondary to melanocytes in the middle to lower dermis that have failed to reach the epidermis during their migration from the neural crest. Melanocytes appear in the dermis in the tenth week of gestation, start to migrate to the epidermis in the following 4 weeks, and disappear from the dermis after the twentieth week. At birth, they are found only on the scalp, dorsa of the hands and feet, and the sacral area. The latter is the most common site for Mongolian spots. The bluish coloration of Mongolian spots results from the Tyndall phenomenon: dermal pigmentation appears blue because of decreased reflectance in the longer-wavelength region compared with the surrounding area. Long wavelengths, such as red, orange, and yellow, are not reflected and continue into deeper parts of the skin compared with the shorter-wavelength blue and violet, which are reflected to the skin surface.

CLINICAL FEATURES

The classic location is the lumbosacral area or the inner aspect of the buttocks (Fig. 8-1). Usually, Mongolian spot is a single lesion, but multiple macules have been described. The lesions are macular and have a round, oval, or angulated shape; some lesions are hair-bearing. The size varies from a few centimeters to lesions measuring 20 cm or more in size. In general, Mongolian spots have poorly delineated borders, but larger lesions tend to

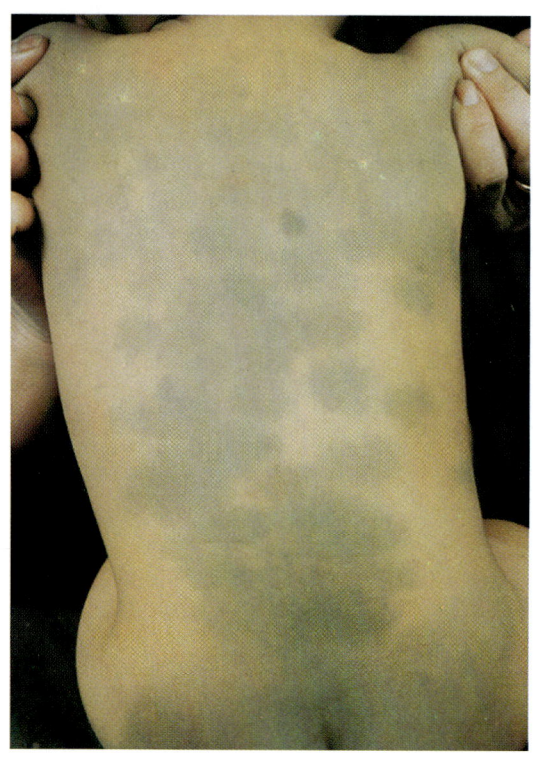

Figure 8-1 *Mongolian spot. This young Japanese child demonstrates extensive Mongolian spots that are not only in the sacral area, the characteristic location, but also extending up the back.* (From TB Fitzpatrick et al (eds): *Dermatology in General Medicine,* 4th ed. New York, McGraw-Hill, 1993, p 978, with permission.)

exhibit better definition. The color varies from uniform light blue to gray and steel blue to grayish green in individuals with dark skin. Persistent variants with darker pigmented spots within the gray-blue macule have been described; they are common in adults with nevus of Ota. Extensive Mongolian spots may occur with bilateral forms of nevus of Ota.

HISTOLOGIC FEATURES

Bipolar dendritic melanocytes are dispersed singly in the lower half or two-thirds of the dermis. These melanocytes are dopa-positive and lie parallel to the epidermis between the collagen bundles without disturbing the normal architecture of the skin. Occasionally, persistent Mongolian spots have the histologic features of a blue nevus with penetration of the subcutis, muscle, and fascia by dermal melanocytes.

On electron microscopy, Mongolian spots show fully developed melanocytes with exclusively mature, electron-dense melanosomes and very few premelanosomes.

SPECIAL INVESTIGATIONS

The Wood's lamp examination is used to distinguish epidermal and dermal hyperpigmentation. In contrast to epidermal pigment, dermal pigment as in the Mongolian spot is not enhanced by Wood's lamp. The Wood's lamp is not helpful in evaluating pigmented lesions in patients who have dark brown or black skin.

BIOLOGIC BEHAVIOR AND PROGNOSIS

As mentioned previously, Mongolian spots are usually present at birth and tend to disappear in early childhood, although variants with late onset and persistent variants have been described. Malignancy in Mongolian spots has not been reported.

DIFFERENTIAL DIAGNOSIS

The differential diagnosis of Mongolian spot includes other dermal melanocytoses such as nevus of Ota, nevus of Ito, dermal melanocyte hamartoma, and blue nevus, as well as a vascular malformation or hemangioma, a contusion, argyria, ochronosis, and fixed drug eruption. The distinctive clinical presentation of Mongolian spot, in particular the characteristic location in the lumbosacral region, presence at birth, occurrence in Asians or other persons of color, and the typical light blue or grayish coloration without surface alteration, generally allows easy distinction from all the entities listed above. Nonetheless, occurrence of Mongolian spots in other anatomic locations may suggest other processes. Histopathologic sampling of such a lesion may be necessary for diagnosis. So-called persistent Mongolian spots may in fact represent variants of nevus of Ota or Ito or related conditions. The findings on histologic examination should allow proper classification of the lesion with attention to the clinical presentation.

MANAGEMENT

Persistent lesions may be treated with cover-up preparations such as Covermark with good cosmetic results. Laser treatment has been used recently with success.

ADDITIONAL READINGS

Burkhart CG, Gohara A: Dermal melanocytic hamartoma. *Arch Dermatol* **117**:102, 1981

Dorsey CS, Montgomery H: Blue nevus and its distinction from Mongolian spot and the nevus of Ota. *J Invest Dermatol* **22**:225, 1954

El Bahrawy A: Ueber den Mongolenfleck bei Europaern. *Arch Dermatol Syphilol* **141**:171, 1922

Gilchrest BA et al: Localization of melanin pigmentation on the skin with Wood's lamp. *Br J Dermatol* **96**:245, 1977

Hidano A: Persistent Mongolian spot in the adult. *Arch Dermatol* **103**:680, 1971

Hidano A et al: Natural history of nevus of Ota. *Arch Dermatol* **95**:187, 1967

Okawa Y et al: On the extracellular sheath of dermal melanocytes in nevus fuscoceruleus acromiodeltiodus (Ito) and Mongolian spot: An ultrastructural study. *J Invest Dermatol* **73**:224, 1979

Zimmerman AA, Becker SW Jr: Precursors of epidermal melanocytes in the Negro fetus; in *Pigment Cell Biology,* edited by M Gordon. New York, Academic Press, 1959, pp 159–170

9. Nevus of Ota and Related Conditions

Nevus of Ota is a persistent, ill-defined, usually unilateral, macular, mottled blue to brown discoloration of the skin and mucous membranes supplied by the first and second branches of the trigeminal nerve.

Synonyms: nevus fuscocaeruleus ophthalmomaxillaris, oculodermal melanocytosis, congenital melanosis bulbi, melanosis bulborum and aberrant Mongolian spots, progressive melanosis oculi, persistent aberrant Mongolian spot, oculomucodermal melanocytosis

EPIDEMIOLOGY

Nevus of Ota occurs predominantly in dark-skinned races, especially in Asians and blacks, but has been described in whites as well. About 80 percent of all reported cases have been in women; however, this is not clear evidence of a female predilection for this anomaly but may simply indicate greater cosmetic concern in women. Nevus of Ota is found in about 0.4 to 0.8 percent of all Japanese dermatologic patients. No epidemiologic studies on the frequency in whites are available at this time.

The lesion has two peaks of onset: the first (about 50 to 60 percent of all cases) in early childhood before the age of 1 year, with the majority present at birth, and the second (40 to 50 percent) around puberty. Onset between the ages of 1 and 11 and after 20 years is rare. Although rare familial forms of nevus of Ota have been reported, the condition is generally not considered hereditary.

ETIOLOGY

Hyperpigmentation in nevus of Ota is due to melanin-producing melanocytes in the dermis that have failed to reach the epidermis during fetal life (see Chap. 8). The larger concentration of melanocytes in nevus of Ota in comparison with Mongolian spots is thought to indicate a hamartomatous nature. According to some patients, the nevus appeared after trauma, contusion, or sunburn. Some women have reported onset around menarche; others have noted postpubertal and postmenopausal onset, which could be secondary to hormonal influence.

CLINICAL FEATURES

Nevus of Ota is usually characterized by a confluence of individual macules varying from pinhead-sized lesions to some several millimeters in diameter (Fig. 9-1). The shape of the individual macule may be round, oval, or serrated, whereas the overall appearance is that of an irregularly demarcated, ill-defined, and often mottled patch that blends with adjacent normal skin (Fig. 9-1*b*). The overall size varies from a few centimeters in diameter to lesions covering almost half the face. The color varies from shades of tan and brown to gray, blue, black, and purple. The lesion usually is unilateral and follows the

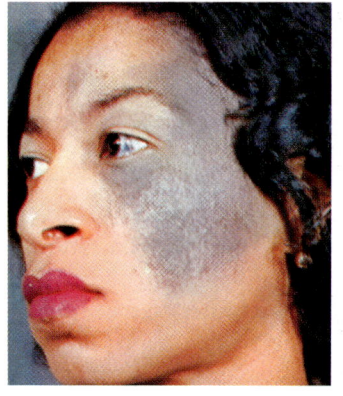
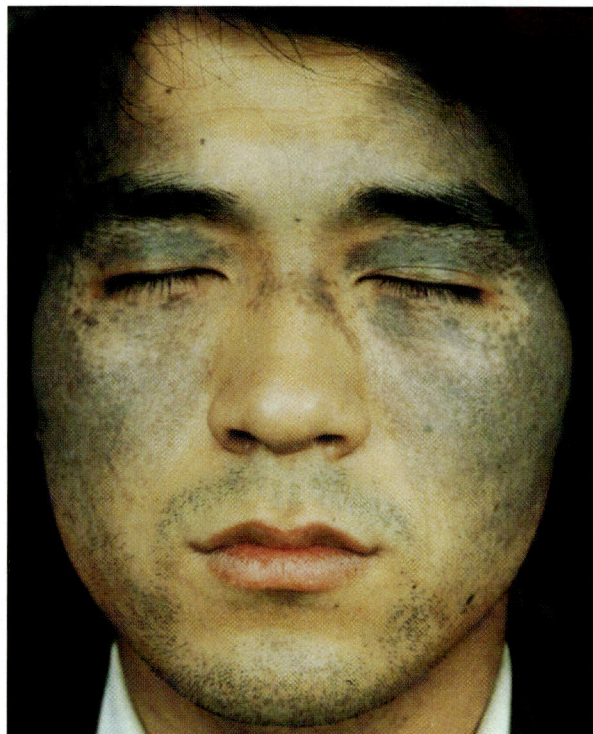

Figure 9-1 *Nevus of Ota. (a) Nevus of Ota in a black; this pigmentation is not usually congenital but rather develops at puberty and does not disappear. Both epidermal and dermal components may coexist. (b) Bilateral type.*

distribution of the first two branches of the trigeminal nerve. The periorbital area, temple, forehead, malar area, earlobe, pre- and retroauricular regions, nose, and conjunctivae are the most common sites affected. A characteristic feature, which is seen in about two-thirds of patients, is the involvement of the ipsilateral sclera (Fig. 9-1c); rarely, nevus of Ota affects the cornea, iris, fundus oculi, optic papilla, retrobulbar fat, periosteum, retina, and optic nerve. Heterochromia of the iris and glaucoma have been reported, but vision is usually not impaired. Other frequent sites of involvement are the tympanum (55 percent), nasal mucosa (28 percent), pharynx (24 percent), and palate (18 percent). Occasionally, the external auditory canal, mandibular area, lips, neck, and thorax are involved. In about 5 to 13 percent of cases, the lesion is bilateral, combined with extensive Mongolian spots. Persistent Mongolian spots are a common finding in adults with nevus of Ota. Bilateral nevi of Ota associated with nevus of Ito (see under "Special Forms and Associated Ab-

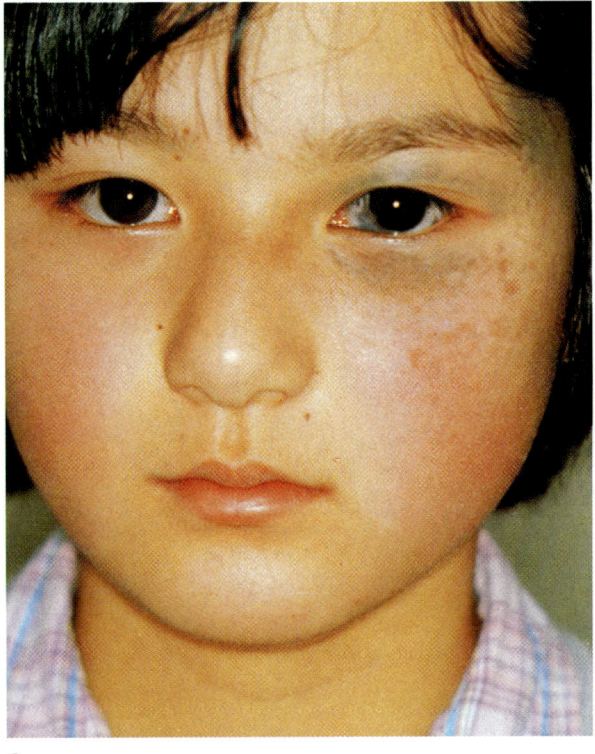

C

Figure 9-1 *Nevus of Ota. (continued)* (c) *Unilateral type with ocular involvement.* (From TB Fitzpatrick et al (eds): *Dermatology in General Medicine,* 4th ed. New York, McGraw-Hill, 1993, p 980, with permission.)

normalities" below) and aberrant and persistent Mongolian spots have been reported. A classification includes four types and two subtypes, according to distribution: mild (orbital and zygomatic), moderate, severe, and bilateral. However, some lesions do not show the classic pattern and may be minor variants or abortive forms with only partial involvement of the skin supplied by the trigeminal nerve. Most common is the moderate type, showing involvement of the eyelid, the zygomatic region, and the base of the nose.

Blue nevi are sometimes found in the lesion itself or in adjacent skin; malignant melanoma arising in association with nevus of Ota have been described (see under "Biologic Behavior and Prognosis" below).

HISTOLOGIC FEATURES

The noninfiltrated areas in nevus of Ota show pigmented, elongated, dendritic melanocytes scattered among the collagen bundles. In comparison with Mongolian spots, the cells are more numerous and are located in the upper third of the reticular dermis; occasionally, cells are found in the papillary dermis or even deep in the subcutaneous fat. Hyperpigmentation of the lower epidermis and an increase in basilar melanocytes may occur. The dopa reactivity of the melanocytes in nevus of Ota varies: slightly pigmented cells are often strongly reactive, whereas heavily pigmented melanocytes often are not reactive. The negative reaction in heavily pigmented melanocytes indicates that all melanogenic enzymes have been consumed. Melanocytes can be found clustering around blood vessels and sweat and sebaceous glands; occasionally, they are seen in vessel walls or in sweat ducts. Raised or infiltrated areas show a larger number of dendritic melanocytes forming cellular aggregates or clumps resembling blue nevi histologically.

BIOLOGIC BEHAVIOR AND PROGNOSIS

As mentioned earlier, nevus of Ota may be present at birth or appear during the first year of life or around puberty but rarely in childhood and adulthood. The lesion shows a tendency toward extension and persists lifelong. Enlargement may be observed in childhood; older patients do not report improvement with advancing age. However, fluctuations of extent and intensity of the color are often described, especially in association with periods of hormonal flux such as menstruation, puberty, or menopause.

Malignancies arising in nevi of Ota are rare. Malignant melanoma has been reported to develop in association with nevus of Ota. Other tumors such as atypical and borderline cellular blue nevi also have been described. Several cases of primary malignant melanoma of the choroid, orbit, iris, chiasma, and meninges have developed in association with nevi of Ota that exhibited eye involvement.

SPECIAL FORMS AND ASSOCIATED ABNORMALITIES

Nevus of Ito (synonym: N. fuscocaeruleus acromiodeltoideus) differs from nevus of Ota mainly in its area of involvement, which corresponds to the distribution of the posterior supraclavicular and cutaneous brachii lateralis nerves (which encompasses the supraclavicular, scapular, or deltoid regions). The clinical and histologic picture is the same as in nevus of Ota. There is a mottled appearance with bluish or brownish macules. Nevus of Ito may occur as an isolated lesion or in association with an ipsilateral or bilateral nevus of Ota. Malignant changes in this lesion have been reported rarely.

Dermal melanocytosis or *dermal melanocyte hamartoma* is a large, diffusely gray-blue pigmented area with several small, well-demarcated darker macules within in it; the lesions are present at birth, but onset in childhood has been reported as well. They have been described on the buttocks and leg in a dermatomal distribution, on the hand gradually extending since childhood, as disseminated macules developing during childhood, or in a generalized form. The histologic features are similar to nevus of Ota.

Acquired nevus of Ota–like macules (nevus fuscocaeruleus zygomaticus, Sun's nevus) are characterized by bilateral bluish macules of the zygomatic area, similar in appearance to nevus of Ota. Mainly Chinese or Japanese women ranging in age from 19 to 69 years have been reported with this process. The eye and oral mucosa are not involved.

Acquired dermal melanocytosis of the face and extremities are very closely related to acquired nevus of Ota–like macules but also involve the extensor aspects of the upper extremities and possibly the palms.

DIFFERENTIAL DIAGNOSIS

The differential diagnosis of nevus of Ota and related conditions includes Mongolian spot, blue nevus, melasma, café au lait macule, nevus spilus, lentigo maligna, contusion, argyria, ochronosis, and drug eruptions, including photosensitivity and fixed drug eruption. The Mongolian spot differs from nevus of Ota and other dermal melanocytoses primarily because of anatomic location in the lumbosacral region, congenital onset, spontaneous regression by age 3 to 4 years, poorly defined clinical appearance, and typical histology of sparsely cellular involvement of the lowermost reticular dermis. Typical blue nevus is distinguished from other dermal melanocytoses because it is a well-circumscribed, slightly elevated or papular lesion measuring less than 1 cm in greatest diameter. Melasma may exhibit both brownish and bluish hyperpigmentation involving the face but is distinguished from nevus of Ota because of the usual bilateral involvement, completely macular surface, and absence of mucous membrane involvement. Café au lait macules are distinguished by a homogeneous light brown or brown color, the absence of bluish coloration, and a completely macular morphology. Nevus spilus is distinguished by typical dark macular or papular speckles superimposed on a café au lait–like macular background. Lentigo maligna on occasion may suggest nevus of Ota because of a unilateral hyperpigmented appearance. However, lentigo maligna usually occurs in older individuals with fair skin and extensive sun exposure. The differential diagnosis for nevus of Ota involving mucous membranes includes melanocytic nevus, mucosal melanotic macules or lentigines, and tattoos. Histopathologic examination may be necessary for definitive diagnosis.

MANAGEMENT AND FOLLOW-UP

Management of the dermal melanocytoses is problematic. Camouflage with opaque makeup is probably favored. Other treatments such as cryotherapy, dermabrasion, or electrodesiccation may cause hypopigmentation or scarring. Successful treatment with a combination of sequential dry ice, epidermal peeling, and argon laser has been described. Nevus of Ota also has been treated successfully by Q-switched ruby laser. Although malignant changes are rare in patients with nevus of Ota, such patients should undergo follow-up especially when eye involvement is evident, since several cases of malignant melanoma have been reported in lesions associated with eye involvement.

ADDITIONAL READINGS

Bashiti HM et al: Generalized dermal melanocytosis. *Arch Dermatol* **117**:791, 1981

Burkhart CG, Gohara A: Dermal melanocyte hamartoma. *Arch Dermatol* **117**:102, 1981

Carleton A, Biggs R: Diffuse mesodermal pigmentation with congenital cranial abnormality. *Br J Dermatol* **60**:10, 1948

Cosman B et al: An effective cosmetic treatment for Ota's nevus. *Ann Plast Surg* **22**:36, 1989

Dorsey CS, Montgomery H: Blue nevus and its distinction from Mongolian spot and the nevus of Ota. *J Invest Dermatol* **2**:225, 1954

Enriquez R et al: Primary malignant melanoma of central nervous system. *Arch Pathol* **95**:392, 1973

Fitzpatrick TB et al: Ocular and dermal melanocytosis. *AMA Arch Ophthalmol* **56**:830, 1956

Hidano A: Persistent Mongolian spot in the adult. *Arch Dermatol* **103**:680, 1971

Hidano A et al: Natural history of nevus of Ota. *Arch Dermatol* **95**:187, 1967

Hidano A et al: Bilateral nevus of Ota associated with nevus of Ito. *Arch Dermatol* **91**:357, 1965

Kopf AW, Bart RS: Malignant blue (Ota's?) nevus. *J Dermatol Surg Oncol* **8**:442, 1982

Kopf AW, Weidman AI: Nevus of Ota. *Arch Dermatol* **85**:195, 1962

Lerner AB et al: Effects of oral contraceptives and pregnancy on melanomas (letter). *N Engl J Med* **301**:47, 1979

Levene A: Disseminated dermal melanocytosis terminating in melanoma. *Br J Dermatol* **101**:197, 1979

Mevorak B et al: Dermal melanocytosis. *Dermatologica* **154**:107, 1977

Mishima Y, Mevorah B: Nevus of Ota and nevus of Ito in American Negroes. *J Invest Dermatol* **36**:133, 1961

Nödl F, Krüger R: Maligner blauer Nävus bei Nävus Ota. *Hautarzt* **35**:421, 1984

Sun C.-C et al: Naevus fuscocaeruleus zygomaticus. *Br J Dermatol* 117:545, 1987.

Taylor CR, Anderson RR: Nevus of Ota treated by Q-switched ruby laser. New England Dermatological Society at Massachusetts General Hospital, Harvard Medical School, Boston, Massachusetts, Spring Meeting, April 13, 1991.

10. Blue Nevus and Its Variants

A blue nevus is an acquired, firm papule, nodule, or plaque-like lesion of blue or blue-gray coloration occurring on the skin and mucous membranes.

Synonyms: blue nevus of Jadassohn-Tièche, nevus bleu, blue neuronevus, dermal melanocytoma

EPIDEMIOLOGY

Blue nevi are usually acquired and have their onset most commonly in childhood and adolescence. They are in rare instances congenital.

ETIOLOGY

Blue nevi consist of dermal melanocytes which are believed to have failed to reach the epidermis during their migration from the neural crest in fetal life. Usually, the melanocytes disappear from the dermis during the second half of gestation, but some residual cells remain in the scalp, sacral region, and dorsa of the hands and feet. These are the sites where blue nevi most commonly occur. The blue coloration of these nevi is the result of the Tyndall phenomenon, which is explained in Chap. 8.

CLINICAL FEATURES

Three types of blue nevi are generally recognized: the common blue nevus, the cellular blue nevus, and the combined blue nevus. The ratio of common blue nevus to cellular blue nevus is at least 5:1. Malignant blue nevus is a rare form of malignant melanoma developing in association with cellular blue nevus.

Common Blue Nevi Common blue nevi are well-circumscribed, dome-shaped papules or nodules of blue, blue-gray, or blue-black coloration (Figs. 10-1 and 10-2). They are usually 0.5 to 1.0 cm in diameter, rarely larger. The lesions may occur anywhere, but about 50 percent of cases are found on the dorsa of the hands and feet. Usually, the lesions are solitary, but they may be multiple or agminated (grouped) or form a plaque *(plaque-type blue nevus)* (Fig. 10-3) composed of multiple papules or nodules with an intervening flat area of blue coloration. Concentric, target-like lesions *(target blue nevus)* have been described as well.

Cellular Blue Nevi Cellular blue nevi are blue-gray or black nodules or plaques, generally 1 to 3 cm in diameter, but sometimes larger (Fig. 10-4). Their surface is smooth but sometimes uneven. In about half the reported cases, they are located on the buttocks or sacrococcygeal area, followed by the scalp and face and the feet. Congenital cellular blue nevi, some with satellite lesions, have been reported, as have benign or malignant cellular blue nevi arising in congenital nevi.

Combined Blue Nevi Histologically, combined blue nevi are composed of a blue nevus and another distinct nevomelanocytic population. Combined nevi are

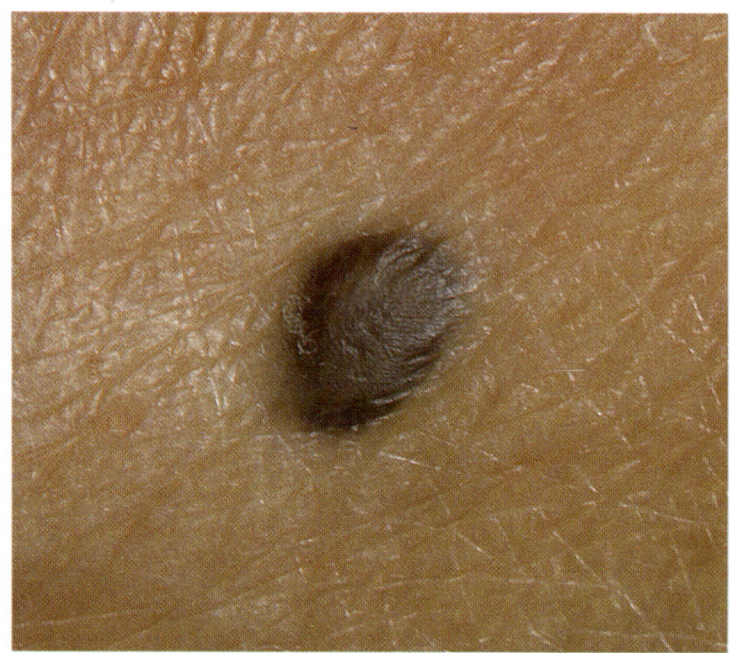

Figure 10-1 *Blue nevus. Pictured is a small, uniformly blue, slightly elevated papular lesion.*

found in about 1 percent of all nevomelanocytic nevi excised for histologic evaluation. The majority of the lesions occur on the face. They usually are nodular, vary in size, show a smooth surface, and are blue-brown to blue-black in color. Some combined nevi exhibit a characteristic discrete blue-black focus within an otherwise typical nevus. Atypical clinical features may suggest melanoma.

Malignant Blue Nevi (Malignant Melanoma) Malignant blue nevi are rare forms of malignant melanoma arising in cellular blue nevi. They tend to show progressive enlargement, often measuring several centimeters in diameter, and have a multinodular or plaque-like appearance. The scalp is the most common site of occurrence, and lymph nodes are the most common sites of metastasis. Malignant blue nevi can arise in a previously benign cellular blue nevus, in a nevus of Ota or Ito, or de novo.

Blue nevi have been described in the vagina, the cervix, the prostate, the spermatic cord, and the lymph nodes.

HISTOLOGIC FEATURES

The common blue nevus is composed of elongated and often slightly wavy melanocytes with long, branching dendrites. The melanocytes, with their long axes parallel to the epidermis, lie grouped or in bundles in the upper and middle dermis. Occasionally, they extend into the subcutaneous tissue or approach the epidermis but do not alter it. Most of the melanocytes

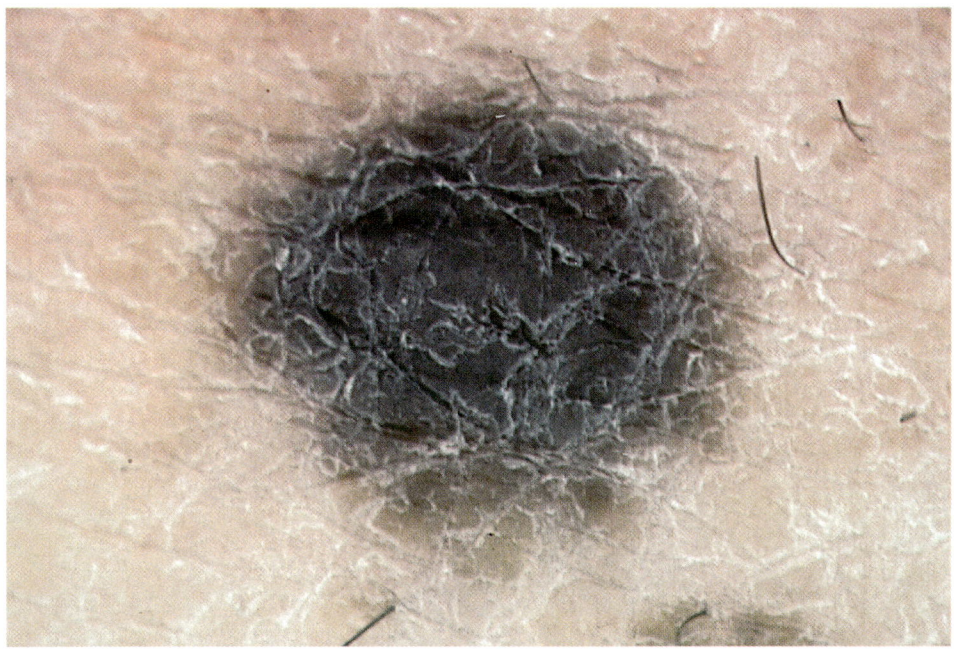

A

Figure 10-2 *Blue nevus. Homogeneous pattern (blue).* (a) *Dark lesion with bluish color. Maximum diameter, 6 mm.* (b, c) *Global features: homogeneous blue pattern without evidence of pigment network.* (a) *Digital clinical surface view (without oil);* (b) *digital epiluminescence microscopic subsurface view (with oil); and* (c) *pigment pattern enhancement of epiluminescence microscopic subsurface view.* (Reprinted with permission from RO Kenet et al: Clinical diagnosis of pigmented lesions using digital epiluminescence microscopy: Grading protocol and atlas. *Arch Dermatol* 129:164-165, 1993.)

are filled with numerous fine melanin granules, often completely obscuring their nuclei and often extending into their dendrites. Variable numbers of melanin-laden macrophages are also present. The amount of collagen is usually increased, giving the lesion a fibrotic appearance.

In the cellular type of blue nevus, one can appreciate deeply pigmented dendritic melanocytes like those in common blue nevi associated with nests and fascicles of spindle-shaped cells with abundant pale cytoplasm containing little or no melanin. The aggregates of spindle cells may be arranged in intersecting bundles extending in various directions, a disposition resembling the storiform pattern of neurofibroma. Penetration of cellular islands into subcutaneous tissue is frequently noted. Some of the cells may appear atypical, with nuclear pleomorphism, accompanied by multinucleated giant cells and inflammatory infiltrates. These "atypical" blue nevi can be difficult to differentiate from malignant melanoma, especially when one of the two above-mentioned components

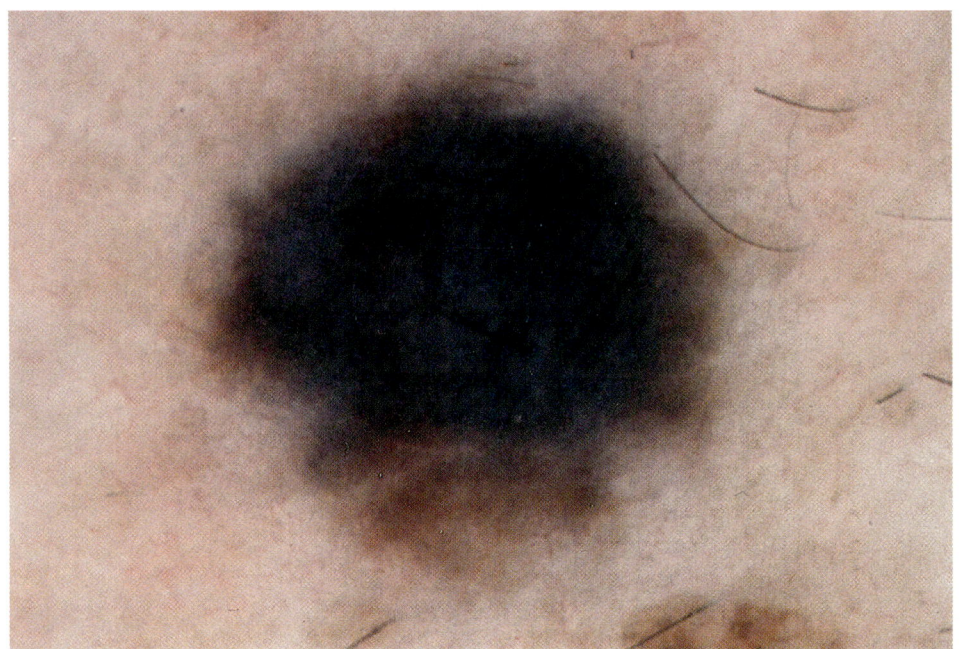

B

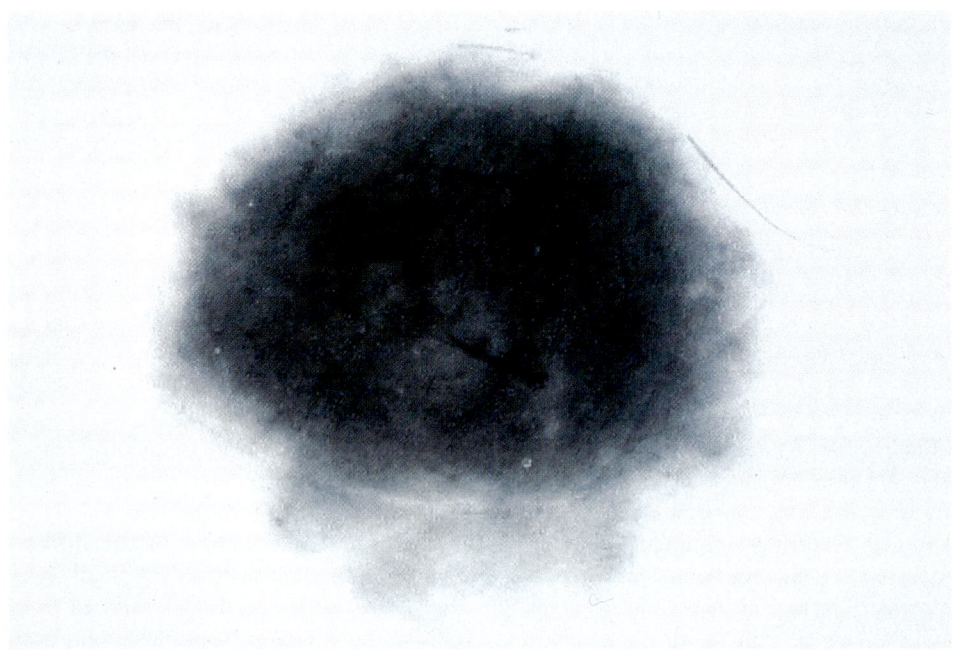

C

Figure 10-2 *(cont.)*

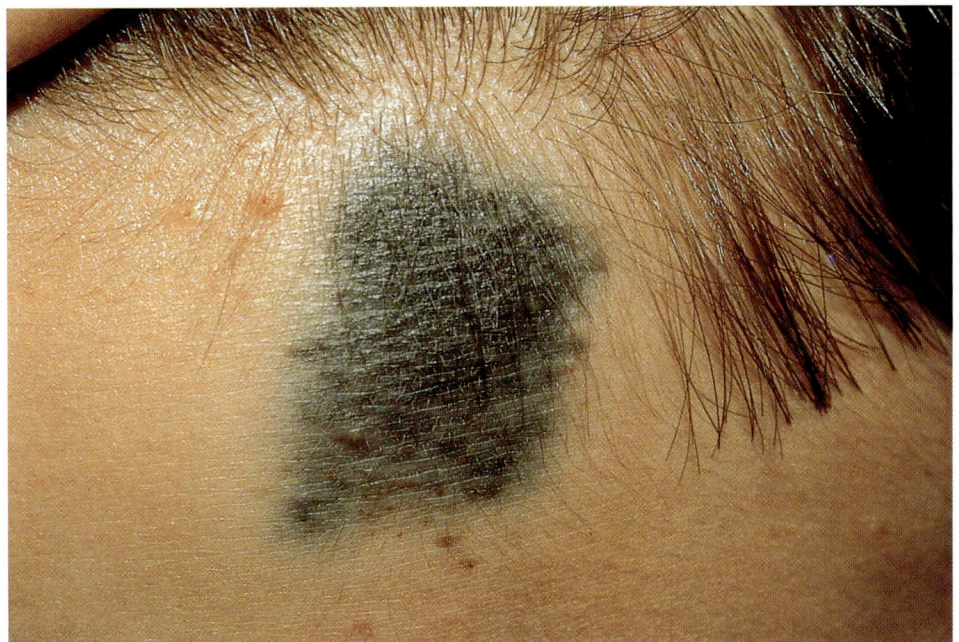

Figure 10-3 *This is a plaque type of blue nevus which is quite distinctively different from the solitary papular lesion customarily seen.*

is missing. Occasionally, lymph nodes draining the anatomic site of a cellular blue nevus contain atypical cells. The foci, found either in the marginal sinuses or in the capsule, are usually small, discrete, and peripherally located. They result from passive transport. These "benign metastases" are found in 5.2 percent of the reported cases of cellular blue nevi.

Electron microscopy reveals that the spindle-shaped cells in cellular blue nevi contain melanosomes with little or no melanization. Melanin production in these cells and transition to bipolar dendritic nevus cells have been documented.

Combined blue nevi have the histologic features of common or cellular blue nevi in combination with a junctional, compound, dermal, or (rarely) spindle and epithelioid nevus. Histologically, the malignant blue nevus resembles the architectural pattern of a benign cellular blue nevus. However, it shows greater cellularity, invasive growth, atypical mitoses, pleomorphism, and in some cases, necrosis. It should be emphasized that biopsies taken from the same lesion may display considerable variance in histology, ranging from benign to malignant.

BIOLOGIC BEHAVIOR AND PROGNOSIS

Little is known about the natural history of common, combined, and cellular blue nevi. Most of them probably remain unchanged or regress. Cellular blue nevi rarely undergo malignant change.

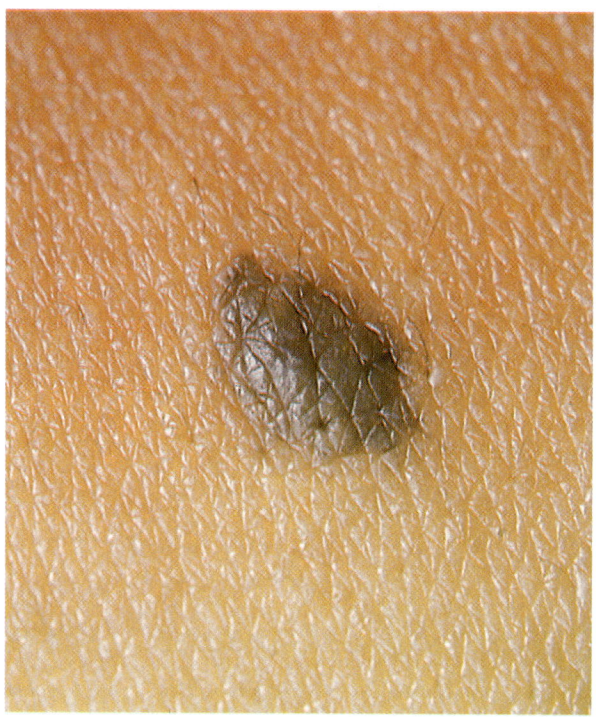

Figure 10-4 *Cellular blue nevus. This lesion is a little more nodular than the typical blue nevus.*

ASSOCIATED SYNDROMES

Blue nevi are sometimes a feature of the LAMB syndrome, which was discussed in Chap. 7.

DIFFERENTIAL DIAGNOSIS

The differential diagnosis of blue nevus and its variants includes primary and metastatic melanoma, dysplastic nevus, pigmented spindle-cell nevus, other hypermelanotic variants of melanocytic nevi, sclerosing hemangioma, dermatofibroma, vascular lesions including angiokeratoma and venous lake, papular pigmented basal cell carcinoma, glomus tumor, and apocrine hidrocystoma. In many instances, the clinical characteristics of blue nevus, particularly the small size (usually < 5 mm in diameter), typical location on the dorsal aspects of the hands and feet, uniform color, symmetry, and well-defined borders, allow distinction from melanoma and other atypical melanocytic lesions. However, in many instances, histopathologic examination will be needed for final diagnosis. In general, cellular blue nevi are often of larger size, i.e., 1 to 2 cm in diameter, and exhibit an irregular surface. The latter features are suspicious for an atypical melanocytic lesion, and histopathologic examination may be needed for differentiation. Combined nevi often exhibit a central black focus that may suggest malignant transformation within a nevus. However, the overall symmetry on gross inspection and the stability of the lesion suggest a benign condition. Excision for histologic examination may nonetheless still be needed to rule out atypicality.

MANAGEMENT

Blue nevi that are < 1 cm in diameter, are clinically stable and without atypical features, and are located in a typical anatomic site do not require removal. On the other hand, histologic evaluation should be strongly considered for lesions appearing de novo, multinodular or plaque-like lesions, or changing lesions.

Cellular blue nevi probably should be resected completely in order to prevent recurrence and misdiagnosis as malignant blue nevus and also because of their risk for malignant transformation (albeit rare). It should be emphasized that cellular blue nevi should be sampled carefully so that a malignant focus is not missed.

ADDITIONAL READINGS

Avidor I, Kessler E: "Atypical" blue nevus—A benign variant of cellular blue nevus. *Dermatologica* **154**:39, 1977

Bogomoletz W: Blue nevus of oral mucosa. *Br J Dermatol* **80**:611, 1968

Bondi EE et al: Target blue nevus. *Arch Dermatol* **119**:919, 1983

Dorsey CS, Montgomery H: Blue nevus and its distinction from Mongolian spot and the nevus of Ota. *J Invest Dermatol* **22**:225, 1954

Gartmann H, Müller HD: Über das gemeinsame Vorkommen von blauem Naevus and Naevuszellnaevus. *Z Hautkr* **52**:389, 1977

Goldenhersh MA et al: Malignant blue nevus. *J Am Acad Dermatol* **19**:712, 1988

Hendricks WM: Eruptive blue nevi. *J Am Acad Dermatol* **4**:50, 1981

Hendrickson MR, Ross JC: Neoplasms arising in congenital giant nevi. *Am J Surg Pathol* **5**:109, 1981

Iemoto Y, Kondo Y: Congenital giant cellular blue nevus resulting in dystocia. *Arch Dermatol* **120**:798, 1984

Jao W et al: Blue nevus of the prostate glad. *Arch Pathol* **91**:187, 1971

Lambert WC, Brodkin RH: Nodal and subcutaneous cellular blue nevi: A pseudometastasizing pseudomelanoma. *Arch Dermatol* **120**:367, 1984

Lamovec J: Blue nevus of the lumph node capsule. *Am J Clin Pathol* **81**:367, 1984

Mishima Y: Cellular blue nevus: Melanogenic activity and malignant transformation. *Arch Dermatol* **101**:104, 1970

Pfaltz M, Schnyder UW: Verlauf und Ultrastruktur beim plaqueartigen Naevus bleu. *Hautarzt* **40**:355, 1989

Pittman JL, Fisher BK: Plaque-type blue nevus. *Arch Dermatol* **112**:1127, 1976

Qizilibash AH: Blue nevus of the uterine cervix. *Am J Clin Pathol* **59**:803, 1973

Reed WB et al: Giant pigmented nevi, melanoma, and leptomeningeal melanocytosis: A clinical and histopathological study. *Arch Dermatol* **91**:100, 1965

Rodriguez HA, Ackerman LV: Cellular blue nevus: Clinicopathologic study of forty-five cases. *Cancer* **21**:393, 1968

Santa Cruz DJ, Yates AJ: Pigmented storiform neurofibroma. *J Cutan Pathol* **4**:9, 1977

Shenfield HT, Maize JC: Multiple and agminated blue nevi. *J Dermatol Surg Oncol* **6**:725, 1980

Silverberg GD et al: Invasion of the brain by a cellular blue nevus of the scalp. *Cancer* **27**:349, 1971

Sterchi JM, Muss HB, Weidner N: Cellular blue nevus simulating metastatic melanoma: Report of an unusually large lesion associated with nevus-cell aggregates in regional lymph nodes. *J Surg Oncol* **36**:71, 1987

Temple-Camp CRE et al: Benign and malignant cellular blue nevus: A clinicopathological study of 30 cases. *Am J Dermatopathol* **10**:289, 1988

Tobon H, Murphy AI: Benign blue nevus of the vagina. *Cancer* **40**:3174, 1977

Tsoitis G et al: Naevus bleu multinodulaire en plaque, superficiel et neuroide. *Ann Dermatol Venereol* **110**:231, 1983

Upshaw E et al: Extensive blue nevus of Jadassohn-Tièche: Report of a case. *Surgery* **22**:761, 1947

Zimmerman AA, Becker SW Jr: Precursors of epidermal melanocytes in the Negro fetus, in *Pigment Cell Biology,* edited by M Gordon. New York, Academic Press, 1959, pp 159–170

11. Common Acquired Melanocytic Nevi

Common acquired nevi range from small, well-circumscribed pigmented macules to raised, flesh-colored lesions, defined by the location of aggregations of "nevus cells" in the skin: junctional nevi have intraepidermal collections of nevus cells, dermal (intradermal) nevi have nevus cells in the dermis, and compound nevi have nevus cells in both areas.

Synonyms: nevocellular nevus, "mole"

EPIDEMIOLOGY

The natural history of acquired melanocytic nevi is poorly documented. The prevalence of nevi is related to age, race, and perhaps genetic and environmental factors. Very few nevi are present in early childhood, but they increase in number, reaching a peak in the third decade of life, and tend thereafter to disappear with increasing age. There is a period of particularly rapid development of nevi at puberty. In general, the greatest numbers of nevi are observed among individuals aged 20 to 29 years. A study in Scotland noted that in the first decade of life females had an average of 3 moles and and males 2 moles. For the age interval 20 to 29 years, women and men had mean nevus counts of 33 and 22, respectively. There was a progressive decline thereafter, with females having a mean of 6 nevi and males 4 nevi in the seventh decade. No substantial differences between men and women have been noted for prevalence of nevi. Caucasians in general have greater numbers of nevi than darker-skinned groups, i.e., blacks and Asians. Furthermore, a greater prevalence of nevi is associated with lighter skin color in Caucasians. The frequency of melanocytic nevi on the palms and soles, nail beds, and conjunctivae is also related to race; nevi on these surfaces are more prevalent in blacks and Asians than in whites. Mean acral nevus counts for blacks in Uganda were 11 versus 2 to 8 for American blacks.

Genetic factors may be operative in the prevalence of nevi: increased numbers of nevi have been shown to cluster in families, especially in families associated with familial melanoma. Although an autosomal dominant mode of inheritance has been postulated for clinically atypical nevi in hereditary melanoma families, the pattern of inheritance may be more complex. Environmental factors such as sun exposure also may influence the development of melanocytic nevi. There is some evidence that individuals residing in sunny climates have a greater prevalence of melanocytic nevi compared with persons living in more temperate zones, but more objective evidence is needed to establish this relationship.

ETIOLOGY

Melanocytic nevi are thought to originate from cells, termed *melanoblasts,* that migrate from the neural crest to the epidermis.

Nevi are hypothesized to result from the proliferation of slightly altered melanocytes or "nevus cells" within the epiermis, producing junctional nevi. It is believed that such nevus cells subsequently migrate into the dermis, giving rise to compound nevi and ultimately dermal nevi when there are no longer residual nevus cells within the epidermis. Nevi are thought to be either developmental malformations (hamartomas) or benign proliferations with some growth advantage over surrounding basilar melanocytes. Factors leading to the onset of melanocytic nevi are poorly understood but could include the genetic influences alluded to earlier and environmental agents, principally solar exposure.

CLINICAL FEATURES

Melanocytic nevi are well-circumscribed, round or ovoid lesions, generally measuring from 2 to 6 mm in diameter. They appear orderly and symmetric overall. Although many nevi display slight asymmetry, the borders are usually regular and well defined. The natural history of melanocytic nevi is believed to be a progression from a junctional nevus to a compound nevus and then to a dermal nevus and subsequent involution. However, this model is based on cross-sectional histologic observations and has not actually been observed. It is also believed that the evolution of a nevus may halt at any point, with a particular lesion remaining a junctional nevus, compound nevus, or dermal nevus. The junctional nevus is a macular lesion with slight accentuation of skin markings visible with sidelighting (Fig. 11-1). Junctional nevi are also characterized by a uniform, medium to dark brown color. Compound nevi show variable degrees of elevation and in general somewhat lighter shades of brown than do junctional nevi (Figs. 11-2 to 11-4). Dermal nevi are usually more elevated and show lighter shades of brown or even flesh tones compared with compound nevi (Figs. 11-5 and 11-6). However, it should be emphasized that there is considerable clinical overlap among all three types of nevi. Dermal nevi and, to a lesser degree, compound nevi may be dome-shaped or papillomatous. Nevi may have a verrucous surface simulating that of seborrheic keratosis. Many nevi contain hairs that are coarse and dark compared with those in surrounding skin.

Nevi on the palms and soles usually are macular or only slightly raised, have regular and well-defined borders, and show uniform brown or dark brown coloration. Melanocytic nevi of the nail bed usually present as uniformly pigmented brown or dark brown longitudinal bands (melanonyhia striata) with regular and distinct margins (Fig. 11-7).

HISTOLOGIC FEATURES

Melanocytic nevi contain intraepidermal or dermal collections of nevus cells or both. The cells within the junctional nests have round, ovoid, or fusiform shapes and are arranged in cohesive nests. In the superficial dermis, the cells in general have epithelioid-cell characteristics and contains amphophilic cytoplasm and, frequently, granular melanin. The nuclei have uniform chromatin with a slightly clumped texture. Deeper in the dermis there is a diminished content of cytoplasm such that the cells resemble lymphocytes; they are frequently arranged in linear cords. There may be a further transition to cells separated by fine connective tissue and assuming a spindled configuration, similar to fibroblasts or Schwann cells.

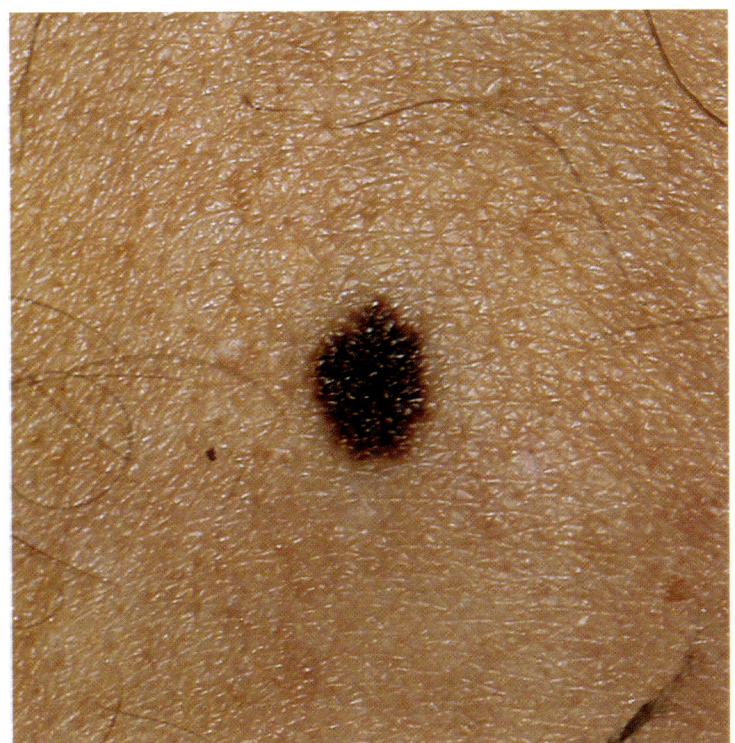

Figure 11-1 *Junctional nevus with slightly irregular borders and uniform dark brown color.*

BIOLOGIC BEHAVIOR

Nevi are thought to begin as junctional nevi, giving place to compound nevi and dermal nevi and finally undergoing gradual regression, perhaps sometimes by way of a fibroepithelial polyp. An important aspect of melanocytic nevi is their relationship to melanoma. A significant proportion of melanoma patients report the prior presence of a long-standing mole at the site of melanoma development. Histologic studies also have documented that approximately one-third of melanomas are associated with nevus remnants. Thus a certain proportion of melanomas are believed to arise from precursor nevi. An increased number of melanocytic nevi also marks increased melanoma risk.

DIFFERENTIAL DIAGNOSIS

The differential diagnosis of melanocytic nevi includes freckle, lentigo simplex, solar lentigo, seborrheic keratosis, lichenoid keratosis, pigmented actinic keratosis, dermatofibroma, neurofibroma, fibroep-

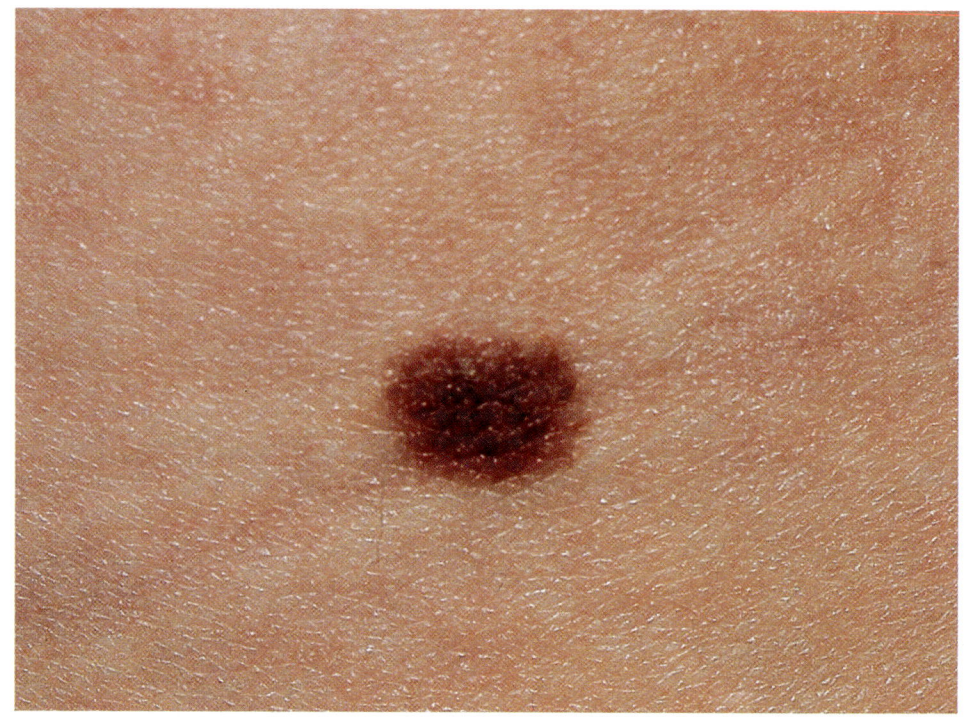

Figure 11-2 *Compound nevus. This slightly elevated papule has an homogeneous reddish-brown color.*

ithelial polyp, CALM, epidermal nevus, atypical (dysplastic) nevus, and melanoma. There may be difficulty in distinguishing a junctional nevus or relatively flat compound nevus from a freckle, CALM, simple lentigo, and solar lentigo. Sidelighting can reveal accentuated skin markings that are present in nevi and not seen in freckles, CALM, or lentigines. In some instances, it is impossible to distinguish a junctional nevus from a simple lentigo without histologic examination. Also, the two entities may overlap (as lentiginous junctional nevus or nevoid lentigo). Raised nevi, potentially confused with seborrheic keratosis, generally do not exhibit the rough, verrucoid surface and pseudo-horn cysts of seborrheic keratosis. Dermatofibromas are usually differentiated from nevi by their very firm consistency, "dimpling," and preference for the lower extremities. Both neurofibromas and fibroepithelial polyps may be indistinguishable from flesh-colored or slightly pigmented, pedunculated dermal nevi. In general, typical melanocytic nevi are dis-

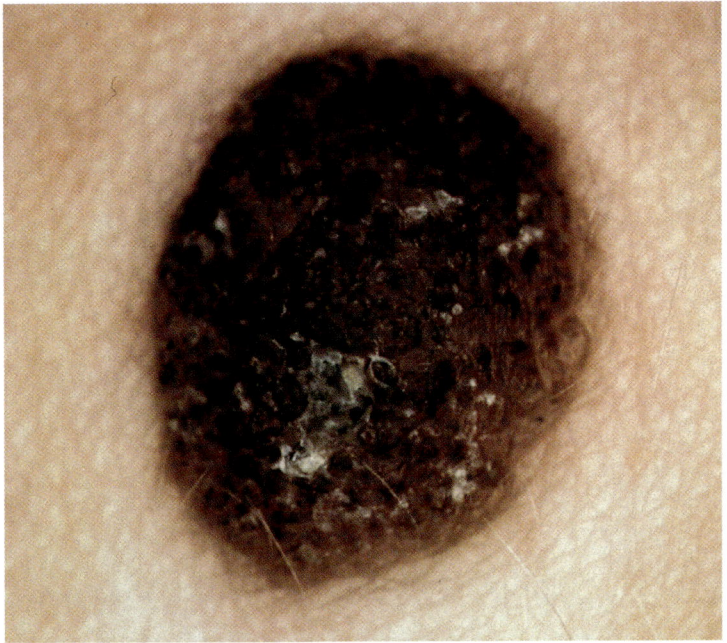

A

Figure 11-3 *Compound nevus. Globular pattern.* (a) *Note the elevation with sharp clinical margins and halo. Maximum diameter, 9 mm.* (b, c) *Global features: globular pattern. Note the absence of sharp network margins (since there is no pigment network) despite sharp clinical margins.* (a) *Digital clinical surface view (without oil);* (b) *digital epiluminescence microscopic subsurface view (with oil) of gross tissue architecture; and* (c) *pigment pattern enhancement of epiluminescence microscopic view.* (Reprinted with permission from RO Kenet et al: Clinical diagnosis of pigmented lesions using digital epiluminescence microscopy: Grading protocol and atlas. *Arch Dermatol* 129:160, 1993.)

tinguishable from atypical (dysplastic) nevi and melanoma by smaller size, overall symmetry and orderly appearance, homogeneous coloration, and regular, well-defined borders. Furthermore, red, blue, white, gray, and black colors are not typically seen in common acquired nevi and should alert one to a potentially atypical lesion.

MANAGEMENT

The indications for removing melanocytic nevi are as follows: (1) a changing lesion, (2) atypical clinical appearance suspicious for melanoma, (3) cosmetic reasons, and (4) repeated irritation. Beyond these indications, there is no reason to remove nevi on a routine basis.

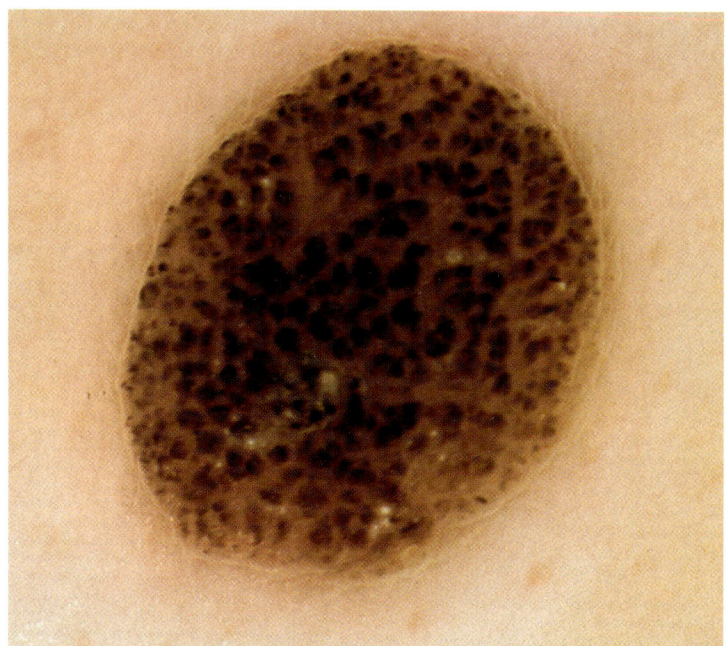

B

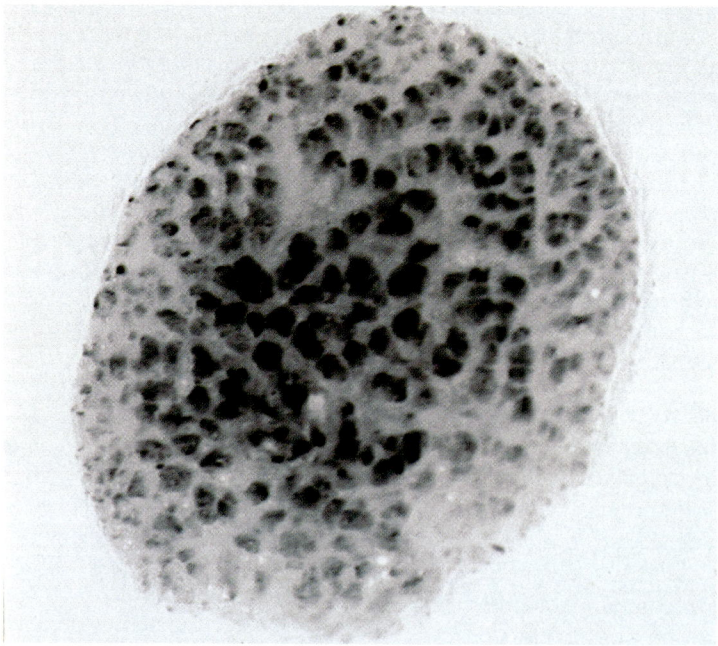

C

Figure 11-3 *(cont.)*

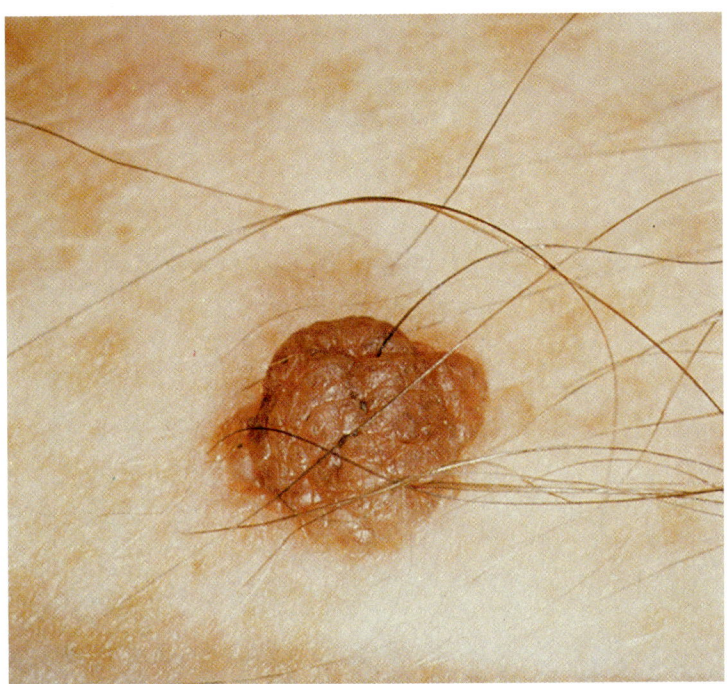

Figure 11-4 *Compound nevus (primarily dermal) exhibits regular borders and papillomatous surface.* (From TB Fitzpatrick et al (eds): *Dermatology in General Medicine,* 4th ed. New York, McGraw-Hill, 1993, p 997, with permission.)

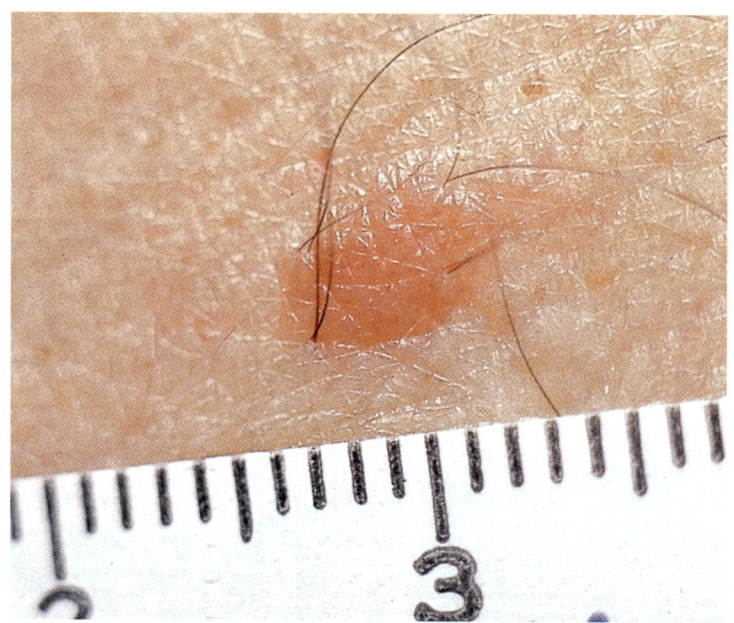

Figure 11-5 *Dermal nevus. This lesion is characterized by well-defined borders, slightly raised papular surface, and a uniform pinkish-tan color.*

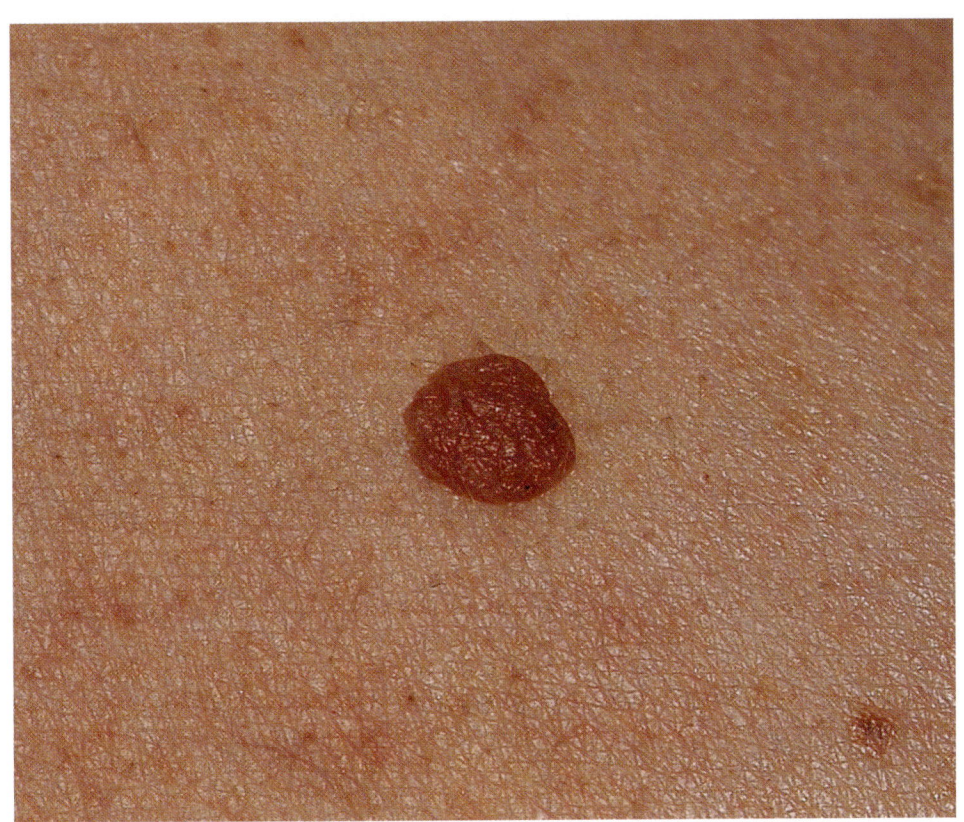

Figure 11-6 *Dermal nevus. Pedunculated lesion with uniform reddish-brown color.*

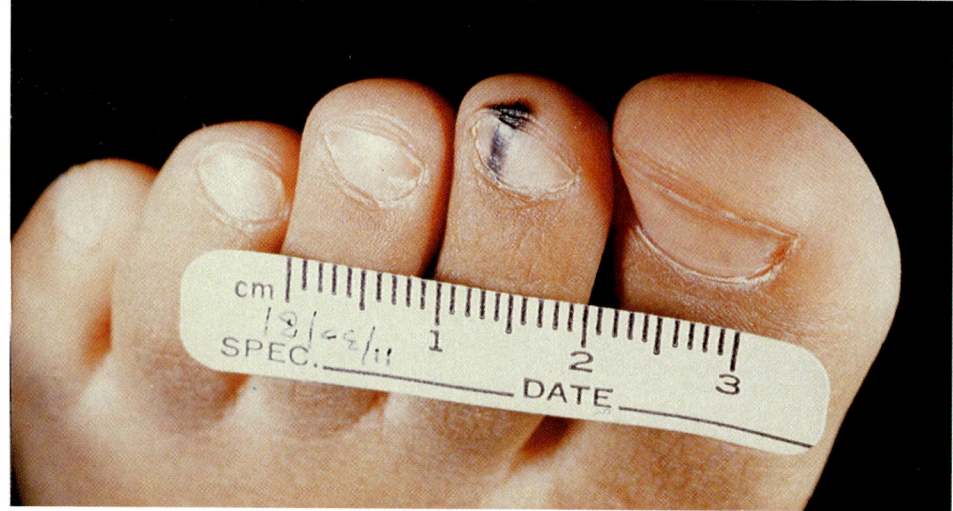

A

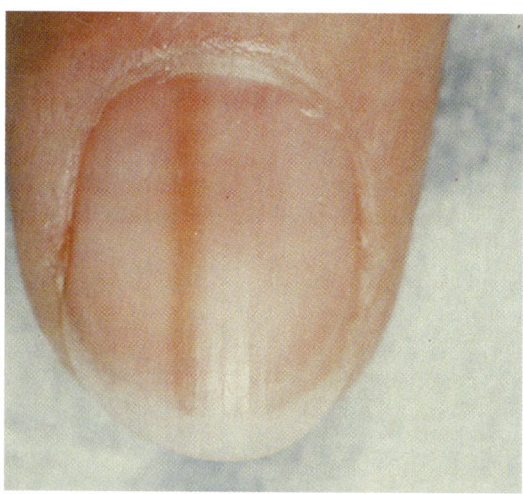

B

Figure 11-7 *Melanocytic nevi of the nail bed. (a) Compound nevus of the nail bed. The dark brown band involving the nail extends onto the distal periungual skin. (b) Melanocytic nevus of the nail bed demonstrating regular light brown pigmented band.* (From TB Fitzpatrick et al (eds): *Dermatology in General Medicine,* 4th ed. New York, McGraw-Hill, 1993, p 998, with permission.)

ADDITIONAL READINGS

Armstrong BK, English DR: The epidemiology of acquired melanocytic naevi and their relationship to malignant melanoma, in *Melanoma and Naevi,* edited by JM Elwood. Basel, Karger, 1988, pp 27–47

Lund HZ, Stobbe GD: The natural history of the pigmented nevus: Factors of age and anatomic location. *Am J Pathol* **25**:1117, 1949

MacKie RM et al: The number and distribution of benign pigmented moles (melanocytic naevi) in a healthy British population. *Br J Dermatol* **113**:167, 1985

Maize JC, Foster G: Age-related changes in melanocytic naevi. *Clin Exp Dermatol* **4**:49, 1979

Nicholls EM: Development and elimination of pigmented moles and the anatomical distribution of primary malignant melanoma. *Cancer* **32**:192, 1973

Pack GT et al: Regional distribution of moles and melanomas. *AMA Arch Surg* **65**:862, 1952

Stegmaier OC: Natural regression of the melanocytic nevus. *J Invest Dermatol* **32**:413, 1959

Stegmaier OC, Montgomery H: Histopathological studies of pigmented nevi in children. *J Invest Dermatol* **20**:51, 1953

Winkelmann RK, Rocha G: The dermal nevus and statistics: An evaluation of 1200 pigmented lesions. *Arch Dermatol* **86**:310, 1962

12. Halo Nevus

The halo nevus is defined as a melanocytic nevus surrounded by a white (hypo- or depigmented) band or halo. The central nevus is almost always a common acquired nevus, but others such as congenital, atypical (dysplastic), and blue nevi may develop halos.

Synonyms: leukoderma acquisitum centrifugum, Sutton's nevus, perinevoid vitiligo

EPIDEMIOLOGY

Halo nevi generally affect individuals under the age of 20 years, with a mean age of approximately 15 years. In one series, the ages ranged from 3 to 42 years. The overall incidence of halo nevi in individuals under age 20 is probably less than 1 percent. There is no difference in incidence between males and females. Approximately 20 percent of individuals with halo nevi have vitiligo, and halo nevi have an association with malignant melanoma and atypical (dysplastic) nevi.

The natural history of halo nevi has not been well documented. However, in general, the onset of a ring of depigmentation is thought to occur over a period of weeks to months. The central nevus may persist or, more likely, undergoes involution over a matter of months to years.

ETIOLOGY

The basis for the development of a halo of depigmentation is thought to be either (1) an immune response against antigenically altered nevus cells associated with tumor progression (dysplasia) or (2) a cell-mediated and/or humoral (antibody-mediated) reaction against nonspecifically altered nevomelanocytes and possible cross-reactivity with nevomelanocytes at a distant site or sites. The first hypothesis holds that all halo nevi are atypical, and thus the immunologic response is one associated with tumorigenesis. The second notion holds that halo nevi are the result of host response directed against nonspecifically altered nevomelanocytes in response to a physical, chemical, or other insult or perhaps result from an autoimmune etiology, as in vitiligo.

The basis for nevus cell destruction in halo nevi is poorly understood. Both humoral and cellular immunologic factors have been implicated. Copeman et al. were the first to show that individuals with regressing halo nevi have antibodies directed against the cytoplasm of melanoma cells. These antibodies also have been noted in patients with primary melanoma who have not developed metastases but not in individuals with other types of conventional nevi. It also has been found that lymphocytes isolated from patients with halo nevi and from melanoma patients are cytotoxic to melanoma cells in culture. It is not known whether the preceding observations are important in the pathogenesis of halo nevi or are merely epiphenomena.

As discussed below, the central nevus component in active halo nevi is usually associated with dense mononuclear—cell infiltrates, while the peripheral white halo has little or no such infiltrate. The mechanisms responsible for the white halo are even less well understood than other aspects of the pathogenesis of halo nevi. Presumably the destruction of melanocytes in this zone is secondary to the diffusion of a cytotoxic factor such as a cytokine.

CLINICAL FEATURES

Halo nevi are characterized by a central melanocytic nevus component that may be relatively flat or raised and dark brown to pink in color. The nevus may exhibit surface scale or crusting. The central nevus is surrounded by a well-circumscribed annulus of hypo- or depigmented skin (Figs. 12-1 and 12-2). In typical halo nevi, the central nevus commonly measures 3 to 6 mm in longest diameter, has regular and well-defined borders, and has homogeneous coloration. The white halo is usually symmetric with a uniform width that may vary from a few millimeters up to several centimeters (uncommon). A Wood's lamp may enhance or discern the halo.

Halo nevi are most typically located on the upper back but may be found in any location. Approximately 25 to 50 percent of affected individuals have two or more halo nevi. Rarely, large numbers of halo nevi occur, sometimes with rapid onset.

After the development of a halo nevus, its subsequent course is variable. The central nevus may persist indefinitely or regress completely, in some cases with the halo remaining (see Fig. 12-1). The coloration of the central nevus may not change or may become irregular or pink or red. Similarly gradually disappear with complete repigmentation of the skin.

HISTOPATHOLOGY

The halo nevus may be junctional, compound, or dermal. In the fully evolved stages, the central nevus is associated with a well-circumscribed, dense, almost band-like infiltrate of mononuclear cells, almost exclusively lymphocytes and histiocytes, that occupies the papillary dermis and permeates nests of nevus cells. The latter change is so prominent that nevus cells are difficult to distinguish from surrounding lymphoid cells. Degenerating nevus cells can sometimes be identified in this zone. Homogeneous eosinophilic bodies, representing degenerated cells, can sometimes be observed near the dermal-epidermal junction. Occasional nevus cells within the infiltrate show prominent eosinophilic cytoplasm and slightly enlarged nuclei. Although most halo nevi demonstrate no obviously atypical nevus cells, some display varying degrees of cytologic atypia. The peripheral zones of the nevus are characterized by diminished or absent basilar melanocytes and melanin in the basal layer. The papillary dermis also may demonstrate slight reparative alteration of the stroma, but usually no inflammatory cell infiltrates are found.

BIOLOGIC BEHAVIOR

As already discussed, the natural history of halo nevi is not well defined and is usually variable. The factors operative in the development of halo nevi are not understood. A relationship to vitiligo, melanoma, and atypical nevi has been well documented.

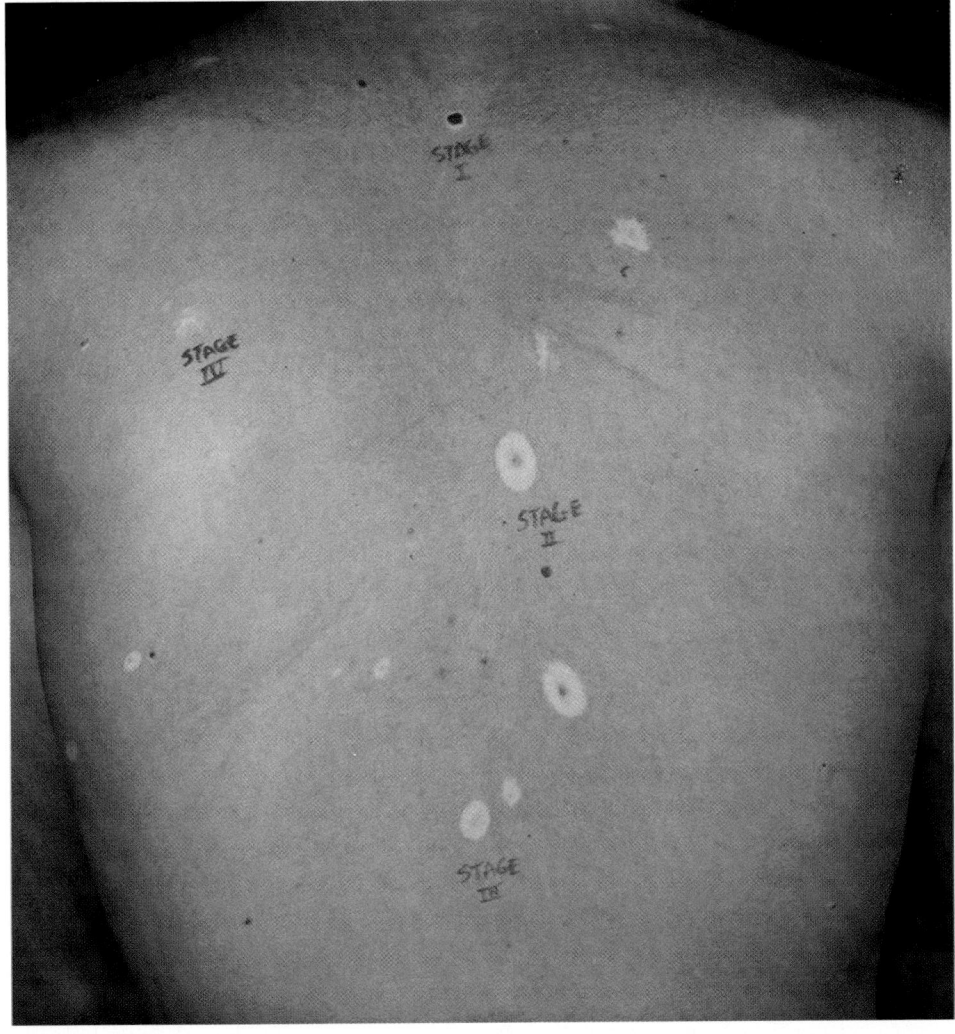

Figure 12-1 *Halo nevi showing the four stages: Stage I where there is a halo forming around a compound nevus, Stage II where the nevus is disappearing, Stage III where the nevus has almost completely disappeared, and Stage IV, the hypopigmented area is beginning to repigment to normal color.*

In some cases, erythema precedes the development of the depigmented halo. As already mentioned, the halo usually develops over the course of weeks to months. The subsequent course of the nevus may vary from complete regression (probably at least 50 percent of cases) to complete repigmentation of the white halo. In some instances, there may be complete regression of the nevus accompanied by the de-

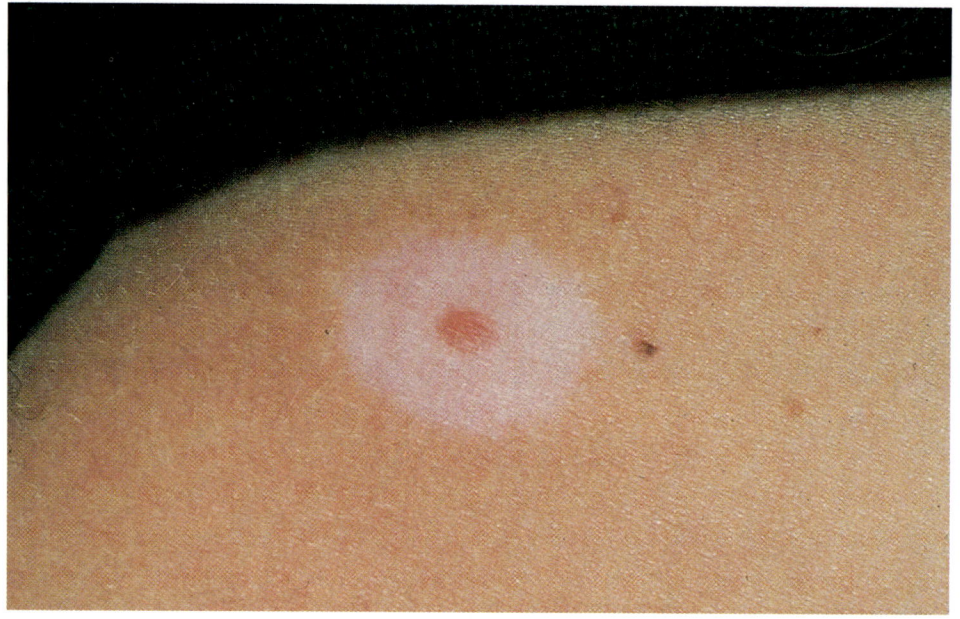

Figure 12-2 *Halo nevus showing a central compound nevus which is slightly hypopigmented itself.*

velopment of a uniform depigmented macule that may persist or exhibit gradual repigmentation. The period associated with nevus regression varies from months to as long as several years.

DIFFERENTIAL DIAGNOSIS

Common acquired melanocytic nevi with the halo phenomenon must be distinguished from (1) other melanocytic proliferations with halos such as congenital nevi, atypical (dysplastic) nevi, blue nevi, spindle and epithelioid cell nevi, and melanoma and (2) nonmelanocytic lesions with halos such as dermatofibromas, seborrheic keratoses, flat warts, molluscum contagiosum, basal cell carcinoma, lichen planus, psoriasis, and sarcoidosis. Congenital halo nevi are distinguished from acquired halo nevi by clinical history of presence at birth or shortly thereafter, large size (usually > 1.5 cm), and supportive histologic features (see Chap. 19). Atypical (dysplastic) nevi measure about 4 to 12 mm or greater in diameter, frequently have irregular or ill-defined borders or both, and show more complexity or irregularity of color in comparison with typical halo nevi. As already mentioned in Chap. 1, malignant melanoma usually has even greater disordered features than atypical (dysplastic) nevi. Furthermore, an asymmetric, irregular halo may be observed with melanoma as compared with the symmetry usually found in halo nevus. Other attributes such as large size (usually > 1 cm), irregular or notched borders, and striking irregularity of color typify melanoma. In general, a halo blue nevus is distinctive because of the central, symmetric, well-circumscribed bluish papule that is so characteristic of blue nevus. However, pigmented spindle-cell nevus, early nodular melanoma, and metastatic melanoma enter into its differential diagnosis. A spindle- and epithelioid-cell (Spitz) nevus with a halo might prove difficult to distinguish from a typical halo nevus because of the rather nondescript appearance of many Spitz nevi, i.e., a pink or reddish papule, possibly with telangiectasia.

MANAGEMENT

The management of patients with halo nevi is individualized and depends on the clinical setting. All persons with halo nevi should be questioned for a personal or family history of malignant melanoma, atypical (dysplastic) nevi, and vitiligo. The individual halo nevus or nevi should be inspected carefully for any asymmetry or atypicality, i.e., features suspicious for atypical (dysplastic) nevus or melanoma. The patient also should undergo a comprehensive skin examination for evidence of other halo nevi, atypical (dysplastic) nevi, melanoma, or vitiligo. A Wood's lamp evaluation is recommended. If no clinical atypicality is observed, the patient should be followed with periodic skin examinations. In general, clinically atypical halo nevi should be excised for histologic examination. Halo nevi with a benign or orderly clinical appearance need not be removed. Individuals beyond age 40 with halo nevi should be examined carefully for melanoma.

ADDITIONAL READINGS

Bergman W et al: Analysis of major histocompatibility antigens and the mononuclear cell infiltrate in halo nevi. *J Invest Dermatol* **85**:25, 1985

Copeman PWM et al: Immunological associations of the halo nevus with cutaneous malignant melanoma. *Br J Dermatol* **88**:127, 1973

Frank SB, Cohen HJ: The halo nevus. *Arch Dermatol* **89**:367, 1964

Kopf AW et al: Broad spectrum of leukoderma acquisitum centrifugum. *Arch Dermatol* **92**:14, 1965

Rhodes AR: Neoplasms: Benign neoplasias, hyperplasias, and dysplasias of melanocytes, in *Dermatology in General Medicine,* 4th ed, edited by TB Fitzpatrick et al. New York, McGraw-Hill, 1993, pp 996–1077

Wayte DM, Helwig EB: Halo nevi. *Cancer* **22**:69, 1968

13. Nevus Spilus

The nevus spilus is defined as a slightly hyperpigmented (tan) macular lesion that contains hyperpigmented foci or speckles that may be either flat or raised. The tan macular area exhibits the histology of a lentigo, while the hyperpigmented foci are usually junctional or compound nevi.

Synonyms: speckled lentiginous nevus, zosteriform lentiginous nevus

EPIDEMIOLOGY

The nevus spilus is usually acquired, but some are congenital. This lesion has been noted to affect approximately 2.3 percent of adult white persons in one series. Males and females are equally affected. Familial cases have not been reported.

ETIOLOGY

The nevus spilus may have a segmental or zosteriform distribution (designated *speckled zosteriform lentiginous nevus* by some), suggesting a localized malformation. Otherwise, it is unclear how nevus spilus might differ in pathogenesis from other melanocytic nevi.

CLINICAL FEATURES

As already mentioned, the nevus spilus may be present at birth but more often develops in childhood. These lesions most commonly affect the trunk and extremities. The tan macular area commonly varies from under 1 to 3 or 4 cm in greatest diameter (Fig. 13-1). This area is completely flat without any distortion of skin markings. The hyperpigmented speckles are approximately 1 to 6 mm in greatest diameter and may be macular or papular. Large varieties of nevus spilus may be unilateral, segmental, or zosteriform and involve a substantial portion of skin, e.g., an entire extremity or half the trunk (Fig. 13-2).

HISTOPATHOLOGY

The tan macule or patch of nevus spilus is characterized by lentiginous melanocytic hyperplasia associated with elongated epidermal rete ridges. The hyperpigmented macular foci are also characterized by lentiginous melanocytic hyperplasia, whereas the papular foci contain junctional or compound nevus elements. In rare instances, the histologic changes of spindle- and epithelioid-cell (Spitz) nevi have been noted in the raised speckled area.

BIOLOGIC BEHAVIOR

In general, the nevus spilus persists indefinitely; however, increased degrees of speckling over time have been documented by serial photography and become more prominent after solar exposure.

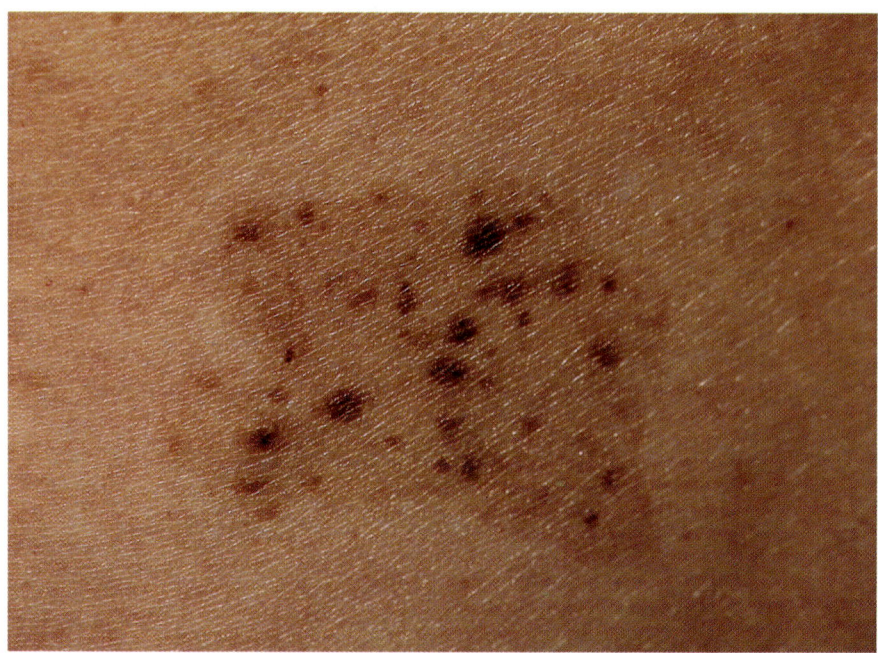

Figure 13-1 *A typical nevus spilus showing scattered pigmented lesions throughout a café au lait macule. Sometimes the café au lait macule cannot be detected without benefit of a Wood's lamp.*

There are several reports of malignant melanoma arising in association with a nevus spilus. In two instances, melanocytic dysplasia has been noted in the nevus spilus adjacent to the site of melanoma development.

DIFFERENTIAL DIAGNOSIS

Relatively flat, lightly pigmented varieties of congenital nevus and Becker's nevus (or melanosis) might on occasion enter into the differential diagnosis of nevus spilus. However, nevus spilus also may be congenital. Typical congenital nevus and Becker's nevus do not have the speckling pattern of nevus spilus.

MANAGEMENT

Because of increasing reports of malignant melanoma developing in nevus spilus, it seems advisable that individuals with congenital or large varieties of nevus spilus should be followed on a periodic basis (photography may be helpful). Areas of change or atypicality in a nevus spilus should be evaluated by biopsy or excision, as is appropriate for other atypical melanocytic lesions.

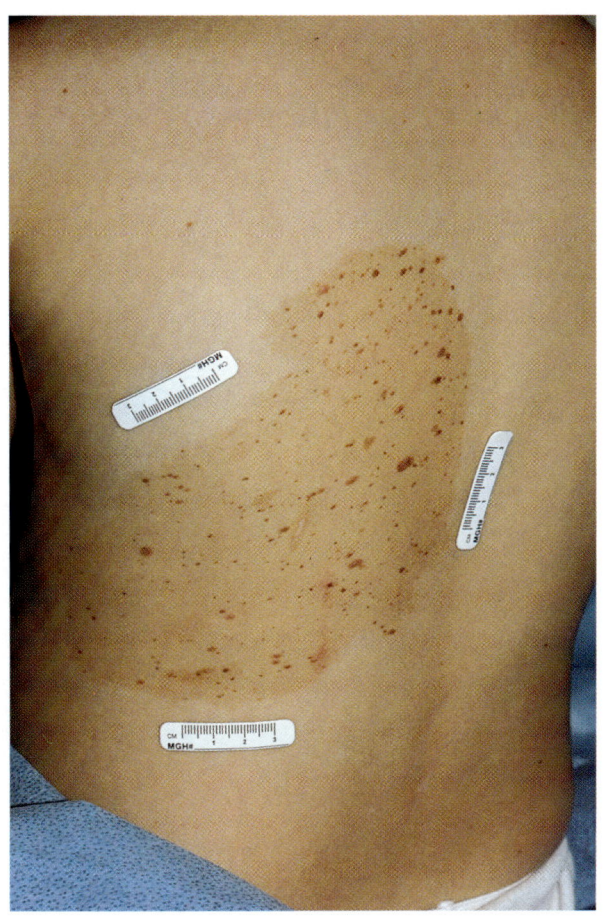

Figure 13-2 *This is a very large nevus spilus showing flat pigmented macules as well as raised lesions.*

ADDITIONAL READINGS

Cohen HJ et al: Nevus spilus. *Arch Dermatol* **102**:433, 1970

Falo LD Jr et al: Evolution of nevus spilus. *Dermatology* (in press)

Kopf AW et al: Congenital-nevus-like nevi, nevi spili, and café-au-lait spots in patients with malignant melanoma. *J Dermatol Surg Oncol* **11**:275, 1985

Kurban RS et al: Occurrence of melanoma in "dysplastic" nevus spilus: Report of case and analysis by flow cytometry. *J Cutan Pathol* **19**:423, 1992

Rhodes AR: Neoplasms: Benign neoplasias, hyperplasias, and dysplasias of melanocytes, in *Dermatology in General Medicine,* 4th ed, edited by TB Fitzpatrick et al. New York, McGraw-Hill, 1993, pp 996–1077

Rhodes AR, Mihm MC Jr: Origin of cutaneous melanoma in a congenital dysplastic nevus spilus. *Arch Dermatol* **126**:500, 1990

Stewart DM et al: Speckled lentiginous nevus. *Arch Dermatol* **114**:895, 1978

14. Segmental Lentiginosis

Segmental lentiginosis is defined by a circumscribed aggregation of individual, small pigmented macules. The overall arrangement may be in a segmental, dermatomal, or zosteriform pattern. The individual macules demonstrate the histology of a lentigo.

EPIDEMIOLOGY

The prevalence of segmental lentiginosis in the general population is not established but is probably rare. There is no known predilection for sex or race.

ETIOLOGY

As with nevus spilus, the segmental distribution of this lesion suggests a developmental abnormality of melanocytes.

CLINICAL FEATURES

The onset of this lesion may be at birth or in childhood. The individual macules are well circumscribed and vary in size from about 2 to 10 mm in greatest diameter. There is no background café au lait–like hyperpigmentation as in nevus spilus. In certain lesions, the café au lait pigmentation can be detected only by use of the Wood's lamp. Large lesions may involve a major anatomic area or have a curvilinear or blotchy pattern, following the lines of Blaschko.

HISTOPATHOLOGY

The individual macules demonstrate lentiginous melanocytic hyperplasia in association with elongated epidermal rete ridges, as in lentigo simplex. Nests of nevus cells are not present. Cytologic atypia of melanocytes has been noted in some lesions.

BIOLOGIC BEHAVIOR

The natural history of segmental lentiginosis is not established. Progression to malignant melanoma has not been reported.

DIFFERENTIAL DIAGNOSIS

Segmental lentiginosis is distinguished from nevus spilus by the absence of a tan macular background and nevus elements. Segmental lentiginosis differs from an agminated nevus by the lack of nevus-cell nesting in the epidermis, dermis, or both.

MANAGEMENT

The same guidelines apply as for nevus spilus (Chap. 13).

ADDITIONAL READINGS

Port M et al: Zosteriform lentiginous naevus with ipsilateral rigid cavus foot. *Br J Dermatol* **98**:693, 1978

Rhodes AR: Neoplasms: Benign neoplasias, hyperplasias, and dysplasias of melanocytes, in *Dermatology in General Medicine,* 4th ed, edited by TB Fitzpatrick et al. New York, McGraw-Hill, 1993, pp 996–1077

Section II

Difficult Diagnostic Lesions

15. Recurrent Melanocytic Nevus

The recurrent melanocytic nevus refers to the clinical and histologic features of a melanocytic nevus recurring in the site of an antecedent nevus that has been partially removed. This circumstance raises the specter of recurrent melanoma.

Synonym: pseudomelanoma

EPIDEMIOLOGY

The frequency with which melanocytic nevi recur has not been clearly established. It would appear that the phenomenon is relatively common among a population of individuals with incompletely removed nevi. According to Park et al., recurrent nevi are noted most often in relatively young females (85 percent of cases, since greater numbers of nevi are removed from women) and on the trunk, followed by the head and neck area. Most of the recurrences have followed a shave excision. Fifty-two percent of cases were noted to recur within 6 months according to Park et al.

ETIOLOGY

The recurrence of melanocytic nevi is thought to result from an intraepidermal proliferation of residual melanocytes, possibly from nearby sweat ducts, hair follicles, or intraepidermal melanocytes. Trophic factors stimulating either melanocyte migration, proliferation, or both may be related to mechanisms of wound healing or scar formation.

CLINICAL FEATURES

These lesions are characterized by circumscribed hyperpigmentation located within a scar from the previous surgical procedure for nevus removal (Fig. 15-1). In most instances, the lesion is macular and exhibits variable irregularity of borders and pigment pattern. Stippling, mottling, and loss of pigment may be observed. Most recurrent nevi measure 4 to 6 mm in diameter, and almost all are < 1.5 cm.

HISTOLOGIC FEATURES

Corresponding to the clinical features, one frequently observes intraepidermal melanocytic proliferation confined to the area above a dermal scar. The epidermis usually exhibits effacement of the rete pattern and variable lentiginous or nested proliferation of melanocytes. Often, the cells contain abundant melanin and relatively uniform nuclei. However, occasionally, low-grade cytologic atypia is noted. Frequently, there are residual dermal nevus cells beneath the superficial dermal scar.

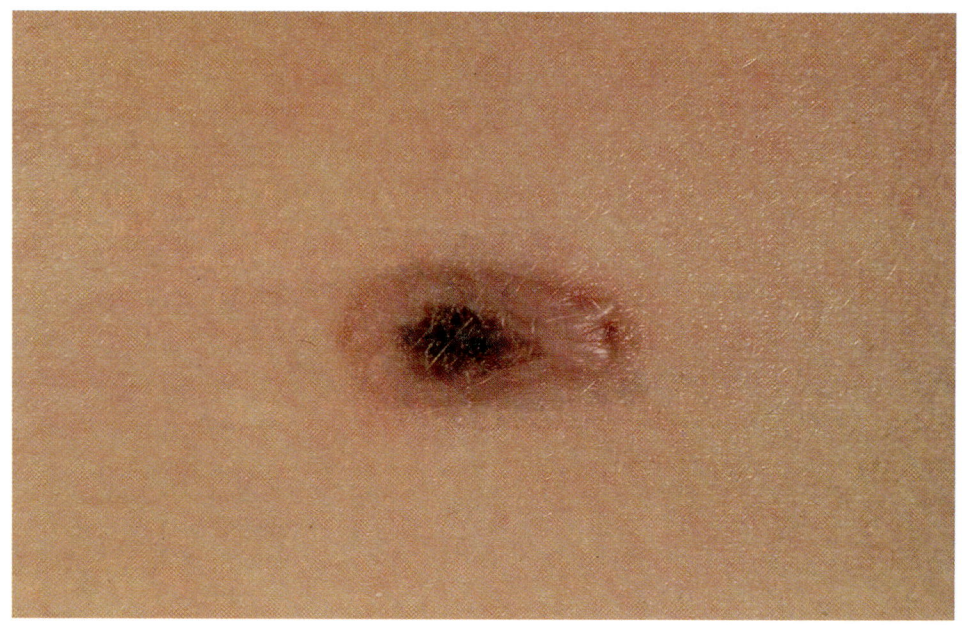

Figure 15-1 *Recurrent melanocytic nevus. Note the slightly irregular hyperpigmented macule located entirely within the surgical scar. The lesion demonstrates variation in the pigmentary pattern.* (Courtesy of A. Bernard Ackerman, M.D.)

BIOLOGIC COURSE

Most recurrent nevi are stable after development and persist indefinitely. No increased melanoma risk has been associated with recurrent nevi.

DIFFERENTIAL DIAGNOSIS

The differential diagnosis of recurrent nevus includes recurrent atypical (dysplastic) nevus, lentiginous melanocytic proliferations developing in melanoma scars, and recurrent melanoma. In general, recurrent melanocytic nevus is confined to the area of the surgical scar, appears within 6 months of surgery, and exhibits a banal histologic picture. Recurrent dysplastic nevi may have greater cytologic atypia than conventional recurrent nevi. Clinical features suggesting melanoma include irregular pigmentation, recurrence beyond the confines of the surgical scar, and a longer interval until recurrence (>6 months).

MANAGEMENT

Establishing that a previous surgical procedure has occurred is integral to the diagnosis. Review of the previous biopsy is mandatory if any atypicality is noted histologically. Excision of a recurrent nevus is not necessary unless abnormal clinical features are present, e.g., extension of the lesion beyond the surgical scar.

ADDITIONAL READINGS

Cox AJ, Walton RG: The induction of junctional changes in pigmented nevi. *Arch Pathol* **79**:428, 1965

Kornberg R, Ackerman AB: Pseudomelanoma. *Arch Dermatol* **111**:1588, 1975

Park HK et al: Recurrent melanocytic nevi: Clinical and histologic review of 175 cases. *J Am Acad Dermatol* **17**:285, 1987

16. Spindle- and Epithelioid-Cell Nevus

The spindle- and epithelioid-cell nevus is a melanocytic nevus, usually acquired, that differs from other common acquired nevi because of distinctive histopathologic features (but a less distinctive gross morphologic appearance). The histologic characteristics that set the spindle- and epithelioid-cell nevus apart from other nevi are the presence of large epithelioid cells and spindle cells in varying proportions. This lesion is frequently misdiagnosed as malignant melanoma.

Synonyms: Spitz nevus, Spitz tumor, Spitz's juvenile melanoma, benign juvenile melanoma, epithelioid cell–spindle cell nevomelanocytic nevus

EPIDEMIOLOGY

The prevalence of spindle- and epithelioid-cell nevi (SECN) in the general population has not been documented accurately. However, among melanocytic lesions that have been surgically excised, approximately 1 percent exhibit the histologic characteristics of SECN. In data from Australia, it has been estimated that SECN account for 1.4 cases per 100,000 population as compared with an annual incidence of 25.4 melanomas per 100,000 population.

SECN are most commonly acquired, but as many as 7 percent may be congenital. SECN occur in all age groups but are uncommon beyond the ages of 40 to 50 years. In the series of Weedon and Little, 33 percent of cases occurred in individuals under 10 years of age, 36 percent of affected individuals were between the ages of 10 and 20 years, and 31 percent were older than 20 years of age. Men and women are equally affected.

ETIOLOGY

The origin of SECN has not been clearly determined, but these proliferations are assumed to be derived from cells taking origin from the neural crest, similar to other melanocytic nevi. No particular etiologic factors that might account for the characteristic histologic changes found in these nevi have been identified.

CLINICAL FEATURES

SECN vary in size from about 2 mm to about 2 cm, with an average diameter of approximately 8 mm. Most commonly, they are well-circumscribed, dome-shaped papules or nodules varying in color from pink to tan to dark brown (Figs. 16-1 and 16-2) (see also Chap. 17). Generally, the color is homogeneous and the margins well defined. The surface topography may be smooth or, in some instances, verrucous. Relatively flat, polypoid, and pedunculated morphologies also have been described. Occasional lesions may exhibit erosions and scale crust. Telangiectasia is also a frequent finding.

Although SECN may involve any part of the body, the head and neck area is probably the most common site, accounting for 42 percent of lesions in one series. There is a rather even distribution of lesions involving the upper extremities, lower ex-

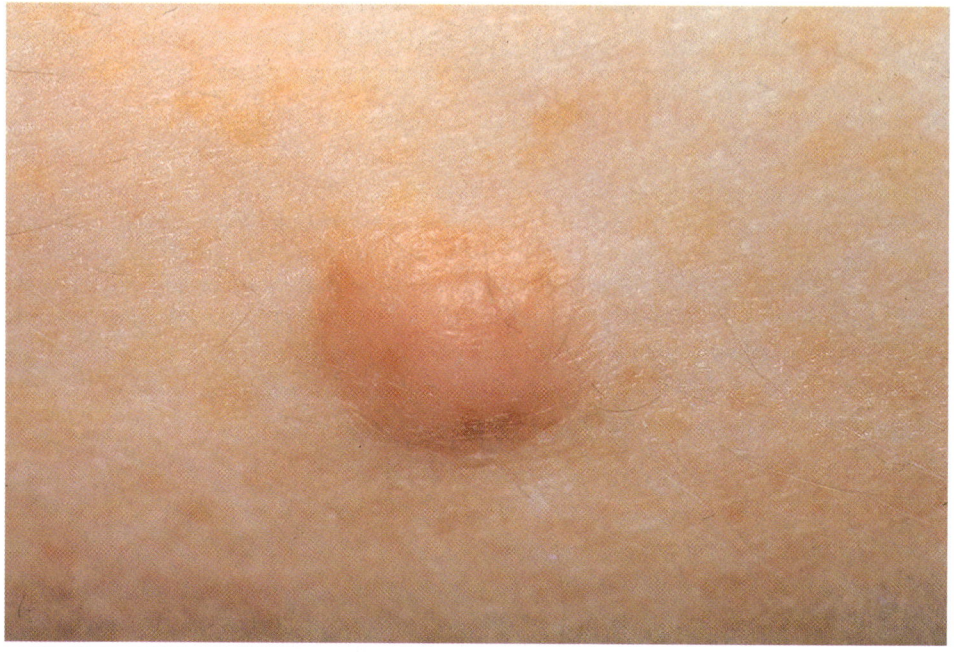

Figure 16-1 *Spitz nevus. Note dome-shaped morphology and pink color.*

tremities, and trunk. In most instances, there is a history of recent onset, but a small percentage of nevi have been present for many years.

HISTOPATHOLOGY

The SECN has a unique histologic appearance. Typically, these lesions display striking nests of large epithelioid cells, spindle cells, or both, usually extending from the epidermis into the reticular dermis in an inverted-wedge configuration. The closely apposed nests of cells within a hyperplastic epidermis often contribute to a so-called raining down appearance. Both mononuclear and multinucleate giant epithelioid cells are frequently observed. These cells extend into the subjacent dermis as both fascicles of cells and single cells. There is orderly infiltration of the dermal collagen by these cells with so-called maturation, i.e., gradual diminution of nuclear and cellular sizes. The individual cells usually have abundant cytoplasm that stains slightly bluish or pink and nuclei with open chromatin patterns. Rather uniform nucleoli are usually also noted. Occasional bizarre cytologic features, necrotic cells, and mitotic figures are found within these lesions and may suggest melanoma.

BIOLOGIC COURSE

The natural history of SECN has not been clearly delineated. As previously mentioned, a small percentage of these lesions

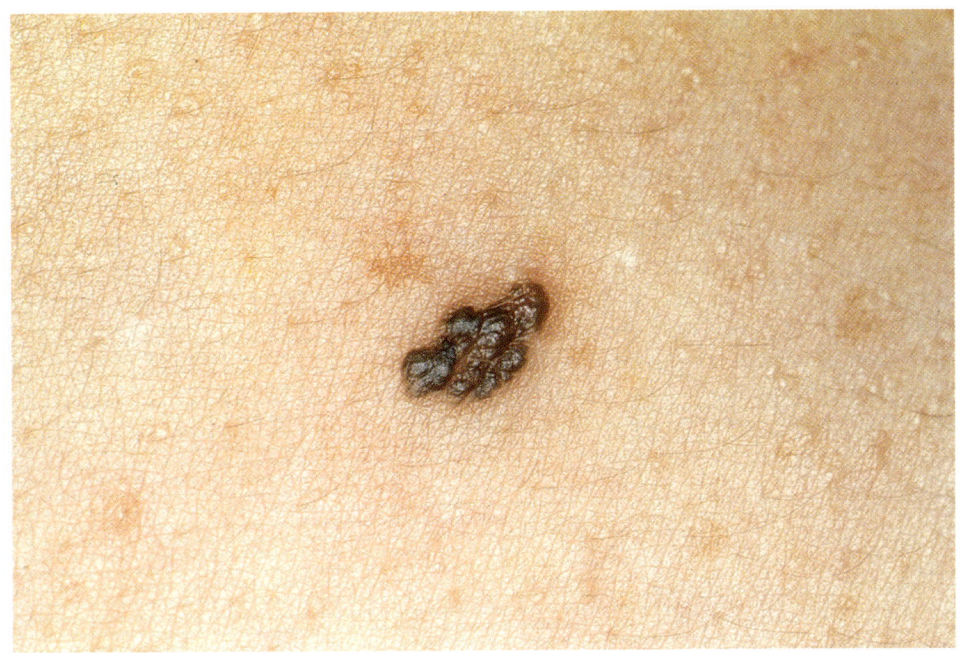

Figure 16-2 *Spitz nevus, pigmented type. The lesion shows slight asymmetry and scalloped borders but has a uniform dark brown color.*

are present at birth, and some acquired ones are long-standing. Although there has been speculation that these lesions involute as do other conventional nevi or possibly evolve to conventional nevi, these courses have not been documented. In most instances, there is a clinical history of recent onset or change. The vast majority of lesions with characteristics of Spitz nevi are benign. However, because of the histologic resemblance of SECN to some melanomas, the presence of atypical variants, and occasional metastases from such lesions, there is some belief that melanoma may in uncommon cases develop in association with SECN. The exact nature and classification of these lesions await definitive clarification. An aggressive variant termed *malignant Spitz nevus* has been reported to result in regional lymph node metastases.

SPECIAL VARIANTS

Agminated (grouped) spindle- and epithelioid-cell nevi are characterized by varying numbers of individual raised nevi occurring in a localized or segmental distribution, often within a background café au lait macule. The latter presentation is usually congenital. *Solitary or multiple spindle- and epithelioid-cell proliferations developing within a large congenital nevi* exhibit the features of typical SECN. *Pigmented spindle-cell nevus* (see Chap. 17) is classified by some authors as a subtype of SECN.

DIFFERENTIAL DIAGNOSIS

The typical nonpigmented types of SECN may suggest a rather wide differential diagnosis most frequently including pyogenic granuloma, other types of hemangioma, verrucae, molluscum contagiosum, juvenile xanthogranuloma, other melanocytic nevi (particularly dermal nevi), dermatofibroma, and mastocytoma. SECN exhibiting varying degrees of pigmentation also may suggest atypical nevi such as dysplastic nevi and melanoma. Histologic examination is usually mandatory for establishing a diagnosis.

MANAGEMENT

Because of the frequent diagnostic difficulty of these lesions, histologic evaluation of the entire lesion is mandatory. Furthermore, recurrence rates as high as 7 to 16 percent have resulted from incompletely excised nevi. Final excision margins of approximately 5 mm are recommended. Margins of approximately 1 cm are advised for atypical variants. It is also advisable that patients with atypical lesions have periodic follow-up every 6 to 12 months.

ADDITIONAL READINGS

Barnhill RL, Mihm MC Jr: The pigmented spindle cell naevus and its variants: Distinction from melanoma. *Br J Dermatol* **121**:717, 1989

Coskey RJ: Spindle cell nevi in adults and children. *Arch Dermatol* **108**:535, 1973

Echevarria R, Ackerman LV: Spindle epithelioid cell nevi in the adult. *Cancer* **20**:175, 1967

Gartmann H: Der pigmentierte spindelzellentumor (PSCT). *Z Hautkr* **56**:862, 1980

Kopf AW, Andrade R: *Yearbook of Dermatology: 1965–1966*. Chicago, Year Book Medical Publishers, 1966, pp 7–52

Lancer H et al: Multiple agminated spindle cell nevi: Unique clinical presentation and review. *J Am Acad Dermatol* **8**:707, 1983

Paniago-Pereira C et al: Nevus of large spindle and/or epithelioid cells (Spitz's nevus). *Arch Dermatol* **114**:1811, 1978

Reed RJ et al: Common and uncommon melanocytic nevi and borderline melanomas. *Semin Oncol* **2**:119, 1975

Sagebiel RW et al: Pigmented spindle cell nevus: Clinical and histologic review of 90 cases. *Am J Surg Pathol* **8**:645, 1984

Smith NP: The pigmented spindle cell tumour of Reed: An underrecognized lesion. *Semin Diagn Pathol* **4**:75, 1987

Spitz S: Melanomas of childhood. *Am J Pathol* **24**:591, 1948

Weedon D, Little JH: Spindle and epithelioid cell nevi in children and adults. *Cancer* **40**:217, 1977

17. Pigmented Spindle-Cell Nevus

The pigmented spindle-cell nevus (PSCN) is characterized by its striking clinical appearance as a solitary, circumscribed, darkly pigmented lesion. The corresponding histologic findings are those of uniform pigmented spindle cells confined to the epidermis and sometimes the papillary dermis. Some authors group this lesion in the general category of spindle- and epithelioid-cell nevi.

Synonyms: pigmented spindle-cell tumor of Reed, pigmented variant of Spitz nevus

EPIDEMIOLOGY

PSCN occur less frequently than spindle- and epithelioid-cell nevi. A few have been noted at birth; however, the mean age at diagnosis is 25 years (the age range in one series was 3 to 66 years). Women are affected more often than men. PSCN are most commonly located on the extremities (69.6 percent of cases in one study), with the thigh the most frequent site. About 20 percent of PSCN are found on the trunk, and 8.8 percent occur in the head and neck area.

ETIOLOGY

As with other melanocytic nevi, the PSCN is thought to be derived from cells migrating from the neural crest. The reasons for the prominent spindle-cell features are not understood.

CLINICAL FEATURES

The PSCN usually is a relatively flat or slightly raised, well-circumscribed lesion averaging about 3 mm in diameter (range 1.5 to 10 mm) (Figs. 17-1 and 17-2). The color is usually dark brown or black and is homogeneous. Irregularity of pigmentation is not common but may be found in atypical variants of PSCN. There is often a history of recent development or alteration. In one study, lesions had been present, on average, about 6 months, but some were of long-standing duration. There is usually no family history of melanoma or dysplastic nevi.

HISTOPATHOLOGY

The PSCN displays a well-circumscribed and orderly appearance. The lesions are usually only slightly raised and are confined to the epidermis but may involve the papillary dermis. The lesion is typified by fascicles of uniform, slender spindle cells that are closely aggregated. The cells usually contain fine, granular melanin. The nuclei contain delicate chromatin and small inconspicuous nucleoli and have an overall monotonous appearance. There may be clefting about the intraepidermal fascicles. Numerous melanophages are usually present in the papillary dermis. Upward migration of nevus cells throughout the epidermis is sometimes noted, but

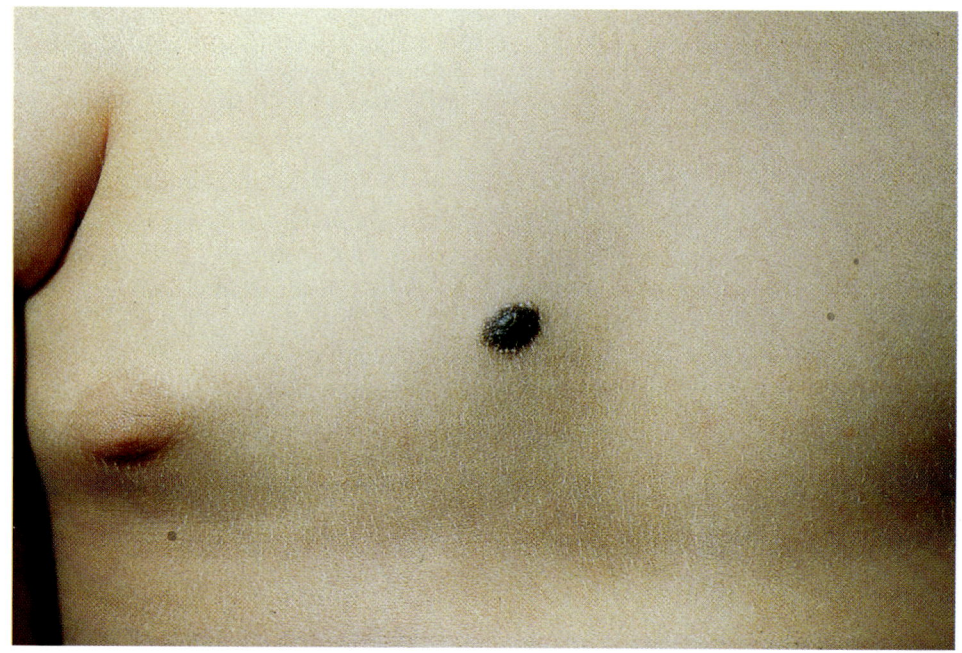

Figure 17-1 *Pigmented spindle-cell nevus. This is a darkly pigmented lesion that might be diagnosed clinically as a blue nevus, Spitz nevus, or a pigmented spindle-cell nevus.*

these are usually confined to the lower half of the epidermis. Atypical variants exhibit prominent single-cell hyperplasia extending peripherally along the basal layer of the epidermis and in a pagetoid pattern throughout the epidermis. Cytologic atypia also may be present in a varying degree in these atypical presentations.

BIOLOGIC BEHAVIOR

The natural history is largely unknown. As has been mentioned, the vast majority of PSCN have been present for only a short time, usually less than a year. Congenital forms of PSCN, although uncommon, have been recognized. The occurrence of atypical varieties of PSCN and the presence of remnants of PSCN in association with malignant melanoma are circumstantial evidence that PSCN can undergo rare transformation to malignant melanoma.

In long-term (mean 8.8 years) follow-up of 15 patients with excised PSCN, there was no evidence of recurrence. In our experience, these lesions have almost never recurred. Thus, unless a lesion has been incompletely excised, recurrence strongly suggests an atypical process, possibly malignant melanoma.

DIFFERENTIAL DIAGNOSIS

The differential diagnosis of PSCN includes early nodular melanoma, dysplastic nevus, blue nevus, a vascular lesion, and pigmented basal cell carcinoma. In general, the borders of PSCN are regular

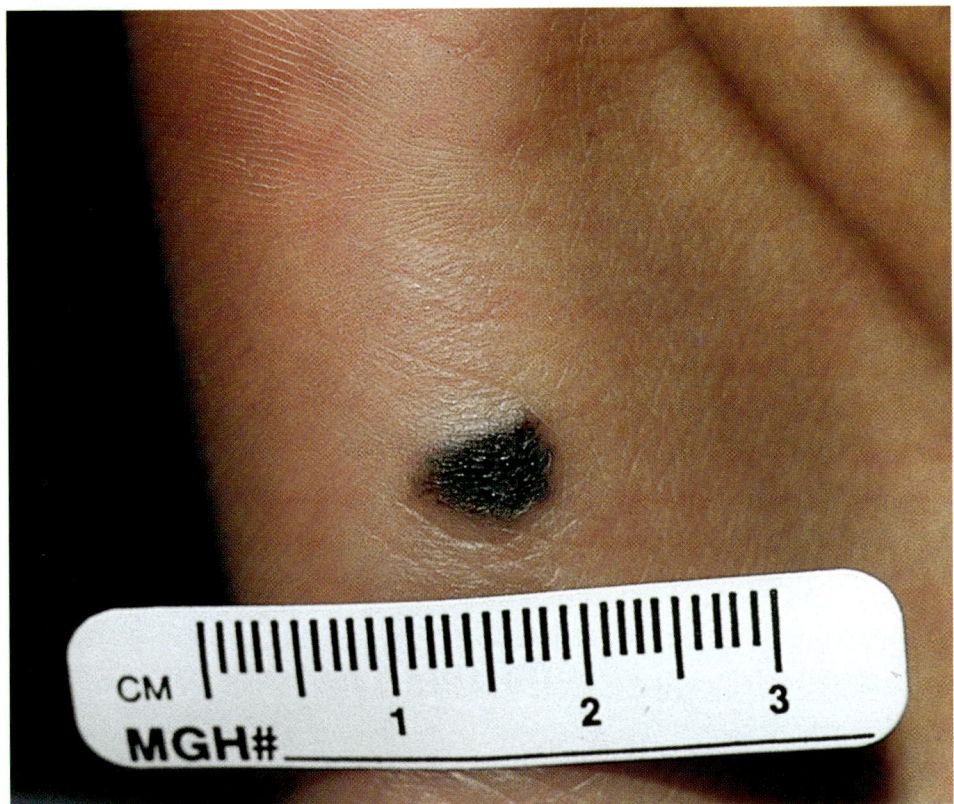

Figure 17-2 *Pigmented spindle-cell nevus. This is a rather typical clinical presentation with a pigmented plaque rather than a dome-shaped lesion, as seen in the Spitz nevus.*

and well defined. The color is also homogeneous in most instances. However, atypical forms of PSCN may exhibit irregularity of borders and color. Histopathologic examination is essential for diagnosis. It must be stressed, however, that the clinicopathologic presentation of typical PSCN is distinctive. Its history is that of a recently developed or changing, small, well-circumscribed, black lesion on the thigh of a young female (usually in her twenties). These lesions are usually conspicuous for the absence of any other pigmented lesions on the body.

MANAGEMENT

The proper management of PSCN is complete excision with clear margins. The reason for this recommendation is to prevent recurrence, since the histologic features of recurring lesions may be alarming and difficult to distinguish from melanoma. For PSCN with atypical features, wider surgical margins are advised. For example, we advocate resection margins of 5 to 10 mm for markedly atypical forms of pigmented spindle-cell nevus. Periodic follow-up, i.e., every 6 to 12 months, is also strongly advised for PSCN with substantial atypia.

ADDITIONAL READINGS

Barnhill RL, Mihm MC Jr: The pigmented spindle cell naevus and its variants: Distinction from melanoma. *Br J Dermatol* **121**:717, 1989

Barnhill RL et al: The histologic spectrum of pigmented spindle cell nevus: A review of 120 cases with emphasis on atypical variants. *Hum Pathol* **22**:52, 1991

Gartmann H: Der pigmentierte Spindelzellentumor (PSCT). *Z Hautkr* **56**:862, 1980

Reed RJ et al: Common and uncommon melanocytic nevi and borderline melanomas. *Semin Oncol* **2**:119, 1975

Sagebiel RW et al: Pigmented spindle cell nevus: Clinical and histologic review of 90 cases. *Am J Surg Pathol* **8**:645, 1984

Smith NP: The pigmented spindle cell tumour of Reed: An underrecognized lesion. *Semin Diagn Pathol* **4**:75, 1987

Section III

Precursors to Primary Melanoma of the Skin

18. Dysplastic Melanocytic Nevus

The dyplastic melanocytic nevus (DMN) of the skin is an acquired (or, in rare instances, congenital) melanocytic lesion that has, by comparison with the common acquired nevus, clinically irregular features of coloration and shape with a size usually 6 mm or greater. Histologically, it exhibits atypical melanocytic proliferation with intraepidermal and often dermal nesting of nevomelanocytes in a setting of abnormal architectural and stromal changes. The DMN has been noted to be a precursor as well as a marker for cutaneous melanoma in the context of familial melanoma; however, it also occurs sporadically—that is, in individuals without such a history. Great difficulties in assessing DMN have resulted from the lack of common clinical and histologic definitions; this lack has significant implications for epidemiology and diagnosis and affects clinical assessment.

Synonyms: B-K mole, atypical nevus, large atypical mole, Clark's nevus, the mole of FAMM (familial atypical mole and melanoma syndrome), nevus with architectural disorder and cytologic atypia. The recent NIH Consensus Conference (January 1992) has recommended the term *nevus with architectural disorder and cytologic atypia* replace *dyplastic melanocytic nevus*. In the following discussion, these two terms will be used interchangeably.

EPIDEMIOLOGY

Estimates of the incidence of DMN cover a wide range, in part because of widely varying definitions, with estimates as high as 53 percent of the U.S. population, but with application of stricter criteria, estimates fall into a range between 1.8 and 9 percent of various populations. The lesions may occur singly or multiply. In the general population, DMN may arise in a "sporadic" fashion, without a history of familial melanoma, or in the setting of a family history of atypical moles or melanoma. In either setting, it appears that they mark some increase in melanoma risk.

Although DMN usually appear around the end of the first decade of life, some congenital melanocytic lesions have been identified as DMN. Sporadic DMN may occur at any time in life, while persons with a family history of DMN and/or melanoma usually manifest their atypical lesions by the end of the second decade. In contrast to common acquired moles that tend to appear in clusters around puberty, DMN may appear in eruptive fashion as late as the sixth decade.

Correlation of the dysplastic nevus with melanoma has been documented in a study of 14 melanoma kindreds. This study followed 401 individuals for an average of 4 years each; 40 new melanomas were noted in family members who had dysplastic nevi. Histologic contiguity of the dysplastic nevi to the melanomas was noted frequently. In another study of 234 melanomas (familial and sporadic), histologic contiguity of dysplastic nevi and malignant melanoma was again observed frequently. These descriptions also tend to corroborate clinical observations of atypical-appearing nevi juxtaposed with melanoma. An estimate of incidence of DMN and melanoma projects that as many as 32,000 people in the United States are members of melanoma-prone families. Further study of the much more common sporadic DMN and their relation to melanoma is likely to be fruitful.

ETIOLOGY

In familial melanoma and familial DMN, genetic analysis has suggested an autosomal dominant mode of inheritance with fairly high penetrance. Linkage analysis has implicated chromosome 1p as a candidate locus for the disease trait. However, other studies have so far failed to confirm this finding, and a polygenic etiology has been suggested by some investigators.

CLINICAL FEATURES

Any darkly and/or irregularly pigmented lesion raises suspicion for the DMN. Nevi meeting the criteria outlined below can occur anywhere on the cutaneous or mucosal surfaces of Caucasians as well as the acral and mucosal surfaces of other races. Others feel that distinct dysplasias other than DMN occur on acral and mucosal sites.

As outlined in Table 1–9, dysplastic nevi occupy an intermediate position on the continuum of common acquired nevi on the one hand and malignant melanoma on the other hand. At each end of the spectrum, DMN overlap with common nevi is diagnostic of DMN; rather, a constellation of clinical findings is required for their recognition (Figs. 18–1 to 18–7). However, the greater the number of clinical abnormalities present, the greater is the confidence that the lesion will prove histologically to be dysplastic. As indicated in Table 1–9, the following gross morphologic features are commonly observed in dysplastic nevi:

ASYMMETRY   DMN often lack mirror-image symmetry. Greater asymmetry suggests greater atypicality.

SIZE   DMN may be of any size but generally range from 4 to 12 mm in greatest diameter. There is generally a positive correlation between increasing size and likelihood of atypia (see Fig. 18–5).

BORDERS   DMN often exhibit irregular and ill-defined borders but not typically the notched or scalloped borders of melanoma (see Fig. 18–3). The DMN with a central raised component and a peripheral macular annulus (the "fried-egg" type of DMN) displays ill-defined or hazy margins most commonly (see Fig. 18–4).

SURFACE TOPOGRAPHY   Many DMN exhibit a relatively flat or plaque-like surface; many are partially macular, particularly at their peripheries (see Fig. 18–5). A "pebbled" or "cobblestone" surface also is common. In general, accentuation of skin margins is visible on sidelighting.

COLORATION   DMN have greater complexity of coloration than common nevi but less than melanoma (see Fig. 18–6). The greater the asymmetry of color and the greater the number of colors, the more probable is cellular atypicality. DMN commonly exhibit irregularity of pigmentation with two or three shades of brown, e.g., tan, brown, and dark brown. The colors flesh, pink, and

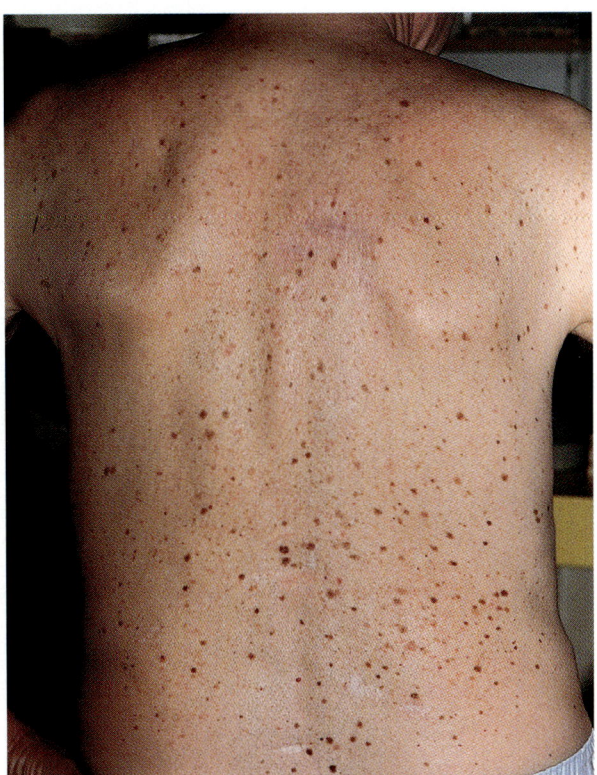

Figure 18-1 *Extensive numbers of clinically atypical nevi on the back. The lesions vary from a few millimeters to over 6 mm in diameter. This patient has developed three primary melanomas.*

brown-black are also often present. Erythema or redness may be present within the lesion or as a perilesional "halo." Some DMN occur with fairly uniform coloration: dark brown, a complex red-brown mahogany, or lacking pigment and displaying a pink-red or erythematous appearance.

CLINICAL SUBTYPES *"Fried-egg" Compound DMN* As mentioned earlier, there is a raised central portion like a compound or dermal nevus and a flat peripheral annulus with ill-defined border (see Fig. 18–4).

"Bull's Eye" or Targetoid Variant Concentric annular zones vary in degree of pigmentation, resulting in this characteristic appearance.

Lentiginous or Lentigo-Like Variant This lesion exhibits a uniform, relatively flat surface and homogeneous dark-brown or brown-black color, suggesting a lentigo and lentiginous nevus.

Seborrheic Keratosis–Like Variant The surface is pebbly and contains pseudo-horn cysts. The coloration is usually brown or dark brown.

Erythematous Variant As previously mentioned, the entire lesion lacks pigment and is uniformly pink-red.

Simulant of Melanoma The degree of asymmetry and irregularity of color

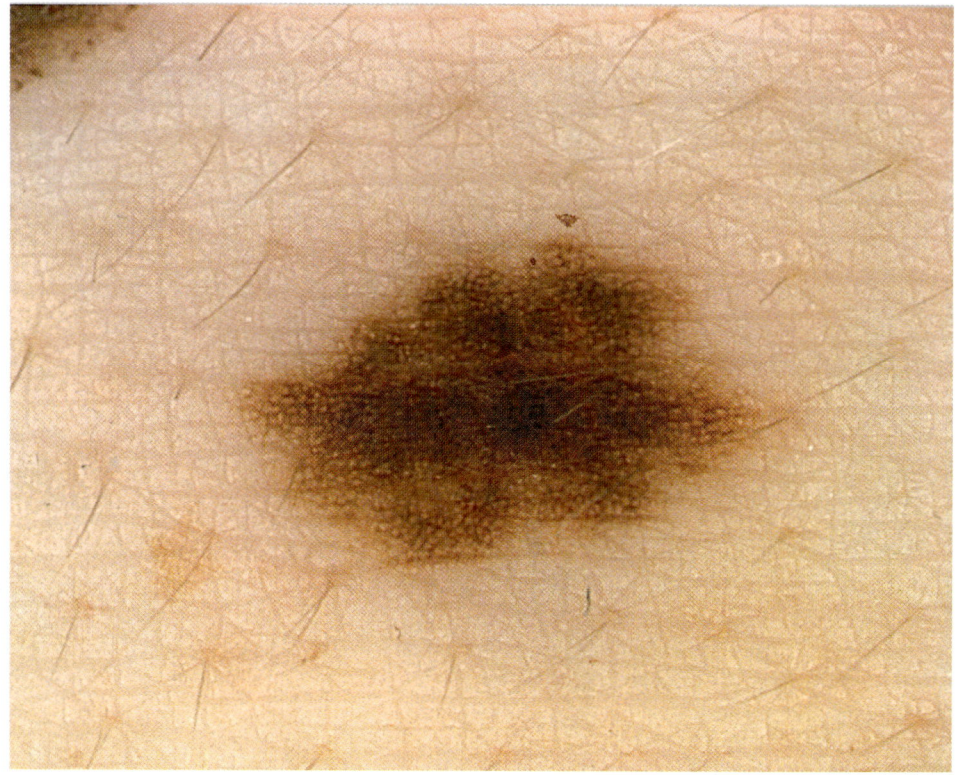

Figure 18-2 *Junctional dysplastic nevus with slight atypia. This is a relatively small brown lesion with some border irregularity and mild patchy pigment variation. Note that a pigment network pattern can be seen in the clinical view (without oil) and that it fades at the periphery rather than having an abrupt cutoff at the lesion border.*

suggest melanoma (see Fig. 18–7). Histologic examination is necessary to exclude melanoma.

DISTRIBUTION DMN may occur anywhere and show considerable heterogeneity. However, they frequently involve the trunk and also show a striking (though less common) predilection for the scalp, doubly covered areas of the body, breasts in women, and bathing trunk area in men. Their numbers may range from one or two to hundreds (see Fig. 18–1). When multiple large lesions are present, their prominence and variation are impressive. When multiple, lesions tend to be randomly and widely dispersed over the body surface, sometimes locally forming patterns such as linear tracts, clusters, or figurate arrays, all helpful in recognizing dysplastic nevi.

HISTOPATHOLOGIC FEATURES

As with their gross morphologic findings, DMN occupy a middle ground between common nevi and melanoma in terms of histologic features. DMN thus exhibit both architectural and cytologic abnormalities. The salient features include lentiginous melanocytic proliferation and/or irregularity of the junctional nesting pattern and variable cytologic atypia of intraepidermal melanocytes. Lymphocytic infiltrates and fibroplasia are also common findings and useful in identifying DMN. Most DMN are compound and exhibit a peripheral "shoulder" or intraepidermal component extending laterally beyond the dermal nevus elements.

BIOLOGIC BEHAVIOR

The overwhelming majority of dysplastic nevi are clinically stable. However, there is definite evidence that some lesions eventuate in malignant melanoma. This evidence comes from the above-cited histologic studies in which direct contiguity between dysplastic nevi and malignant melanoma has been observed. There are, furthermore, a number of studies documenting alterations in DNA content and reactivity of the dysplastic nevus with monoclonal antibodies directed against various melanocyte-associated antigens. The progressive abnormalities in DNA content and the increased reactivity with melanocyte-associated antigens have been correlated with progressive degrees of histologic atypia. These findings imply a progression of the dysplastic nevus toward melanoma.

DIFFERENTIAL DIAGNOSIS

The diagnosis of pigmented lesions approximately 4 to 12 mm in size includes both melanocytic and keratinocytic lesions. Among nevomelanocytic proliferations, the principal differential diagnostic considerations lie among common acquired nevi, small congenital nevi, pigmented spindle-cell nevi, nevus spilus, and malignant melanoma. The dysplastic nevus can be identified successfully because of its haphazard, irregular coloration—including hues of pink, tan, brown, and even black—and its irregularity in shape. The other nevic lesions either show symmetry and/or uniformity of coloration or, when irregularly colored, show orderly gradations or patterns of pigmentation.

Malignant melanoma is distinguished from DMN by the presence of greater asymmetry, irregular margins often with prominent notching, and striking variations in color: shades of gray, white, and blue-black are often admixed with brown and tan (see Table 1–9).

As far as keratinocytic lesions are concerned, both pigmented seborrheic keratoses and pigmented actinic keratoses may exhibit pink, tan, brown, or dark brown coloration. Both lesions have dull surface reflectance to incident light, and both exhibit hyperkeratosis, sometimes evident as scale. The seborrheic keratosis has small punctate horn cysts and, often, a waxy appearance. It usually lacks the peripheral macular annulus of pigmentation associated with the dysplastic nevus. The actinic keratosis has a rough hyperkeratotic surface and, when pigmented, usually does not exhibit striking color variegation.

MANAGEMENT

Management depends, first, on whether the patient in question presents with one or a few nevi or with numerous nevi, a personal history of melanoma, and then on

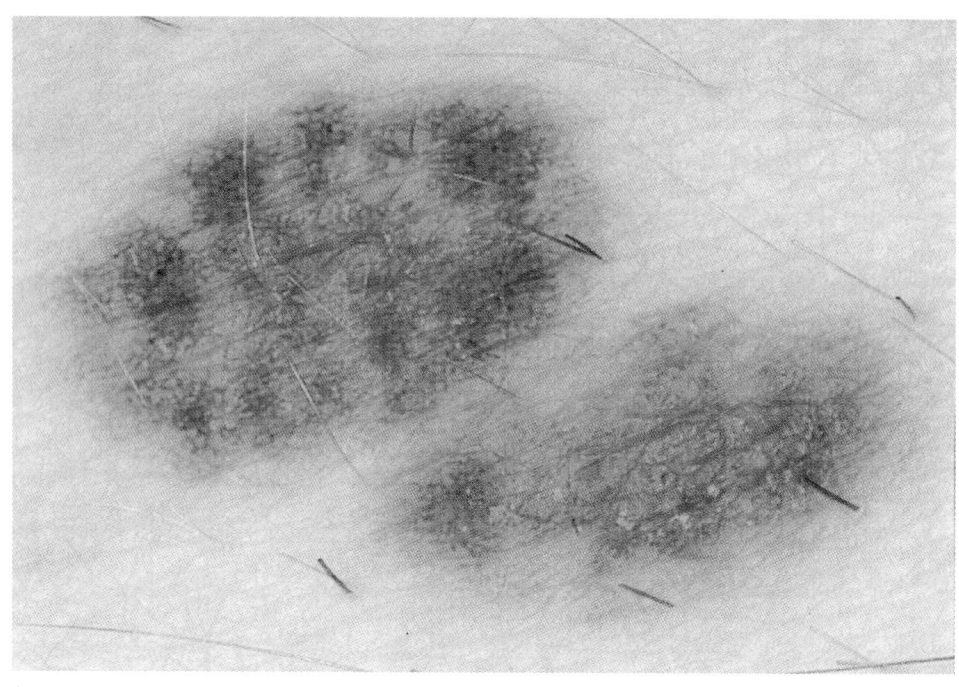
A

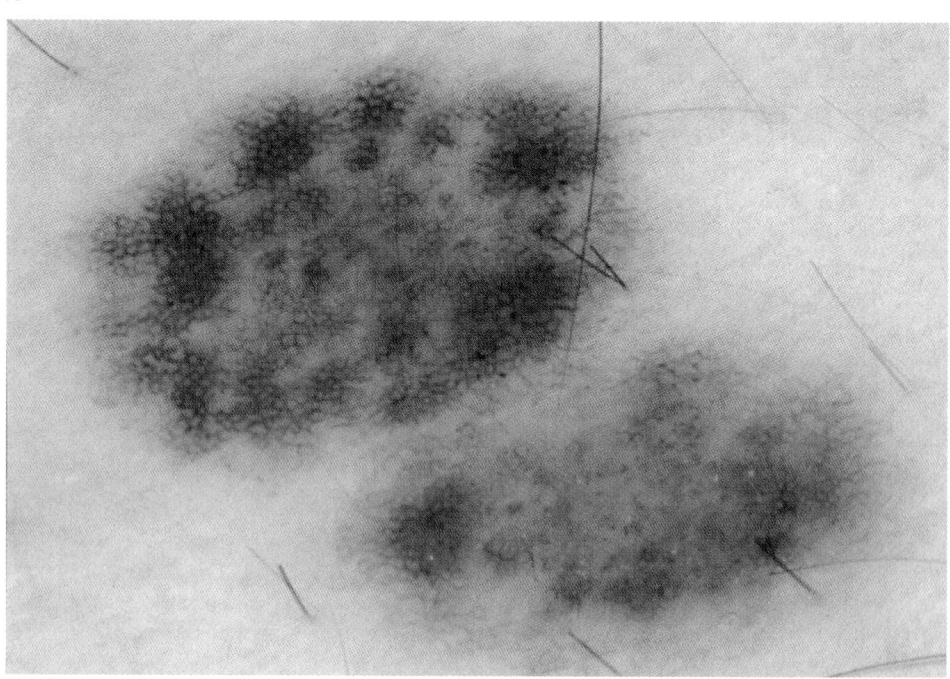
B

Figure 18-3

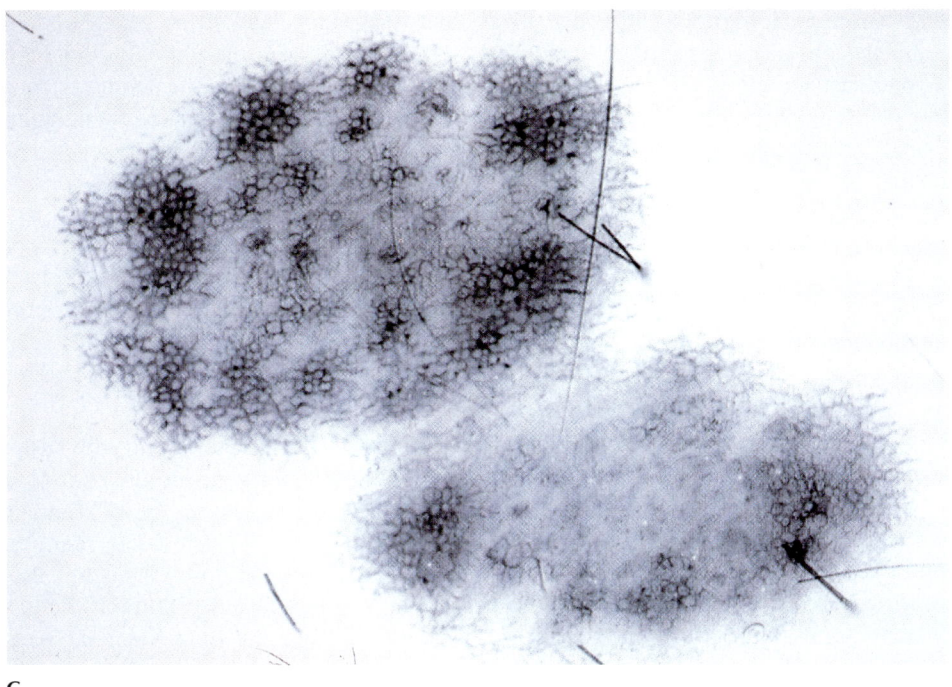

c

Figure 18-3 *Compound dysplastic nevus. Network patches.* (a) *Symmetric lesion with pigment variegation. Maximum diameter 9 mm.* (b, c) *Global features: network pattern. Network features: peripheral dark patches (regions of relatively darker network lines), marked; central light patches (relative hypopigmentation), moderate.* (a) *Digital clinical surface view (without oil);* (b) *digital epiluminescence microscopic subsurface view (with oil) of gross tissue architecture; and* (c) *pigment pattern enhancement of epiluminescence microscopic subsurface view.* (Reprinted with permission from RO Kenet et al: Clinical diagnosis of pigmented lesions using digital epiluminescence microscopy: Grading protocol and atlas. *Arch Dermatol* 129:169, 1993.)

whether there exists a familial setting of dysplastic nevi and/or melanoma. A gradient of melanoma risk has been clearly established for these various subsets of patients. Melanoma risk probably is continuous and increases with progressive increases in numbers of nevi, clinical atypia of nevi, and familial occurrence of atypical nevi and melanoma.

Regardless of the risk group, all pigmented lesions suspicious for melanoma and changing lesions should be excised completely for histopathologic examination. At present, it is not considered mandatory to remove clinically atypical nevi simply to confirm or exclude DMN histologically. An acceptable practice is to follow such patients on a regular schedule with baseline photography as needed. The frequency of follow-up examinations is individualized and is based on the preceding risk factors, i.e., number of nevi, lesional stability, and personal and family history of melanoma (Table 18–1).

For patients having clinically suspicious lesions removed, initial surgical margins of no more than 5 mm are advised. If lesions are slightly atypical, no reexcision is recommended, as long as no residuum of the nevus is clinically apparent. If lesions are moderately atypical and present in margins, even when no residual lesion is clinically obvious, a reexcision with clear margins is recommended. If severe atypia is present, reexcision with up to 5- to 10-mm margins is preferred. Any newly appearing lesion that has suspicious clinical features should be excised.

Follow-up of patients with multiple atypical nevi, especially in the context of a family history of melanoma, should be carried out every 3 to 6 months. Documentation, either by clinical photography or by body charts, should be made and periodically updated. If a patient is considered unreliable for follow-up, a more aggressive approach to surgical removal of any suspicious lesions is appropriate. Clinically atypical nevi located on sites difficult for the patient to examine, e.g., the scalp or back, should be considered for excision.

Finally, each person presenting with DMN should have a family history taken for the presence of dysplastic nevus and/or melanoma. First-degree blood relatives should be examined both for documentation and to assess and potentially diminish their own risks of developing melanoma.

Table 18-1 Follow-Up Schedule and Photography for Clinically Atypical Nevi

RISK CATEGORY	FOLLOW-UP INTERVAL	PHOTOGRAPHY
Few clinically atypical nevi, sporadic	12 months*	Baseline 1:1 Polaroid photos, most atypical nevi
Numerous atypical nevi, sporadic	6 months	Total-body 35-mm slides,*,[†] 1:1 Polaroid photos, most atypical nevi
Few atypical nevi, family history of positive melanoma	6–12 months	Baseline 1:1 Polaroid photos, most atypical nevi
Few atypical nevi, personal history of melanoma	6 months	Baseline 1:1 Polaroid photos, most atypical nevi
Numerous atypical nevi, personal or family history of melanoma	3–6 months	Baseline total-body 35-mm slides[†], 1:1 Polaroid photos, most atypical nevi

*Follow-up intervals and photography individualized.
[†]Total-body photos are optional.

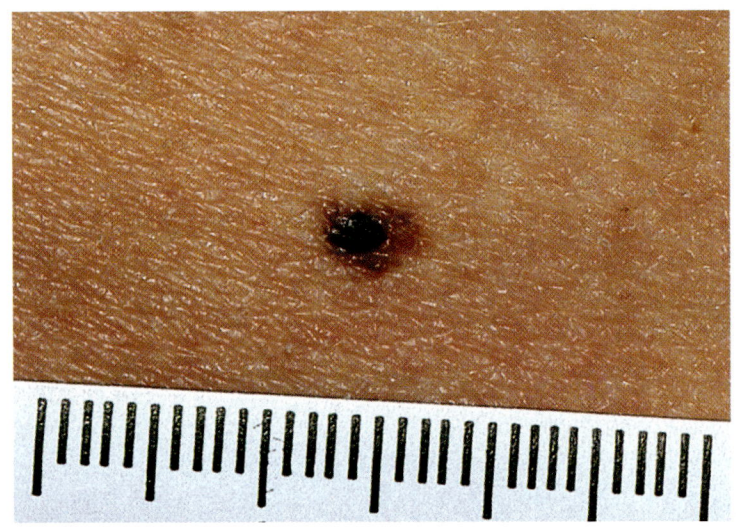

Figure 18-4 *This is a compound dysplastic nevus showing a dark brown eccentric papule surrounded by a lighter brown annulus.*

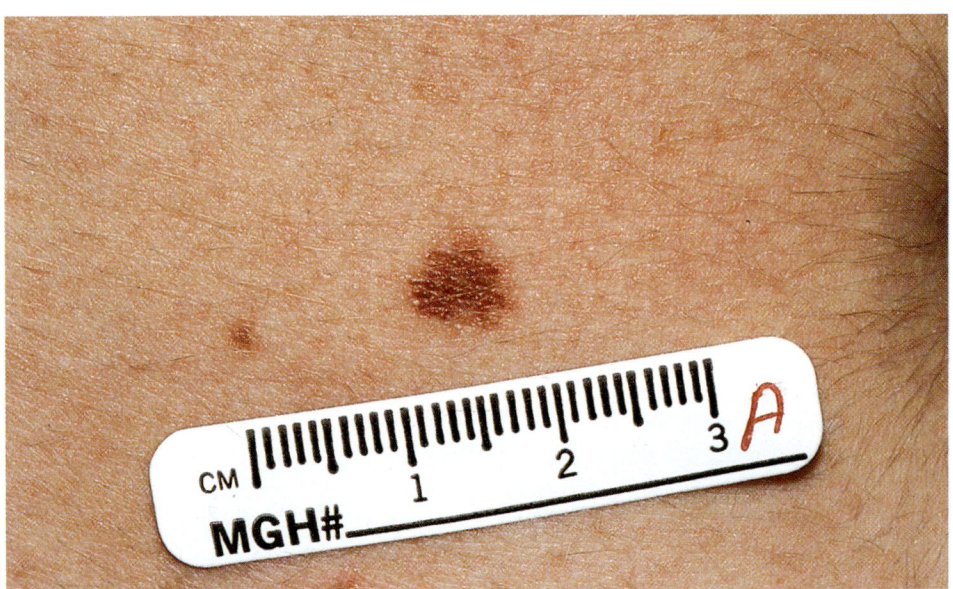

Figure 18-5 *A relatively flat dysplastic nevus with variegation of color and irregular borders. The lesion is considerably larger than most common acquired nevi. The surface elevation in such dysplastic nevi usually can only be detected usually by the use of sidelighting.*

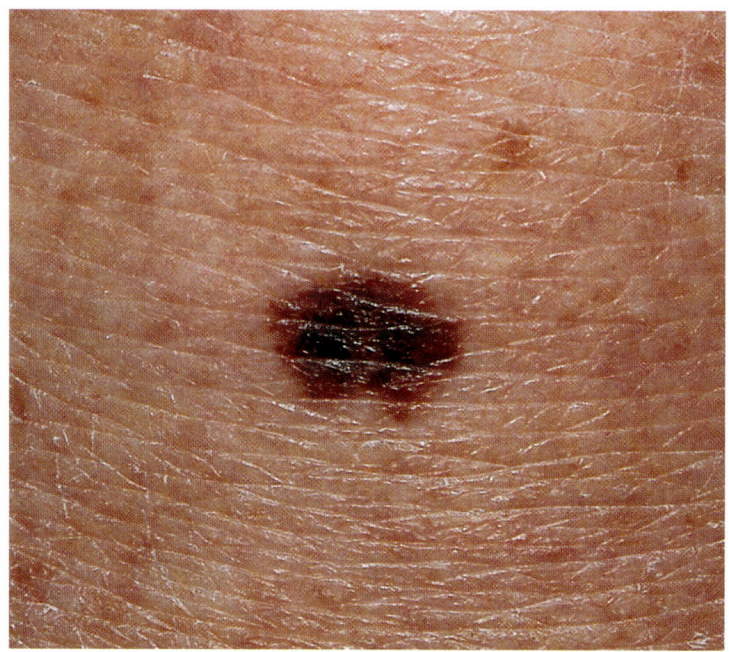

Figure 18-6 *A dysplastic melanocytic nevus with irregular borders and variegation of color. This lesion showed a moderate to severe atypia on histologic examination.*

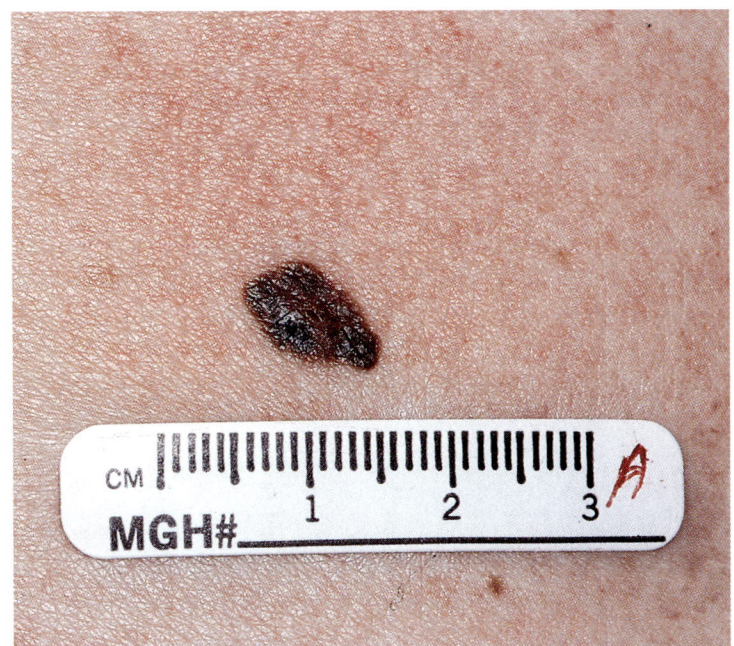

Figure 18-7 *Dysplastic melanocytic nevus. This lesion is variegated with a suggestion of bluish color in the lower left portion of the nevus. This lesion proved to be a dysplastic nevus with moderate to severe atypia. Clinically, this lesion is worrisome for melanoma.*

ADDITIONAL READINGS

Ackerman AB, Mihara I: Dysplasia, dysplastic melanocytes, dysplastic nevi, the dysplastic nevus syndrome, and the relation between dysplastic nevi and malignant melanomas. *Hum Pathol* **16**:87, 1985

Bale SJ et al: Mapping the gene for hereditary cutaneous malignant melanoma—Dysplastic nevus to chromosome 1p. *N Engl J Med* **320**:1367, 1989

Bale SJ et al: Cutaneous malignant melanoma and familial dysplastic nevi: Evidence for autosomal domination and pleiotropy. *Am J Hum Genet* **38**:188, 1986

Barnhill RL: Current status of the dysplastic melanocytic nevus. *J Cutan Pathol* **18**:147, 1991

Barnhill RL et al: Correlation of histologic architectural and cytoplasmic features with nuclear atypia in atypical (dysplastic) nevomelanocytic nevi. *Hum Pathol* **21**:51, 1990

Barnhill RL, Roush GC: Correlation of clinical and histopathologic features in clinically atypical melanocytic nevi. *Cancer* **67**:3157, 1991.

Clark WH Jr et al: A study of tumor progression: The precursor lesions of superficial spreading and nodular melanoma. *Hum Pathol* **15**:1147, 1984

Clark WH Jr et al: Origin of familial malignant melanomas from heritable melanocytic lesions: "The B-K mole syndrome." *Arch Dermatol* **114**:732, 1978

Clemente C et al: Histopathologic correlation in the diagnosis of dysplastic nevi: Concordance among pathologists convened by the World Health Organization Melanoma Programme. *Hum Pathol* **22**:313, 1991

Elder DE et al: Dysplastic nevus syndrome: A phenotypic association of sporadic cutaneous melanoma. *Cancer* **46**:1787, 1980

Friedman RJ et al: The dysplastic nevus: Clinical and histologic features. *Dermatol Clin* **3**:239, 1985

Greene MH et al: High risk of malignant melanoma in melanoma-prone families with dysplastic nevi. *Ann Intern Med* **102**:458, 1985

Kelly JW et al: Clinical diagnosis of dysplastic melanocytic nevi. *J Am Acad Dermatol* **14**:1044, 1986

Kraemer KH et al: Dysplastic nevi and cutaneous melanoma risk. *Lancet* **2**:1076, 1983

Mihm MC Jr, Googe PB: *Problematic Melanocytic Lesions: A Case Method Approach.* Philadelphia, Lea & Febiger, 1990

Piepkorn M et al: The dysplastic melanocytic nevus: A prevalent lesion that correlates poorly with clinical phenotype. *J Am Acad Dermatol* **20**:407, 1989

Rhodes AR et al: Dysplastic melanocytic nevi in histologic association with 234 primary cutaneous melanomas. *J Am Acad Dermatol* **4**:563, 1983

Van Haeringen A et al: Exclusion of the dysplastic nevus syndrome (DNS) locus from the short arm of chromosome 1 by linkage studies in Dutch families. *Genomics* **5**:61, 1989

19. Congenital Melanocytic Nevus

Congenital melanocytic nevi (CMN) are melanocytic nevi present at birth. They consist of proliferations of benign nevomelanocytes that may be intraepidermal, dermal, or both. Rarely, lesions appear after birth or within 2 years that are not otherwise remarkably different from congenital nevi and are therefore referred to as *congenital nevus tardive*. Some CMN may be just a few millimeters in size and appear clinically indistinguishable from common acquired nevi. In general, CMN fall into the categories small and large, but some authors classify these nevi as small, intermediate, and giant.

For practical purposes, small congenital nevi are < 1.5 cm in diameter. Intermediate- or medium-sized congenital nevi are from 1.5 to 10 or 19.9 cm in diameter. Large (or giant) congenital nevi cover large areas of the body such as the arm, scalp, or even the entire dorsal surface from scalp to feet.

Some authors base the distinction between small and large congenital nevi on their ease of removal. In this scheme, small congenital nevi generally can be removed by simple excision, intermediate congenital nevi often require a skin graft for closure, and giant nevi often cannot be removed or require staged excisions.

Synonyms: congenital nevomelanocytic nevus, giant pigmented nevus, garment nevus, nevus pigmentosus et pilosus, giant hairy nevus, bathing-trunk nevus

EPIDEMIOLOGY

Estimates of the incidence of congenital nevi when histologic confirmation is a criterion range as low as 0.64 percent; another series based on clinical criteria found an incidence of 2.7 percent. Giant hairy nevi are rare, with an estimated incidence of 0.005 percent from one study. Patients with giant nevi often have multiple smaller nevi as well. Familial aggregation of congenital nevi also has been reported.

ETIOLOGY

Melanocytes develop by differentiation from neural crest cells and begin to appear in fetal skin before 40 days gestation. Given the observation of congenital divided nevi of the eyelid and the fact that eyelids reopen in the sixth uterine month, it appears that CMN develop sometime during this interval from 40 days to 6 months gestation.

CLINICAL FEATURES

CMN of the small and intermediate types are usually round or oval and symmetric (Figs. 19-1 to 19-3). They are usually slightly raised at birth and exhibit a light tan background of coloration, often highlighted by fine speckling—speckles often correlate with perifollicular hyperpigmentation. The lesions may be hairy or hairless. Some CMN have very rugose, pebbly, or coarse surfaces (see Fig. 19-2).

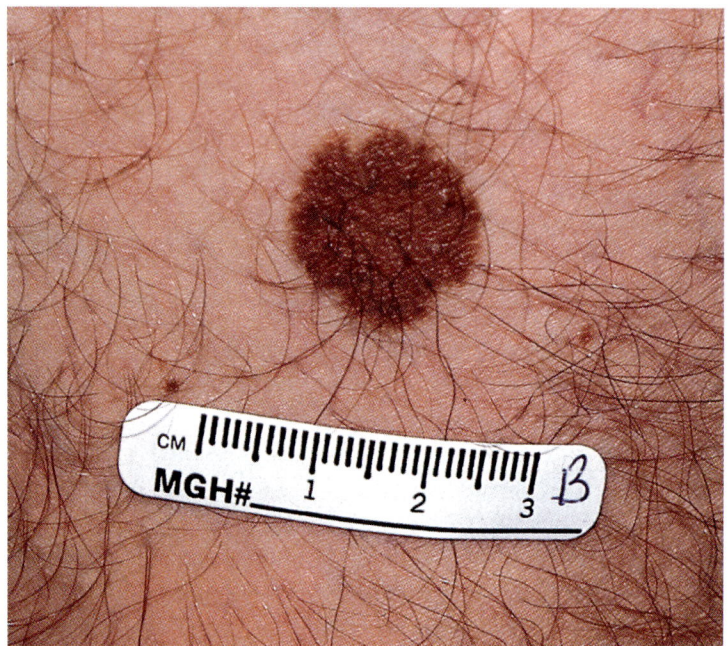

Figure 19-1 *Small congenital nevus. Note the large size; acquired nevi do not achieve this size. This lesion has somewhat irregular borders, but the overall pigment pattern is relatively uniform.*

Lesions that begin as slightly raised tend with age to become more elevated; darkening coloration and the assumption of a verrucous appearance are also common. However, congenital nevi containing areas of very dark pigmentation or manifesting dramatic surface irregularities are suspicious for cytologic atypia.

Giant nevi may present with features identical to those described for small nevi (Figs. 19-4 to 19-6). However, in general, the giant nevus exhibits a panoply of coloration and surface features. By and large, the borders of giant CMN are smooth and have regular contours, though some have strikingly irregular configurations. Again, as patients with giant nevi age, these variations become more prominent, and again, it is the areas of marked variegation of color and surface features that may indicate atypia. Nodules in giant congenital nevi should be considered for histologic evaluation.

Giant CMN are notable for varying numbers of so-called satellite CMN on the skin beyond the giant nevus. Such lesions typically have characteristics of small congenital CMN (see Fig. 19-6).

While CMN change in size with the growth of the individual, they do not

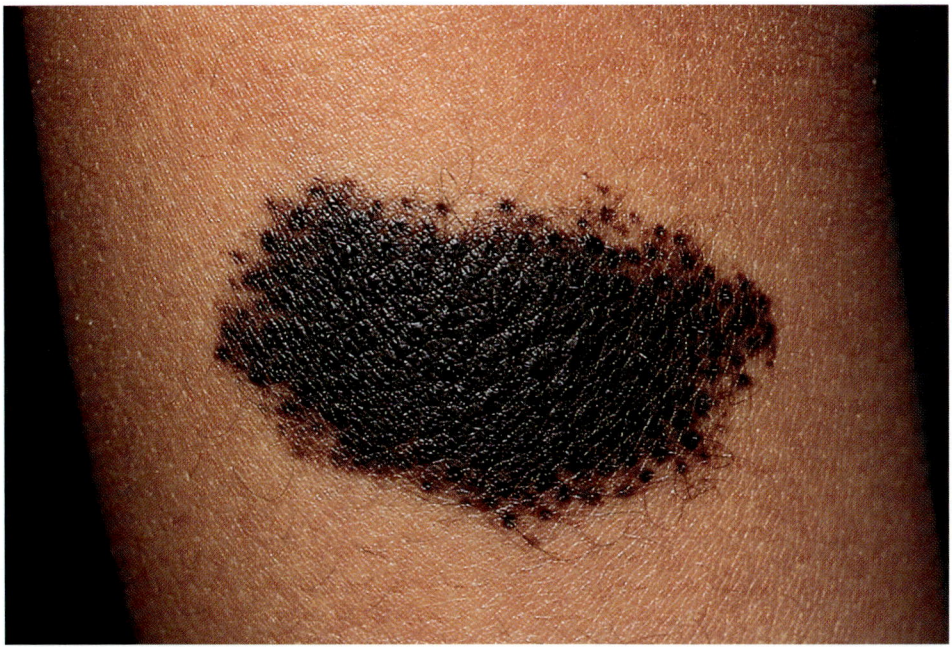

Figure 19-2 *Medium-sized congenital nevus: This lesion exhibits symmetry, a pebbled surface, and an homogeneous brown-black color.*

spread to cover proportionately larger areas than those defined at their congenital (or tardive) origin. Any extension into previously unaffected normal skin must be viewed with concern.

HISTOPATHOLOGIC FEATURES

Histologically, the congenital nevus is composed of the same types of nevus cells as are acquired nevi. (Some lesions can be indistinguishable not only clinically but also histologically from common acquired nevi. Thus, though a nevus may be congenital by history, its entire nevic cell ulation may be confined to the epidermis and/or papillary dermis.)

There are certain features of congenital nevi that usually permit their diagnosis under the microscope. In contrast to common acquired nevi, which are confined to the papillary and upper reticular dermis, congenital nevi may exhibit infiltration of the lower reticular dermis or subcutaneous fat. It is characteristic to observe nevus cells in a single-cell, or "Indian-file", array throughout the middle or lower dermis and even extending into the septa of the subcutis. Especially helpful is the presence of nevus cells surrounding (cuffing) and

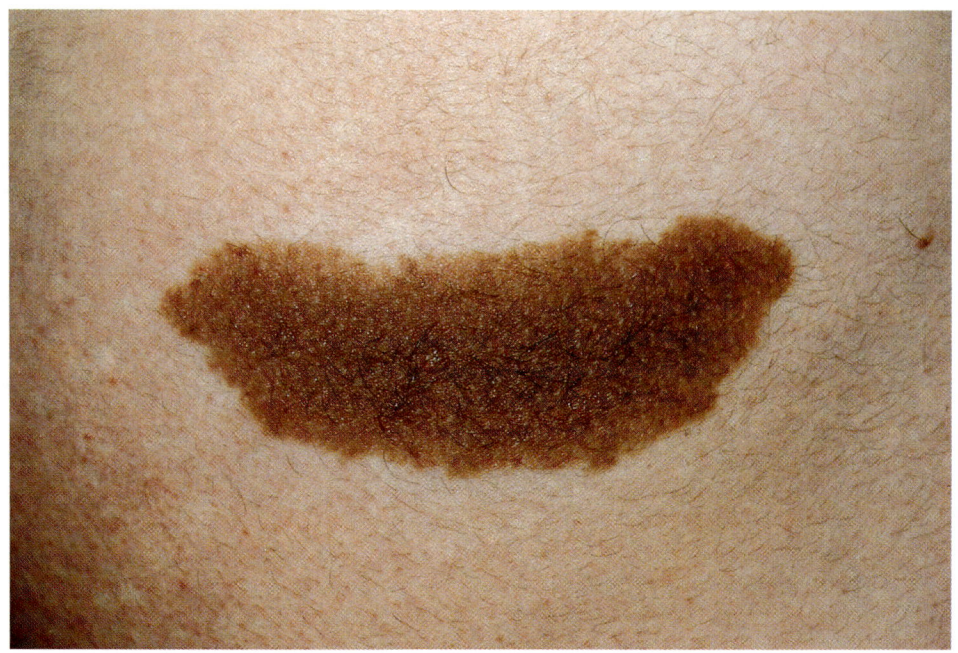

Figure 19-3 *This is a medium-sized congenital nevus which has a regular pigment pattern without variegation of color. This lesion could easily be excised without a graft, either performed serially or possibly with primary closure.*

within the walls of blood vessels, within appendages such as hair follicles and sweat glands, and within cutaneous nerves, particularly when observed in the lower half of the reticular dermis. Nevus cells may be found in the papillae and epithelium of hair follicles, in the sebaceous glands, in arrectores pili muscles, and in the eccrine ducts of the lower dermis.

BIOLOGIC BEHAVIOR

Congenital nevi, as indicated above, do not increase out of proportion to the anatomic area they occupy. An enlarging lesion may be evidence of a focus of atypia or melanoma supervening in the nevus.

CMN can become raised, exhibit changing surface characteristics, or develop halos of hypopigmentation; in rare instances, CMN may regress completely. Giant nevi which darken in childhood may display lightening of coloration over the decades.

Important in the biologic behavior of CMN is their potential for malignant degeneration, most importantly their relationship to malignant melanoma. Melanocytic atypia in congenital nevi ranges from slight atypicality to outright, fully evolved malignancy. More rarely, a variety of other malignant tumors may oc-

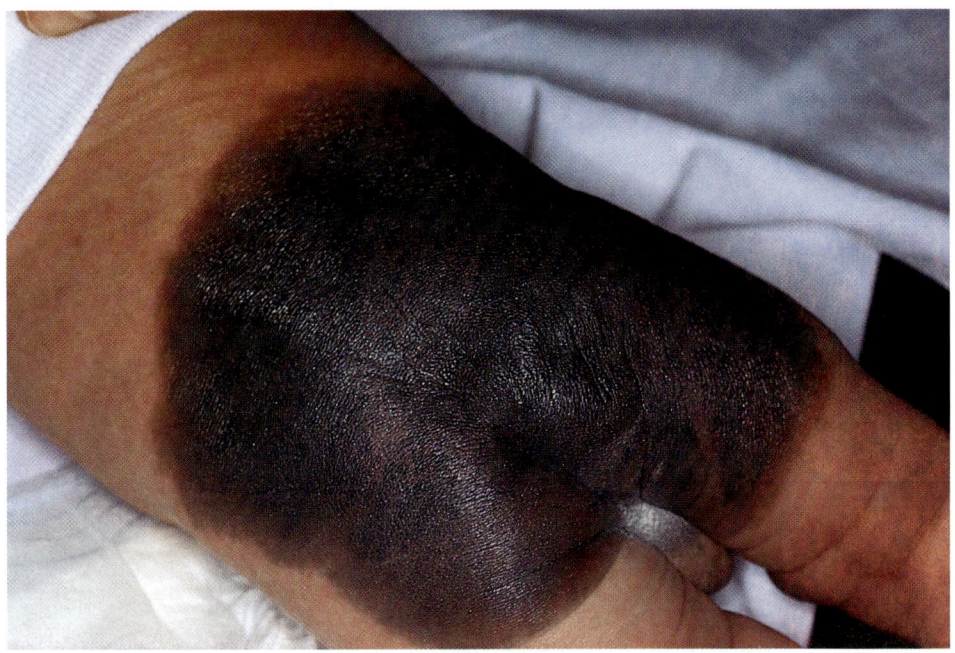

Figure 19-4 *Large congenital nevus in a newborn.*

cur in these lesions; these malignancies include a variety of soft-tissue tumors such as neurogenic sarcomas, fibrosarcomas, leiomyosarcomas, rhabdomyosarcomas, osteogenic sarcomas, and liposarcomas.

All sizes of CMN are susceptible to malignant transformation (Fig. 19-7). Estimates of the association of melanoma with nevi diagnosed as congenital by history range from 9 to 58 percent. Documented occurrence of melanoma in CMN defined as such by pathologic examination is 1 to 8 percent. The calculated risk overall is approximately 5 to 10 percent. The association of melanoma with small congenital nevi has been estimated to be about 5 percent or less (see Fig. 19-7). Estimates for malignant degeneration in large congenital nevi also vary but probably also are near 5 percent.

When a malignant melanoma develops in a congenital nevus, it appears histologically as a distinct invasive nodule, lacking maturation. Thus it differs from the type of superficial atypia that some congenital nevi show early in life.

DIFFERENTIAL DIAGNOSIS

The giant hairy nevus is distinctive. Rarely, nevus spilus may mimic its "garment" distribution. Any nevus > 1.0 cm

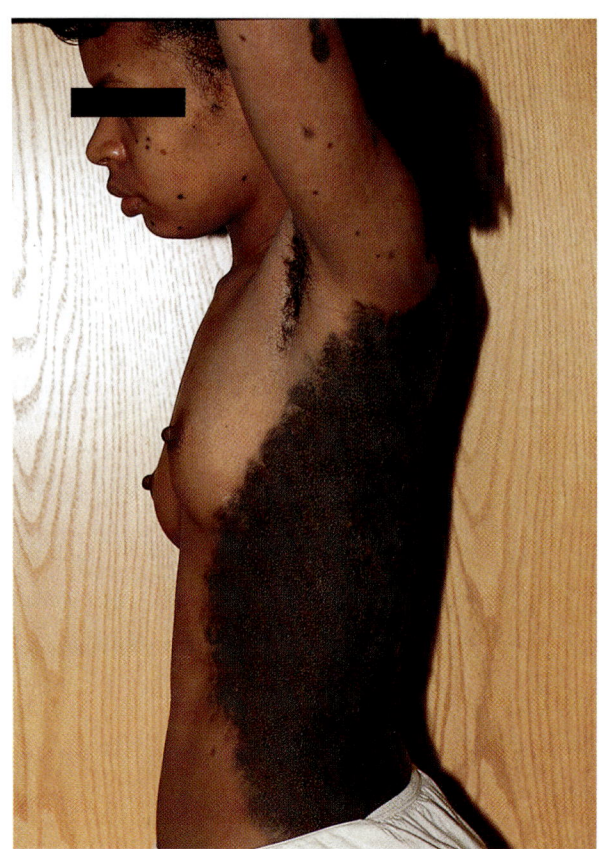

Figure 19-5 *This is a giant congenital nevus covering most of the back. This patient also has scattered satellite lesions on the extremities. A spindle-cell melanoma was noted to develop in the sacral area of this nevus. There has been no evidence of recurrence with 5 years of follow-up.*

raises possibilities of a dysplastic nevus, malignant melanoma, congenital nevus, or a pigmented keratinocytic lesion such as an epidermal nevus, Becker's nevus, a large pigmented seborrheic keratosis, and the rare instance of a pigmented squamous cell carcinoma or Paget's disease, either mammary or extramammary, with pigmentation. History is important, and often histology is essential in resolving this differential diagnosis.

MANAGEMENT

The management of CMN is primarily related to two factors: their increased risk for progression to melanoma and their cosmetically disfiguring appearance. The decision to remove a congenital nevus is individualized and based on melanoma risk, age of the individual, anatomic location (proximity to vital structures), cosmetic outcome, and complexity of removal. Excision of small congenital nevi can usually be delayed until later child-

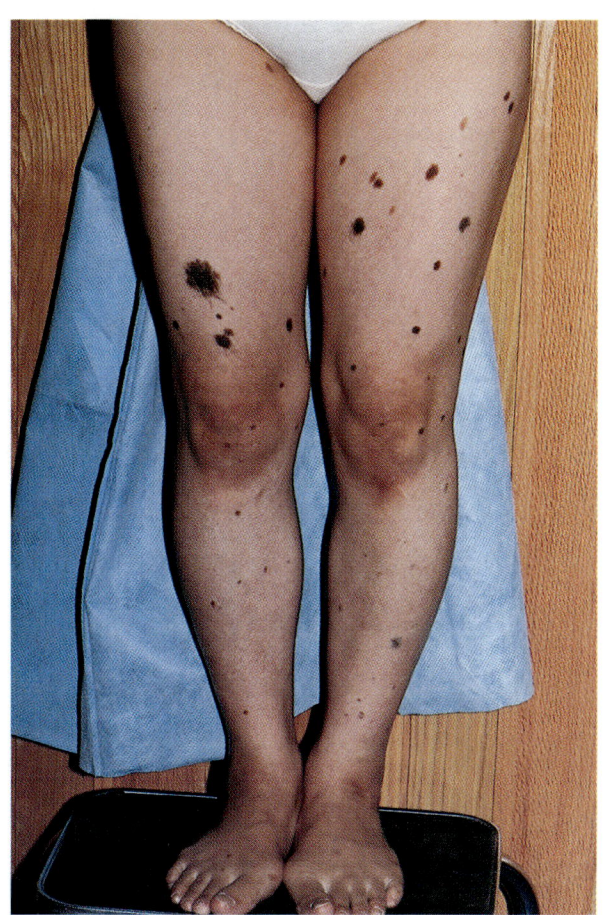

Figure 19-6 *These are satellite lesions in a patient who has a giant nevus on the trunk. Some of them have coarse, dark hairs, particularly the one on the right thigh.*

hood but should be performed before puberty, since this is when melanoma risk increases; an acceptable alternative to surgical excision is baseline photography and yearly follow-up. The management of giant congenital nevi is more problematic, since melanoma risk is present at birth, but general anesthesia presents significant risk at that time. If such giant nevi are to be removed, most authorities recommend delaying the procedure for a few months so that the risk from general anesthesia is not so great as in the perinatal period.

Follow-up of small and large congenital nevi is a reasonable minimum course of action until the risk of malignancy arising in these lesions can be more definitely determined by prospective, randomized, and statistically valid studies.

When melanoma supervenes in a large congenital nevus, it may involve the dermal or subcutaneous component and be difficult to detect early. Malignant melanoma of the small CMN type usually begins in the epidermis and can be detected more readily.

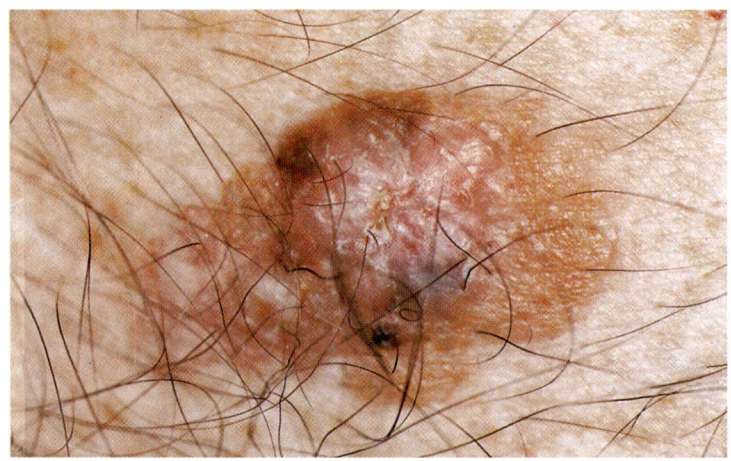

Figure 19-7 *Melanoma arising in a small congenital nevus. A 2.0-cm tan lesion with a 1.0-cm central nodule with pinks, grays, blues, and browns within it. The lesion was on the anterior pectoral area of a 40-year-old white man.* (From TB Fitzpatrick et al: *Color Atlas and Synopsis of Clinical Dermatology,* 2nd ed. New York, McGraw-Hill, 1992, p. 681, with permission.)

ADDITIONAL READINGS

Castilla EE et al: Epidemiology of congenital pigmented nevi: Incidence rates and relative frequencies. *Br J Dermatol* **104**:307, 1981

Everett MA: Histopathology of congenital pigmented nevi. *Am J Dermatopathol* **11**:11, 1989

Hidano A et al: Statistical survey of skin changes in Japanese neonates. *Pediatr Dermatol* **3**:140, 1986

Illig L et al: Congenital nevi less than or equal to 10 cm as precursors to melanoma. *Arch Dermatol* **121**:1274, 1985

Lanier VC et al: Congenital giant nevi: Clinical and pathological considerations. *Plast Reconstr Surg* **58**:48, 1976

Lorentzen M et al: The incidence of malignant transformation in giant pigmented nevi. *Scand J Plast Reconstr Surg* **71**:163, 1977

Mark GJ et al: Congenital melanocytic nevi of the small and garment type: Clinical, histologic, and ultrastructural studies. *Hum Pathol* **4**:395, 1973

Pers M: Naevus pigmentosus giganticus: Indikationer for operative behandling. *Ugetskr Læger* **125**:613, 1963

Reed WB et al: Giant pigmented nevi, melanoma, and leptomeningeal melanocytosis. *Arch Dermatol* **91**:100, 1965

Rhodes AR: Congenital nevomelanocytic nevi: Histologic patterns in the first year of life and evolution during childhood. *Arch Dermatol* **122**:1257, 1986

Rhodes AR et al: A histologic comparison of congenital and acquired nevomelanocytic nevi. *Arch Dermatol* **121**:1266, 1985

Rhodes AR et al: The malignant potential of small congenital nevocellular nevi: An estimate of association based on a histologic study of 234 primary cutaneous melanomas. *J Am Acad Dermatol* **6**:230, 1982

Santa Cruz DJ, Bashiti H: Bathing trunk nevus with extensive vascular involvement. *J Cutan Pathol* **6**:513, 1979

Walton RG et al: Pigmented lesions in newborn infants. *Br J Dermatol* **95**:389, 1976

Section IV

Cutaneous Malignant Melanoma

Cutaneous malignant melanoma results in most instances from the malignant transformation of intraepidermal melanocytes of sun-exposed skin. However, some melanomas also seem to develop in association with precursor lesions such as congenital or atypical acquired melanocytic (dysplastic) nevi. At present, the incidence rates for cutaneous melanoma among Caucasian populations worldwide are rising more precipitously than for any other type of cancer.

Synonyms: cutaneous melanoma, malignant melanoma, melanosarcoma (archaic), and melanocarcinoma (archaic)

EPIDEMIOLOGY

Currently, approximately 35,000 patients develop cutaneous melanoma annually in the United States, and over 6000 deaths are attributed to this malignancy each year. It is primarily a disorder of light-complexioned Caucasians, especially those who sunburn easily, tan poorly, freckle, or have a family history of melanoma and various precursors of melanoma such as the dysplastic nevus. MacKie et al. have developed a risk-factor algorithm that allows individual assessment of melanoma risk. In this four-factor model, the probability of incidence can vary 600-fold for men and 175-fold for women and depends on the number of nevi, presence and number of dysplastic nevi, occurrence and number of severe sunburns, and presence sunburns, and presence or absence of freckling. In the United States and Australia, the sex ratios are approximately 1:1. However, in northern Europe, there is a preponderance of women over men that may reach 2:1. Melanomas are rare in childhood, with rates of approximately 1 per million per year, and are nearly 100 times more frequent after age 15. The incidence rate in the United States overall is approximately 10 per 100,000 per year, but incidence rates as high as 25 per 100,000 per year have been reported from the southwestern United States. Melanoma incidence increases with age, and two subtypes of melanoma, lentigo maligna melanoma and acral lentiginous melanoma, are especially frequent in older individuals. The disease is much less common in individuals of black or Asian ancestry, with rates 1/7 to 1/20 that of Caucasians. The site distribution also differs in blacks and Asians in that the common sites are palms, soles, nail beds, and mucous membranes.

CLASSIFICATION OF CUTANEOUS MELANOMA

Four subtypes of melanomas have been described. Three have initial phases of lateral (mainly intraepidermal) growth in the skin (radial growth). These include *superficial spreading melanoma* (the most common type of melanoma) (70 percent), *acral lentiginous melanoma* (10 percent), and *lentigo maligna melanoma* (5 percent). One type of melanoma appears without a discernible radial growth phase and is designated *nodular melanoma* (15 percent). All four types of melanoma can produce confluent nodules or plaques that expand and infiltrate beyond the papillary dermis, at which point they are considered to have entered the vertical growth phase and have become potentially capable of metastasis.

The classification of melanoma outlined above has not been universally accepted. Some authors maintain that histologic differences among the three forms of radial growth are primarily related to anatomic site. See chapters 20 through 23.

NATURAL HISTORY

Cutaneous melanoma is thought to evolve through a series of relatively well-characterized phases. The initial lesion may show atypical melanocytes throughout the full thickness of the epidermis; when confined to the epidermis, the lesion is termed *melanoma in situ*. Radial growth phase melanoma includes superficially invasive lesions that can extend into the papillary dermis. The vertical growth phase is present when there is nodule formation clinically and microscopically and discrete nests of tumor cells are seen in the papillary dermis that are larger than those in the epidermis. Capacity for metastasis seems to correlate with the presence of the vertical growth phase. A number of factors have been identified that affect the likelihood of metastasis and ultimate death from primary melanoma. These factors include the vertical thickness of the primary tumor measured from the granular cell layer down to the deepest tumor cells (using an ocular micrometer and measurements expressed in millimeters), Clark's anatomic levels of invasion (level II—penetration into the papillary dermis; level III—filling the papillary dermis; level IV—penetration into reticular dermis; level V—penetration into subcutaneous fat), mitotic rate, presence of an ulcer on microscopic examination, and microscopic satellites in the specimen where the thickest portion of the tumor is measured (*microscopic satellites* are defined as nests of tumor cells 0.05 mm or greater in diameter separated from the main body of tumor by either reticular dermal collagen or subcutaneous fat). These factors can be used to estimate prognosis. There is a direct relationship between tumor thickness and the likelihood of metastatic disease. There is also a correlation between the thickness of the tumor and the time to recurrence: the thicker the tumor, the sooner the recurrent disease will present. A six-factor model for vertical growth phase melanoma has been developed by Clark et al. and is depicted in Table 1. This six-factor model includes

Table 1 Probabilities of 8-Year Survival (Multivariable Logistic Regression Model)

MITOTIC RATE AXIAL/SUBVOL†	TILS*	TUMOR REGRESSION	FEMALE EXTREMITIES		FEMALE AXIAL, SUBVOL†		MALE EXTREMITIES		MALE AXIAL/SUBVOL†	
0.0/mm²	Brisk	Absent	1.00	**0.99**	1.00	**0.98**	1.00	**0.98**	0.99	**0.95**
		Present	1.00	**0.99**	0.99	**0.95**	0.99	**0.96**	0.96	**0.86**
	Nonbrisk	Absent	1.00	**0.98**	0.98	**0.94**	0.99	**0.95**	0.96	**0.84**
		Present	0.99	**0.95**	0.96	**0.85**	0.97	**0.88**	0.89	**0.66**
	Absent	Absent	0.99	**0.94**	0.95	**0.82**	0.96	**0.85**	0.86	**0.60**
		Present	0.96	**0.86**	0.87	**0.61**	0.89	**0.67**	0.69	**0.35**
0.1–6.0/mm²	Brisk	Absent	1.00	**0.98**	0.98	**0.94**	0.99	**0.95**	0.95	**0.84**
		Present	0.99	**0.95**	0.96	**0.84**	0.97	**0.87**	0.88	**0.65**
	Nonbrisk	Absent	0.99	**0.95**	0.95	**0.82**	0.96	**0.86**	0.87	**0.61**
		Present	0.96	**0.86**	0.87	**0.62**	0.90	**0.68**	0.70	**0.36**
	Absent	Absent	0.95	**0.83**	0.84	**0.57**	0.87	**0.63**	0.65	**0.31**
		Present	0.88	**0.64**	0.66	**0.32**	0.71	**0.38**	0.40	**0.14**
>6.0/mm²	Brisk	Absent	0.99	**0.94**	0.95	**0.81**	0.96	**0.85**	0.86	**0.60**
		Present	0.96	**0.85**	0.86	**0.61**	0.89	**0.67**	0.68	**0.35**
	Nonbrisk	Absent	0.95	**0.84**	0.84	**0.57**	0.88	**0.63**	0.65	**0.31**
		Present	0.88	**0.64**	0.66	**0.32**	0.72	**0.38**	0.40	**0.14**
	Absent	Absent	0.85	**0.59**	0.61	**0.28**	0.67	**0.33**	0.34	**0.12**
		Present	0.68	**0.34**	0.35	**0.12**	0.42	**0.15**	0.16	**0.04**

*Tumor-infiltrating lymphocytes.
†Axial/subvol includes head, neck, trunk, volar, and submucosal locations.
NOTE: Data for lesions <1.70 mm thick (i.e., vertical growth phase, clinical stage I cases) are in regular type; data for lesions ≥1.70 mm (vertical growth phase, clinical stage I cases) are in boldface.
SOURCE: Clark WH Jr et al: Model predicting survival in stage I melanoma based on tumor progression. *J Natl Cancer Inst* **81**:1893, 1989.

thickness greater than or less than 1.70 mm, sex, anatomic site (axial, plus palms and soles, versus other locations on extremities), presence of tumor-infiltrating lymphocytes (absent, moderate, or marked), presence of regression (yes/no), and mitotic rate (0, 0.1 to 6, and >6 mitoses per square millimeter). High-, intermediate- and low-risk profiles can be created by combinations of these factors.

STAGING

There are several staging systems in use for cutaneous melanoma. The simplest system, which has been in wide use for a number of years, is a three-stage system: stage 1, localized disease; stage 2, disease in lymph nodes; stage 3, disseminated disease. Recently, a four-stage system has been adopted jointly by the UICC/AJCC and will probably become dominant. It divides *localized* melanoma into two stages: stage 1, primary tumors <1.5 mm thick; stage 2, primaries >1.5 mm thick. Stage 3 is regional nodal disease, and stage 4 is disseminated disease. Table 2 compares these two staging systems.

MANAGEMENT

Tables 3 and 4 list those factors which are relevant in the history and physical examination. The primary goal of early treatment is surgical elimination of the primary tumor prior to metastatic spread. In asymptomatic patients, extensive radiologic examinations have generally not been of value in altering management de-

Table 2 Melanoma Staging Systems

	THREE STAGE	
STAGE	CLINICAL	PATHOLOGIC
I	Localized disease*	Absence of histologic evidence of tumor in regional nodes
II	Suspicious palpable regional lymph nodes	Histologic evidence of melanoma in regional nodes (microscopic or macroscopic)
III	Presence of distant metastases by history, physical, or laboratory examination	Histologic documentation of distant metastases
	FOUR STAGE (AJCC/UICC)	
I	Primary tumor <1.5 mm	
II	Primary tumor >1.5 mm	
III	Suspicious palpable regional lymph nodes	Histologic evidence of melanoma in regional nodes (microscopic or macroscopic)
IV	Presence of distant metastases by history, physical, or laboratory examination	Histologic documentation of distant metastases

*May also include rare cases of local recurrence, satellitosis, or in-transit metastases.

cisions, nor are routine blood studies normally worthwhile in detecting early metastatic disease. Table 5 lists the surgical margins currently recommended for the management of primary melanoma.

Elective regional nodal dissection for primary melanoma is a controversial procedure. Randomized studies now in progress should establish its benefit or lack thereof within the next 5 years. At present, whether or not to perform nodal dissection is an individualized decision based on the tumor thickness, anatomic site, patient, and surgeon. Adjuvant therapies for high-risk patients are all experimental, with no proven benefit at the present time.

For disseminated melanoma, therapy is problematic, and management decisions

Table 3 Guide to Clinical Evaluation of a Suspected Melanoma: History

VARIABLE	COMMENT
Age	Melanoma frequency peaks at age 20–45 years, although age-specific rates continue to rise with age; prepubertal melanoma is uncommon; when it occurs in first few years of life, it is usually in association with congenital nevi.
Sex	Effect of pregnancy or sex hormones on melanoma causation and behavior is controversial; lower legs are common sites for melanoma in white female subjects.
Race	Decreased frequency of melanoma in dark-skinned persons; melanomas of the soles, palms, nail beds, mucous membranes are most common in this group.
Onset and duration	Of interest to know whether melanoma arose from a precursor lesion, how fast it developed, and the time to diagnosis.
Increased size or color change	Noted frequently in early melanomas.
Pruritus, tenderness, ulceration, bleeding	Important warning symptoms for melanoma, and except for pruritus, are often indicative of late disease.
Sun exposure	Increased exposure, especially history of severe sunburns, in fair-skinned persons (skin phototypes I and II) associated with increased risk.
Past history of melanoma	Increases risk for developing melanoma ninefold.
Family history of melanoma	Increases risk for developing melanoma eightfold.
Family history of dysplastic nevi	Family history of dysplastic nevi, especially in setting of familial melanoma, increases risk of developing melanoma.

must be individualized. Factors that are favorable in patients with disseminated disease are (1) disease at a single site, (2) noninvolvement of liver, and (3) nodal or soft-tissue disease in contrast to visceral metastases.

PREVENTION

Efforts to increase patient and professional education and awareness of the diagnostic features of melanoma are ongoing. A simple system for public education is the ABCDE concept (see Table 1-10). Complete skin examination at the time of physical examination is also recommended. Efforts to reduce sun exposure by shifting time of activity, using protective clothing, and applying sunblocks of high sun-protection factor are thought to be of potential value, especially in individuals under age 20. Screening of families in which one family member has melanoma or dysplastic nevi is also thought to be of value. Until better therapy is developed for metastatic disease, all efforts should be focused on early detection or prevention.

Table 4 Guide to Clinical Evaluation of a Suspected Melanoma: Physical Examination

VARIABLE	COMMENT
Lesion location	Record exact location of lesion.
Lesion color	Variegation of red, pink, gray, white, and blue in a brown or black lesion is highly suspect for melanoma.
Lesion size	Measure the greatest two dimensions at right angles.
Configuration	Irregular border, notching, asymmetry should heighten suspicion of melanoma.
Topography	Melanoma usually raised, except thin acral lentiginous lesions; and lentigo maligna; surface often irregularly raised. (Use sidelighting.)
Depigmentation	Suggests immunologic response with destruction of melanocytes and/or melanoma cells. (Wood's lamp may aid evaluation.)
In-transit lesions	Inspect and palpate around lesion and over lymphatic drainage areas for satellite or in-transit lesions.
Lymph nodes	Palpate regional nodes for presence of tumor.
Dysplastic/congenital nevi	May be precursor lesion for melanoma. Presence of these nevi increases risk for having second primary melanoma.

Table 5 Surgical Guidelines for Patients with Clinical Stage I Melanoma*

TUMOR THICKNESS (MM)	EXCISION MARGIN (CM)	CLOSURE	ERLND†
<1.0	1	Primary	No
1.0–1.5	2.0	Primary	No
1.5–4.0	2.0	Primary, flap or graft‡	Optional§
>4.0	2–3	Primary, flap or graft‡	No

*These are arbitrary guidelines. They should be modified for individual patients depending on overall assessment of prognosis.
†Elective regional lymph node dissection.
‡Primary closure is used except over the distal half of extremities or head and neck, where flap or graft may be required.
§Offered as patient option; done only when lymphatic drainage pattern of the melanoma is well defined.

INTRODUCTION

20. Lentigo Maligna and Lentigo Maligna Melanoma

Lentigo maligna melanoma (LMM) is relatively uncommon among the major types of melanoma and occurs in older individuals on the most sun-exposed areas—the head, neck, and forearms. There is general agreement that sunlight is a major etiologic factor in the development of LMM. Lentigo maligna (LM) is an intraepidermal melanocytic proliferation that encompasses a spectrum from a slightly atypical precursor to fully developed melanoma in situ (radial growth phase.)

Synonyms: Hutchinson's melanotic freckle, Dubreuilh's melanosis

EPIDEMIOLOGY AND ETIOLOGY

LMM comprises approximately 5 to 10 percent of all cutaneous melanomas. LM, the initial phase of LMM, may evolve over a long period of time (up to 20 years) and eventuates in LMM in 5 to 30 percent of cases. LMM affects the sexes equally, and median age at diagnosis is 65 to 70 years. LMM is more prevalent in persons with skin phototypes I, II, or III and is directly related to cumulative sun exposure.

CLINICAL FEATURES

LM begins as a flat (macular) lesion that slowly extends laterally and has the appearance of a "stain." There is commonly prominent variation in hues of tan, brown, and black (Figs. 20-1 to 20-5). Even greater complexity of color is often associated with the phenomenon of regression and is represented by varying admixtures of pink, gray, blue, and white (see Figs. 20-1 and 20-2). The borders are frequently highly irregular and notched. The overall size may range from 1.0 to 20.0 cm or larger. It is important to emphasize that the entire lesion or any portion of it may be amelanotic and may resemble superficial basal cell carcinoma and other erythematous lesions. The presence of raised or papular foci usually indicates the development of LMM. Such papular areas may be brown, black, blue, or amelanotic (pink). The development of grossly evident papules or nodules often correlates with the onset of the vertical growth phase (Fig. 20-6).

LM and LMM occur virtually exclusively on sun-exposed, chronically sun-damaged skin of older individuals. The most common locations are the cheeks, nose, and forehead.

HISTOPATHOLOGIC FEATURES

The radial growth phase of LMM is characterized by a mainly basilar proliferation of atypical melanocytes that often involves adnexal epithelium. There is usually a background of marked solar elastosis and flattening of the epidermal rete ridges. The dermal invasive component of LMM is most commonly composed of spindle cells. Desmoplastic and neurotropic forms of melanoma occasionally are associated with the invasive elements of LMM.

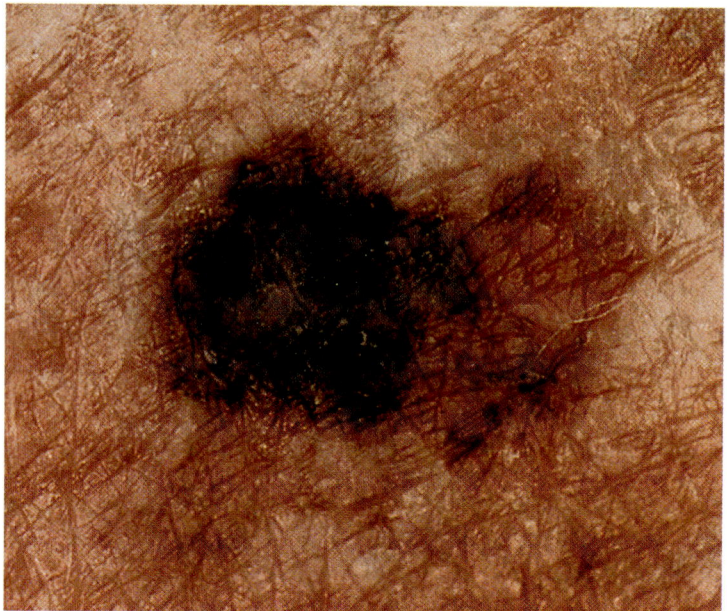

A

Figure 20-1 *Lentigo maligna melanoma in situ with regression. (a) (Clinical surface view, without oil): This lesion exhibits asymmetry, irregular borders, and pigment and color variability on a region of "sun-damaged" skin (many lentigines and telangiectasia). (b) (Gross subsurface tissue morphology as seen with ELM, with oil): There is an irregular pigment network pattern with small dark regions of pigment confluence overlying the network. [Small regions of dark pigment confluence in the setting of an irregular pigment network may be an early (sensitive but not necessarily specific) sign of melanoma. This feature is presently under investigation.] There is also central hypopigmentation and erythema, with a subtle blue-gray veil. This constellation of features may suggest but is not diagnostic of early melanoma. (c) (Digital enhancement of subsurface morphology): Digital contrast enhancement of the ELM view emphasizes that there is a subtle reticular pigment network pattern that is perturbed by other features. Note the small, dark, irregular regions of pigment confluence overlying the network.*

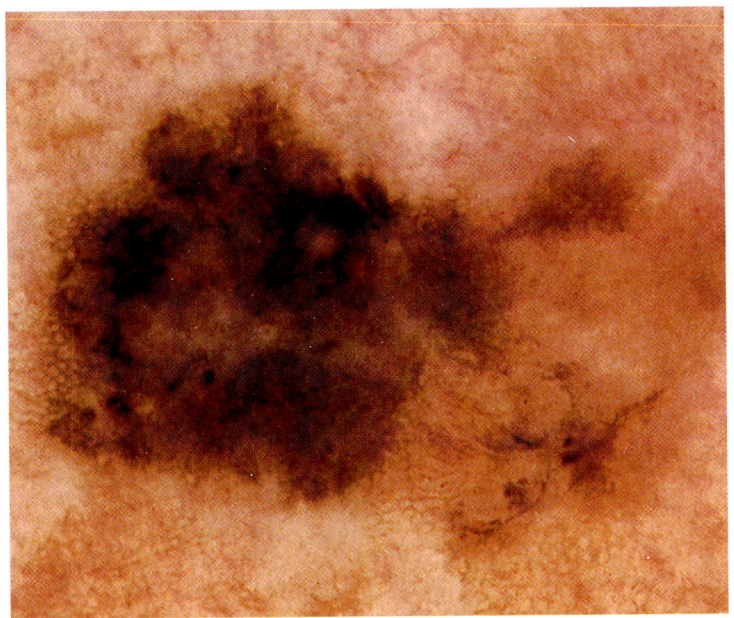

B

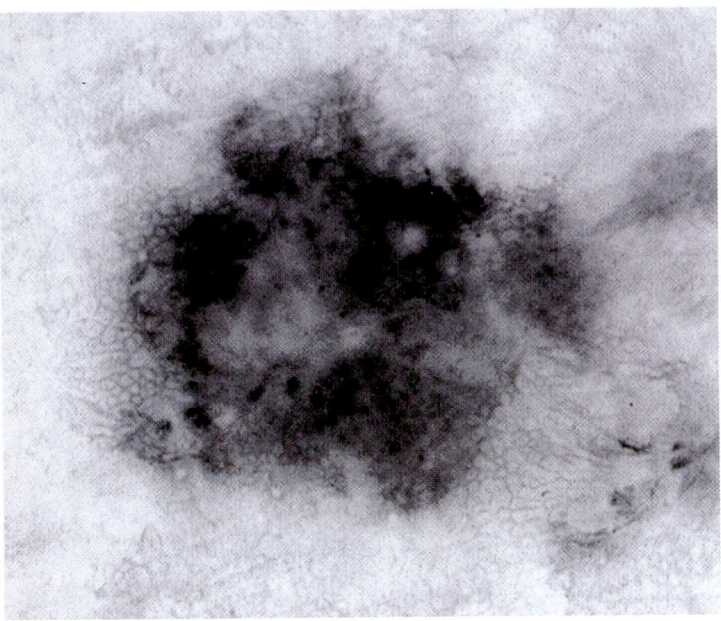

C

Figure 20-1 *(cont.)*

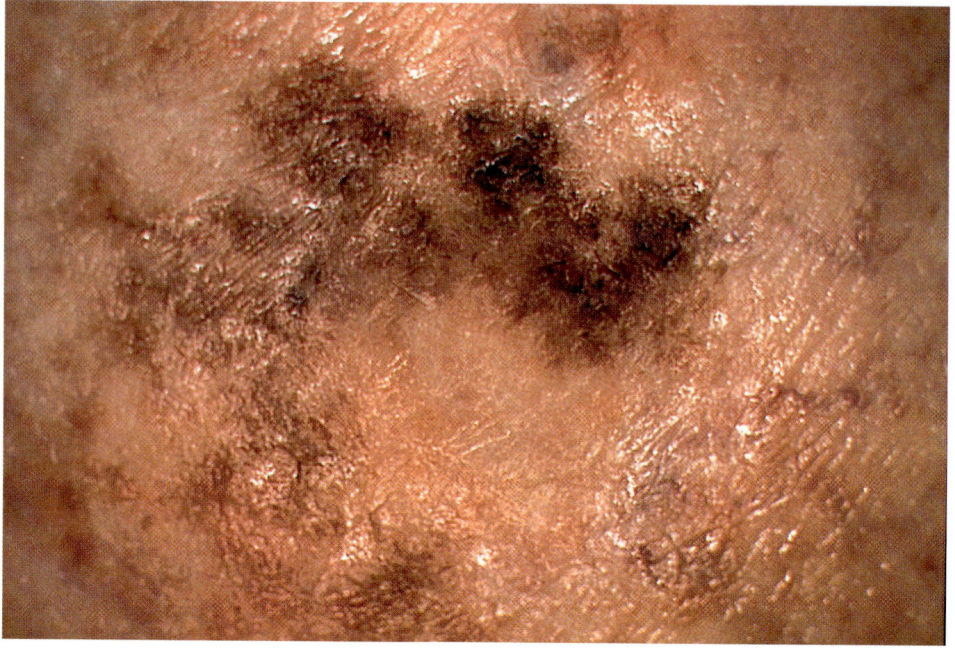

A

Figure 20-2 *Lentigo maligna melanoma in situ with regression. (a) (Clinical surface view, without oil): This is a crescent-shaped brown lesion with asymmetry, border irregularity, color variability, and large diameter (greater than 6 mm). (b) (Gross subsurface tissue morphology as seen with ELM, with oil, upper right portion of lesion): Pigment network pattern with marked irregularity with small regions of dark pigment confluence overlying network. [Small regions of dark pigment confluence in the setting of an irregular pigment network may be an early (sensitive but not necessarily specific) sign of melanoma that is presently under investigation.] (c) (Digital enhancement of subsurface morphology): Digital image enhancement of the ELM view emphasizes that there is a markedly irregular reticular pigment network pattern. Note the small dark irregular regions of pigment confluence overlying the network.*

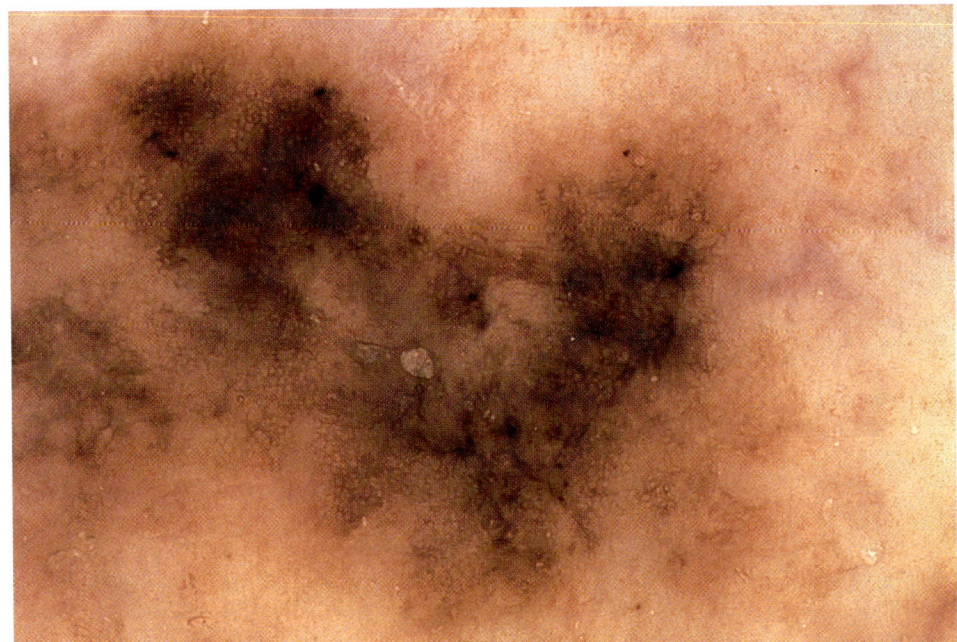

B

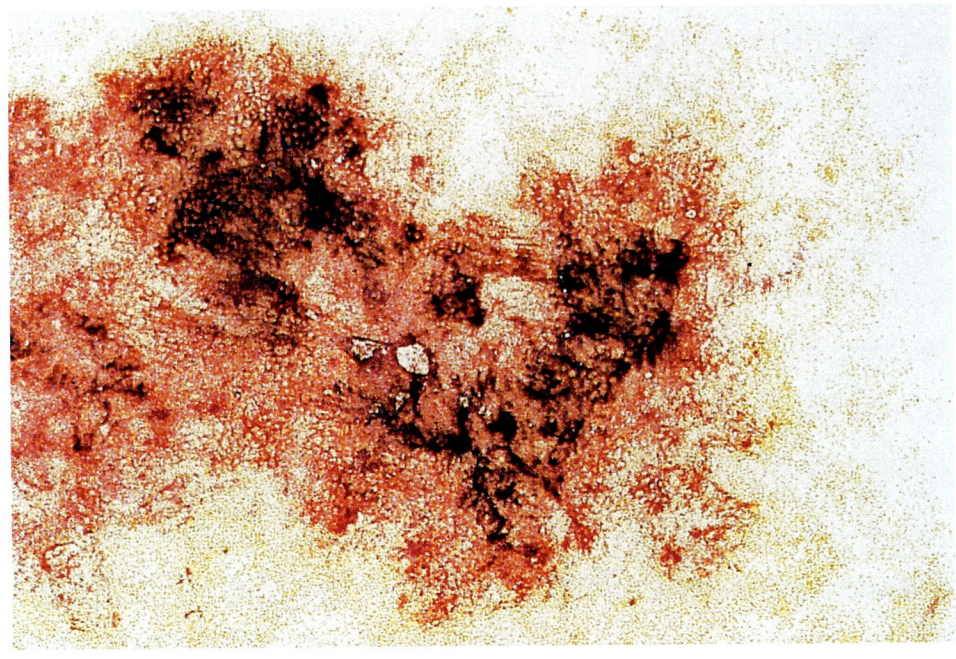

C

Figure 20-2 *(cont.)*

BIOLOGIC COURSE

There has been a debate in the literature concerning whether LMM has a more favorable prognosis than other types of melanoma. When matched for tumor thickness and anatomic site, LMM appears to have no better prognosis than other types of melanoma. However, most LMM are diagnosed while still thin, usually having been present for years and possibly indicating a more indolent course.

DIFFERENTIAL DIAGNOSIS

The differential diagnosis for LM and early LMM primarily includes solar lentigo, relatively macular forms of seborrheic keratosis, and pigmented actinic keratosis (Fig. 20-7). In general, LM and LMM are larger, show more variation in color, and have more irregular borders than the latter lesions, which also tend to show surface scaling as opposed to the smooth surface of LM. However, histopathologic examination is necessary for definitive diagnosis.

Amelanotic forms of LM and LMM are exceedingly difficult to diagnose without heightened clinical suspicion. Such lesions may suggest basal cell carcinoma, lichenoid keratosis, and other inflammatory skin conditions.

ADDITIONAL READINGS

(See Chapter 23.)

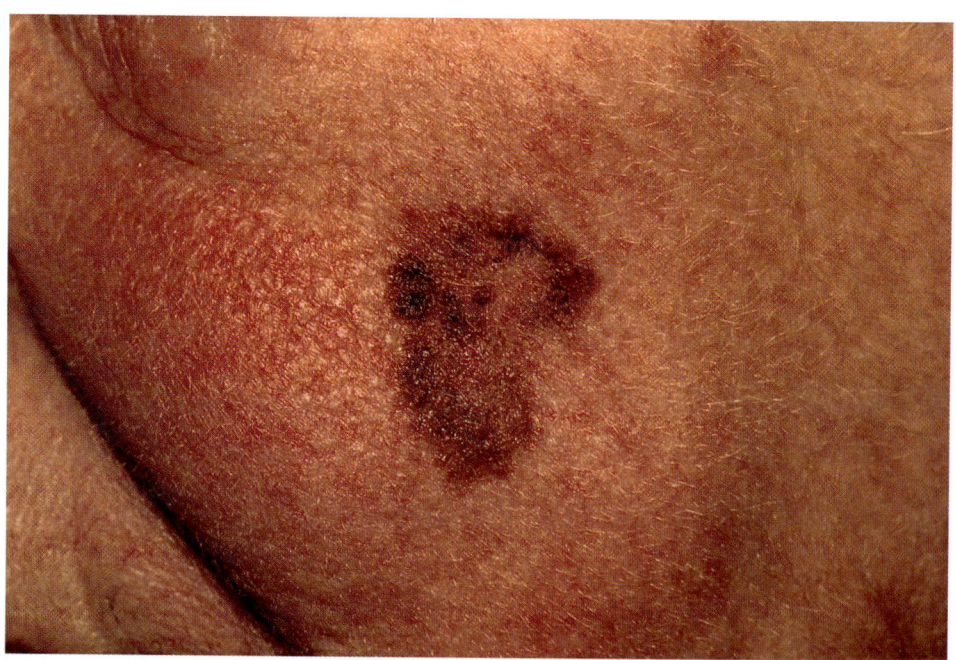

Figure 20-3 *Lentigo maligna melanoma, radial growth phase. The lesion exhibits asymmetry, irregular borders, and variegation of color.*

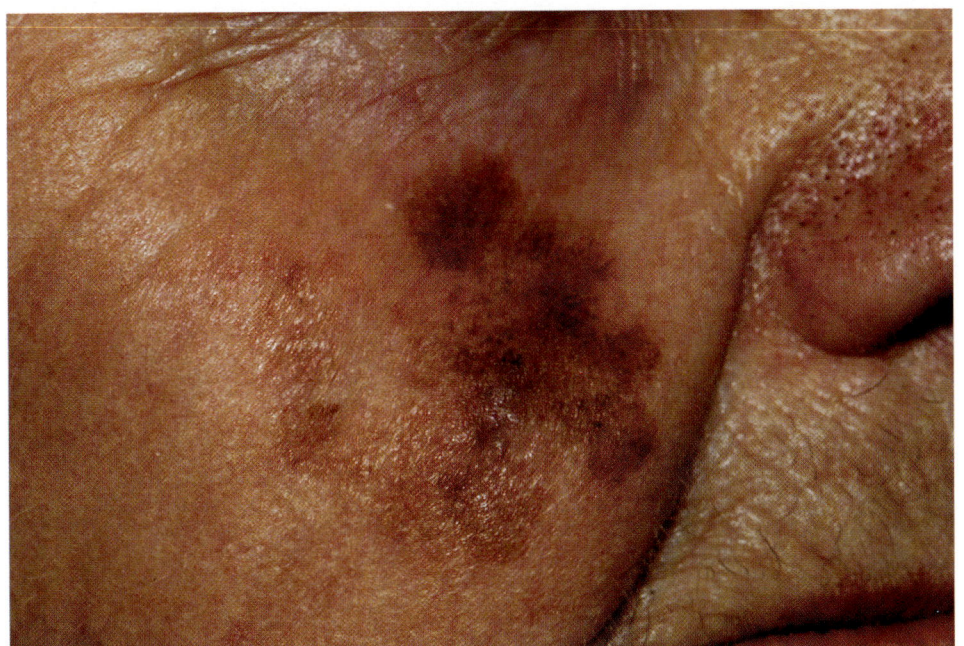

Figure 20-4 *Lentigo maligna melanoma, radial growth phase. This lesion shows rather prominent notching of borders and a complex admixture of tan, brown, and dark brown speckles.*

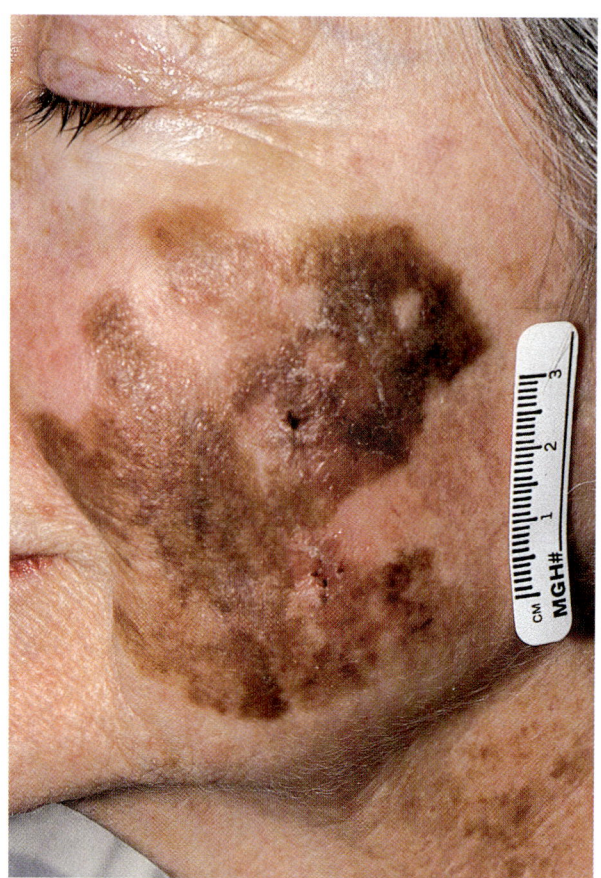

Figure 20-5 *Lentigo maligna melanoma. This is a very large lesion demonstrating striking asymmetry, notching of borders, and prominent variegation of color.*

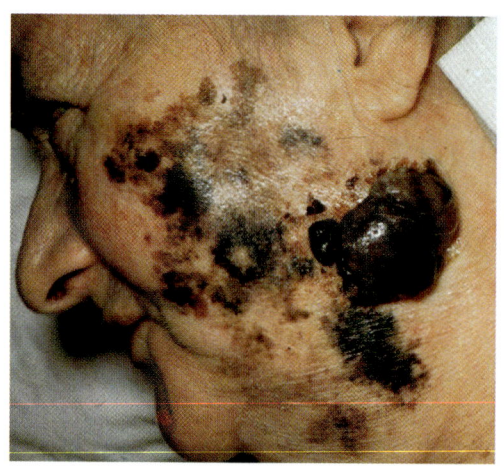

Figure 20-6 *Lentigo maligna melanoma with development of vertical growth phase. A large brown nodule has developed immediately beneath the ear in this extensive lentigo maligna melanoma.* (From TB Fitzpatrick et al. (eds.): *Dermatology in General Medicine,* 4th ed. New York, McGraw-Hill, 1993, p 1088, with permission.)

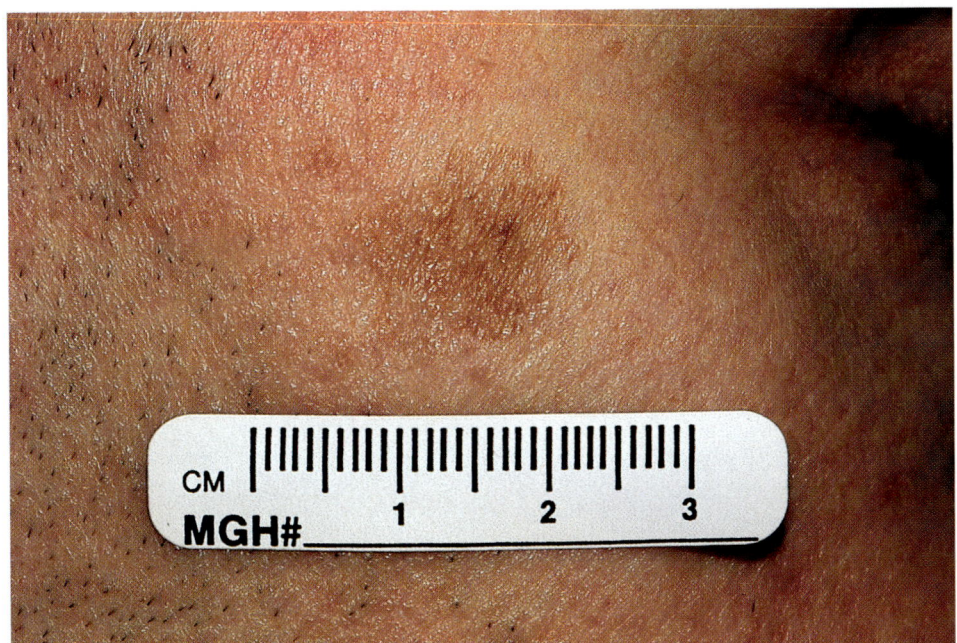

Figure 20-7 *Pigmented actinic keratosis. This tan macular lesion measures slightly more than 1 cm in diameter. With sidelighting, one can detect a slight alteration of the surface texture. This lesion enters into the differential diagnosis of lentigo maligna and solar lentigo. Biopsy of this lesion, however, revealed actinic keratosis.*

21. Superficial Spreading Melanoma

Superficial spreading melanoma (SSM) is the most common type of cutaneous melanoma developing in white populations and most commonly affects the upper back of men and lower extremities of women. The rapid increase in incidence of melanoma is primarily accounted for by the increasing incidence of SSM.

Synonym: pagetoid melanoma

EPIDEMIOLOGY AND ETIOLOGY

SSM primarily affects persons 30 to 50 years of age, with possibly a slightly greater incidence in females. Although SSM may involve any anatomic site, it seems to occur primarily on sites of intermittent sun exposure, e.g., the trunk of both sexes and the lower extremities of women. SSM is almost exclusively a cancer of white-skinned persons, with only 2 percent of SSM occurring in darkly pigmented races. Approximately 20 to 50 percent of SSM are reported to develop in association with a precursor melanocytic nevus, a proportion of which shows fea-

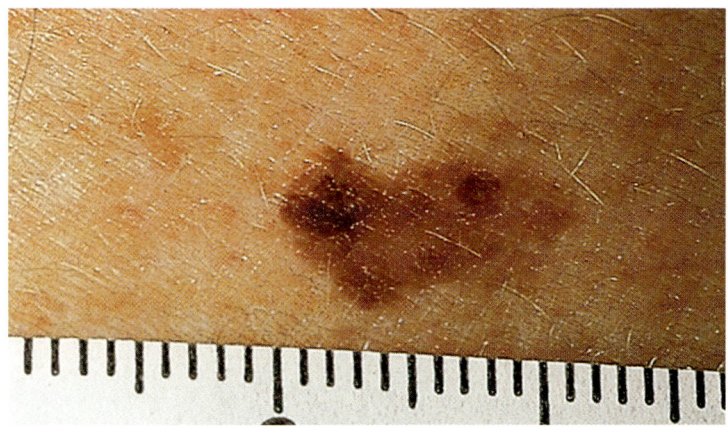

Figure 21-1 *Malignant melanoma in situ. This lesion is relatively flat, measures approximately 12 mm in greatest diameter, and exhibits asymmetry, irregularity of borders, and variation in the pigmentary pattern.*

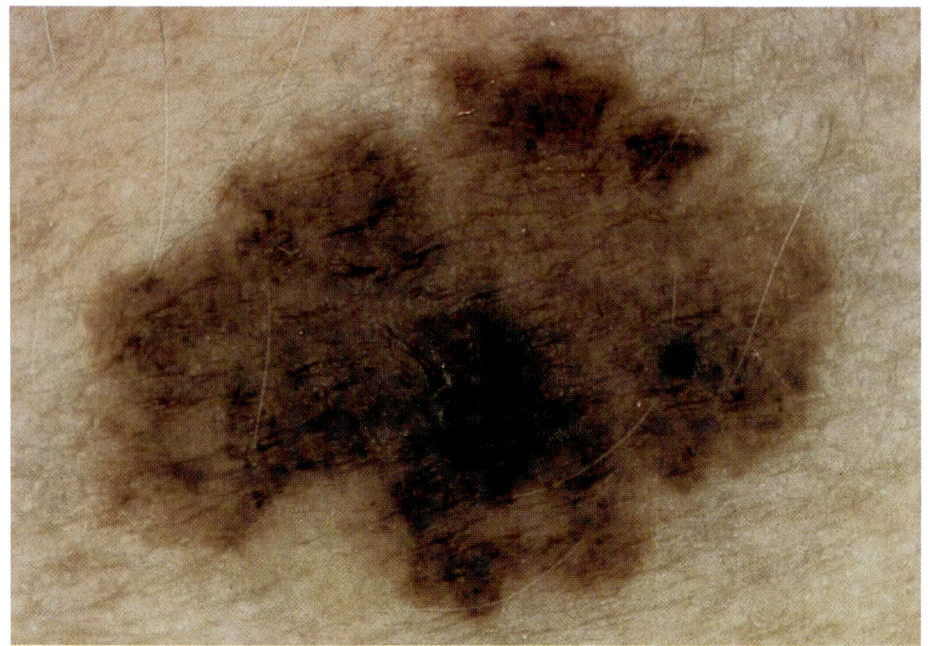

A

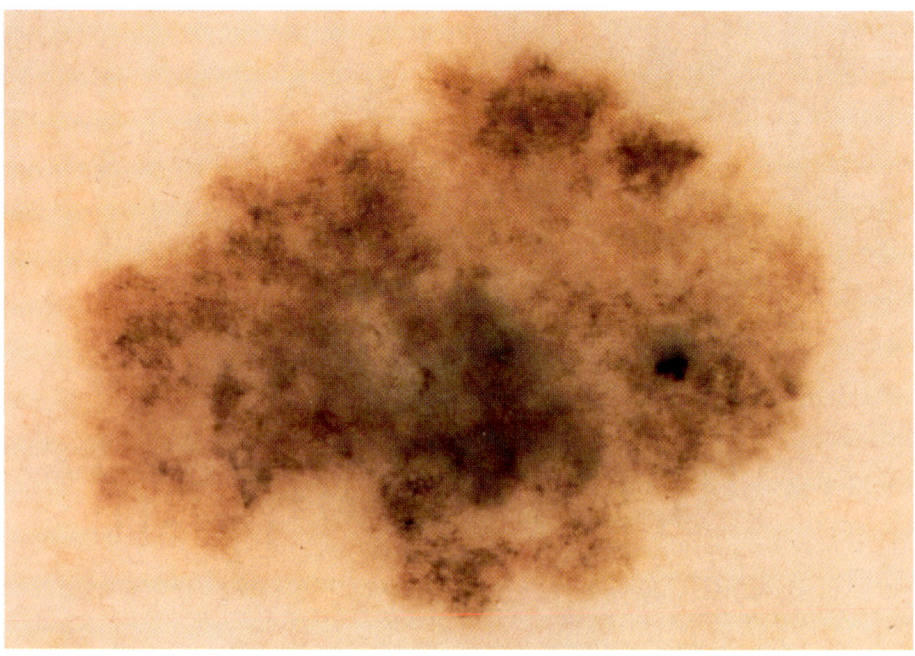

B

Figure 21-2

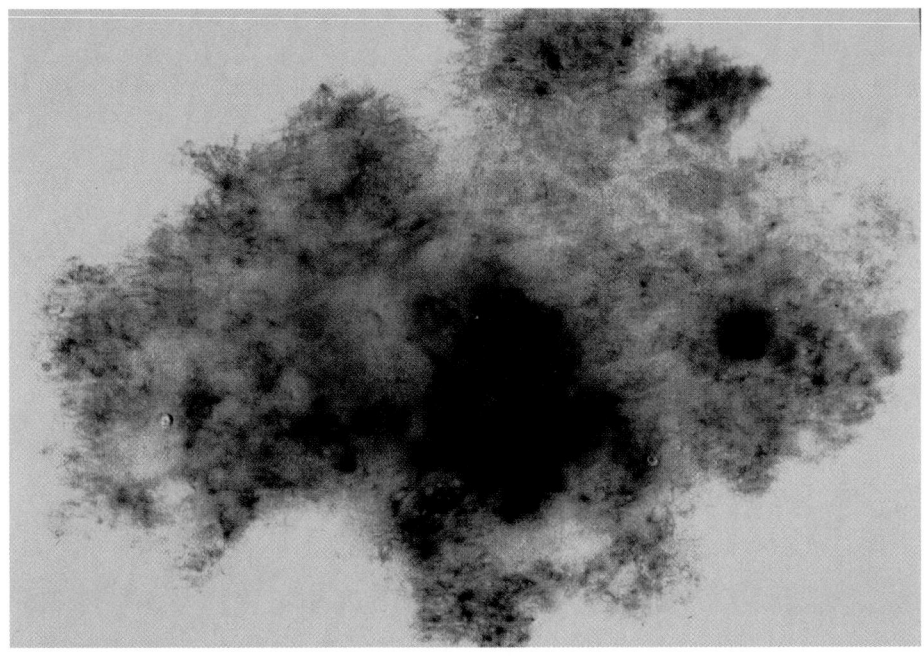

C

Figure 21-2 *Superficial spreading melanoma, 0.45 mm in depth. Mean network irregularity, marked.* (a) *Asymmetric lesion with irregular borders, marked pigment variegation, and dark foci with suggestion of blue color. Maximum diameter 12 mm.* (b, c) *Global features: network pattern [with small nodular focus at 3 o'clock position (b)], peripheral dots [6 o'clock position in enhancement (c)]. Network features: mean network irregularity, marked; peripheral dark patches, marked.* (a) *Digital clinical surface view (with oil), and* (c) *pigment pattern enhancement of epiluminescence microscopic subsurface view.* (Reprinted with permission from RO Kenet et al: Clinical diagnosis of pigmented lesions using digital epiluminescence microscopy: Grading protocol and atlas. *Arch Dermatol* 129:157, 1993.)

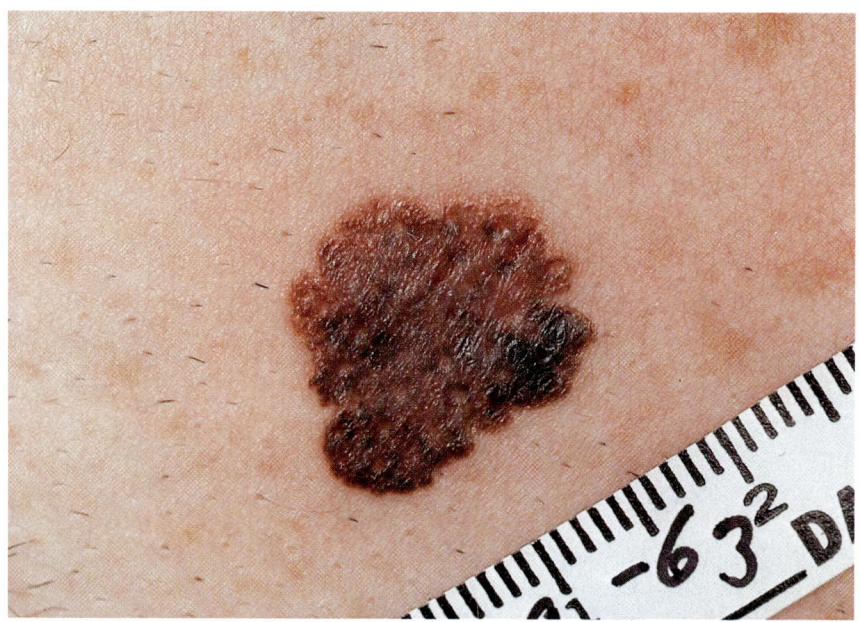

Figure 21-3 *Superficial spreading melanoma, radial growth phase. This lesion is a slightly raised plaque with asymmetry, irregularity of borders, and striking complexity of color. Note the scalloping of the borders.*

tures of the so-called dysplastic nevus. Patients with SSM also may develop multiple primary melanomas, particularly those individuals with a history of familial melanoma.

CLINICAL FEATURES

SSM usually develops as an asymmetric plaque with variation in color and pigment pattern and irregularity or notching of borders (Figs. 21-1 to 21-11). During its period of lateral (radial growth phase) growth, when abnormal melanocytes are confined to the epidermis and upper papillary dermis, the lesion may be flat with minimally elevated borders. This period may last from approximately 1 to 7 years. The coloration of SSM is characterized by varying shades of brown admixed with complex hues of red, blue, gray, white, and black. Frequently, foci of regression may be evident clinically as areas of white, pink, gray, or blue. The mean diameters are usually 0.8 to 1.2 cm, but early lesions may be as small as 0.4 cm and thick lesions may be 4.0 cm or larger. The vertical growth phase is heralded by the presence of an elevated area (papule or nodule) within the radial growth plaque (see Figs. 21-9 to 21-11).

HISTOPATHOLOGIC FEATURES

This form of melanoma is most commonly characterized by a dispersion of epithelioid melanoma cells throughout the epidermis (*pagetoid*) spread) in the radial growth phase. With tumor progression, microinvasion of the papillary dermis oc-

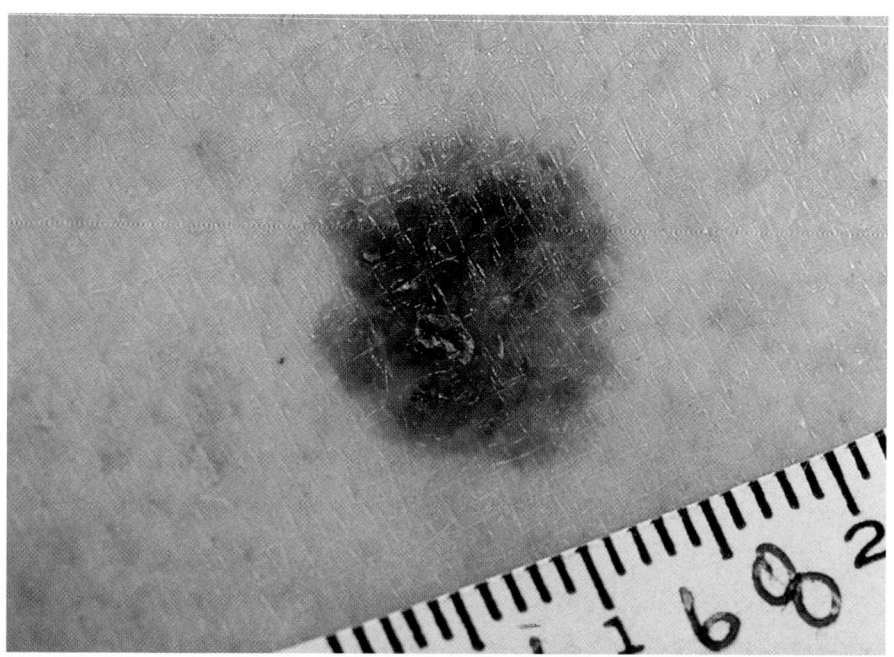

Figure 21-4 *Superficial spreading melanoma, radial growth phase. This melanoma measures approximately 10 mm in diameter and displays asymmetry, slight scalloping of borders, and irregularity of color.*

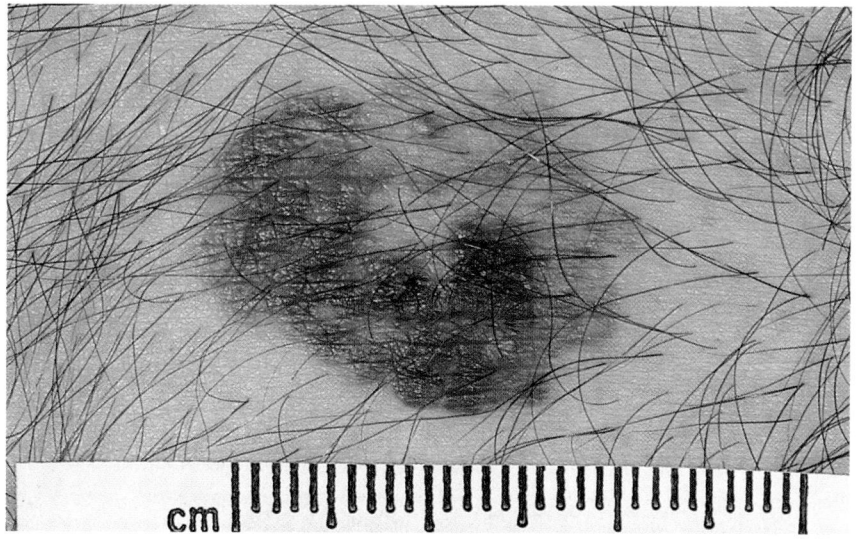

Figure 21-5 *Superficial spreading melanoma, radial growth phase. This lesion is notable for asymmetry, some irregularity of borders, and prominent variegation of color with central hypopigmentation.*

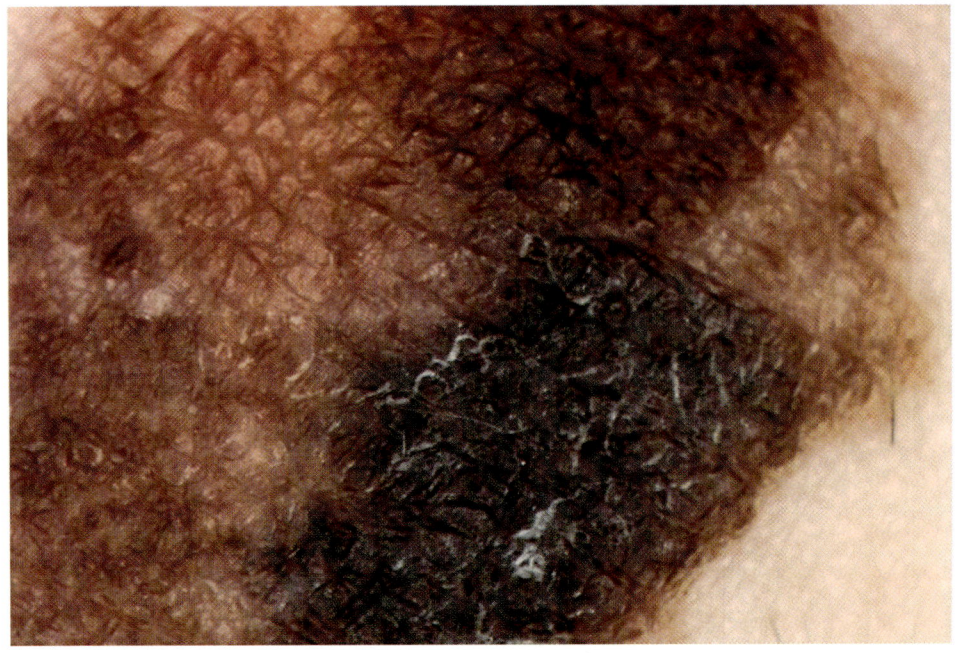

A

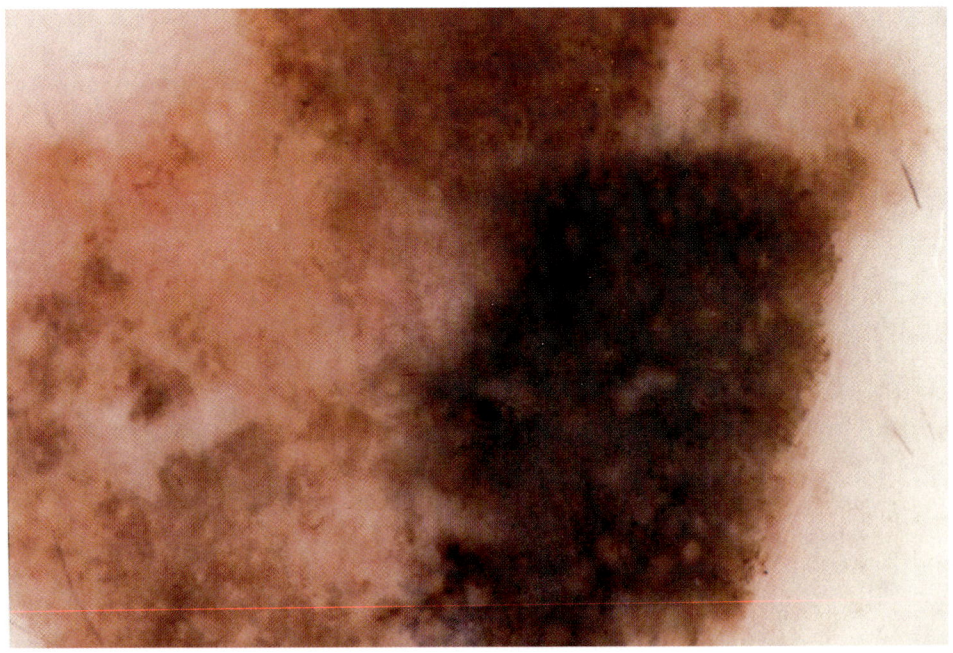

B

Figure 21-6

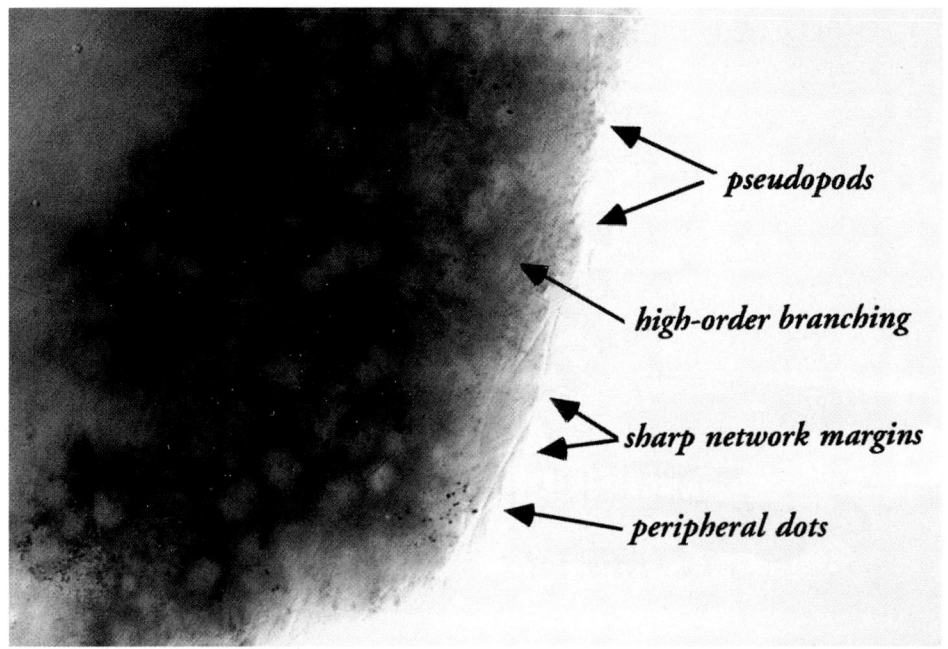

C

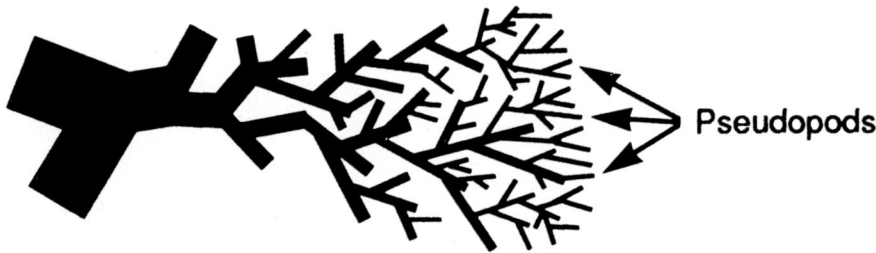

High-Order (Treelike) Branching

D

Figure 21-6 *(cont.)*

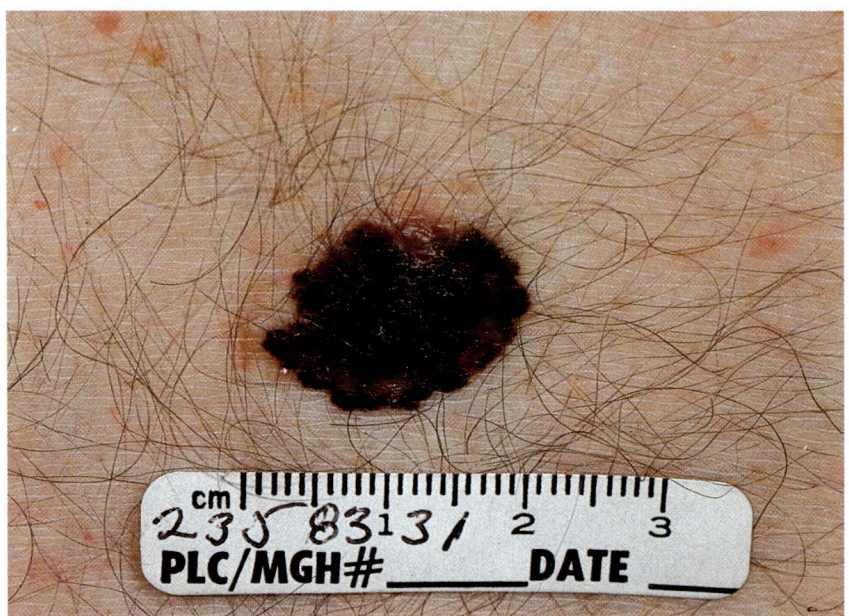

Figure 21-7 *Superficial spreading melanoma, radial growth phase. This lesion exhibits asymmetry, somewhat scalloped borders, and an overall brown-black color.*

Figure 21-6 (See pages 168 and 169) *Superficial spreading melanoma, 0.65 mm depth. Multicomponent pattern. (a) Note dark region with sharp clinical margin. Maximum diameter 2 cm. (b, c) Global features: multicomponent pattern (three or more discrete regions with one dark region with broadened network lines). Local features: pseudopods (arrows), peripheral dots (arrow), whitish veil (milky way)/blue-gray veil [subtle blue haze over dark region (b)], and erythema [upper left quadrant (b)]. Network features: sharp network margins (margin of dark network, arrows), markedly thick and dark network lines (dark region), high-order "tree-like" network branching (d) [e.g., arrow in (c)]. (a) Digital clinical surface view (without oil); (b) digital epiluminescence microscopic subsurface view (with oil); and (c) pigment pattern enhancement of epiluminescence microscopic subsurface view. (Reprinted with permission from RO Kenet et al: Clinical diagnosis of pigmented lesions using digital epiluminescence microscopy: Grading protocol and atlas. Arch Dermatol 129:157, 1993.)*

curs and may eventuate in an expansile plaque or nodule (the vertical growth phase).

DIFFERENTIAL DIAGNOSIS

SSM must be distinguished from clinically atypical (dysplastic) nevi, pigmented basal cell carcinoma, pigmented Bowen's disease (Fig. 21-12), and unusual solar lentigines and seborrheic keratoses. In general, SSM shows an overall greater size and atypicality than atypical nevi (see Table 1-9). The presence of more complexity of color, evidence of regression, and notching or scalloped borders usually favors SSM. In most instances, the size and plaque-like character of SSM allow discrimination of it from basal cell carcinoma. Usually, solar lentigo and seborrheic keratosis tend to be well circumscribed and do not show the complexity of color notable in SSM. Seborrheic keratoses usually are also distinguished by the "waxy, stuck-on" or keratotic surface alteration. However, verrucous forms of SSM may be impossible to diagnose without histopathologic examination.

ADDITIONAL READINGS
(See Chapter 23.)

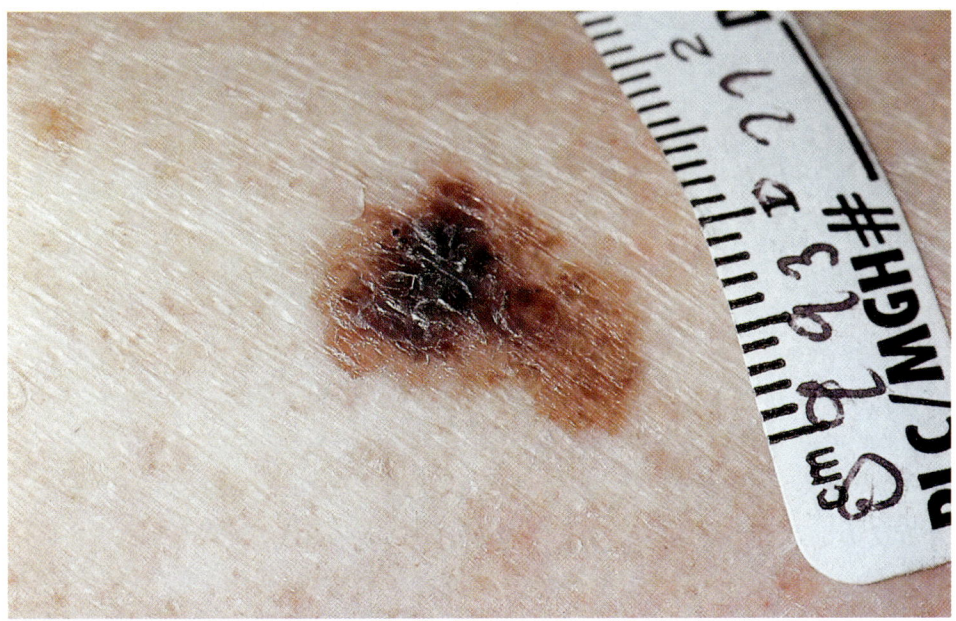

Figure 21-8 *Superficial spreading melanoma, radial growth phase. This lesion is remarkable for asymmetry, slight irregularity of borders, and a central, almost translucent blue-black area.*

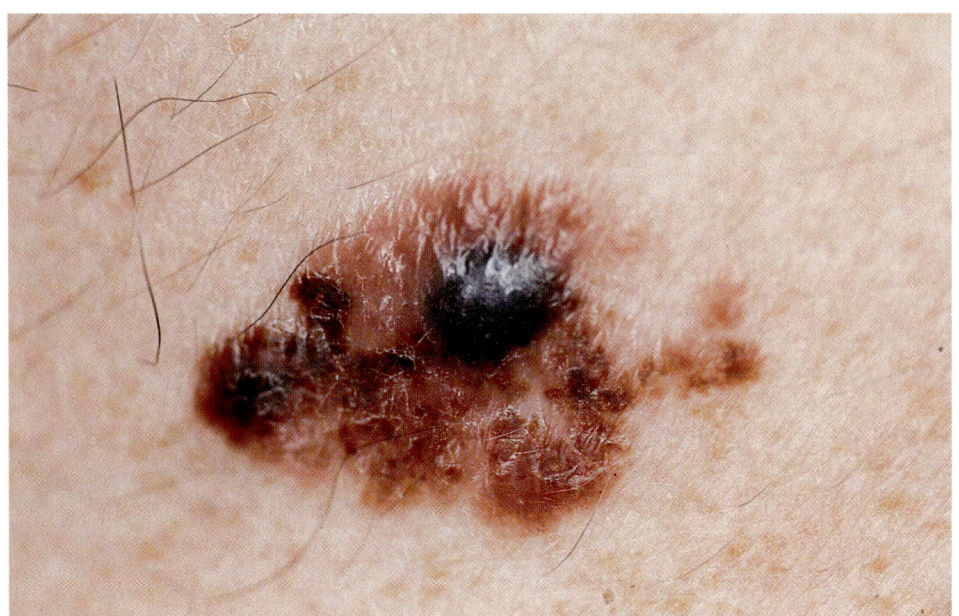

Figure 21-9 *Superficial spreading melanoma with development of the vertical growth phase. This lesion is notable for striking asymmetry, scalloping of borders, variegation of color, and a central, slightly raised blue-black papule. The latter lesion heralds the development of the vertical growth phase.*

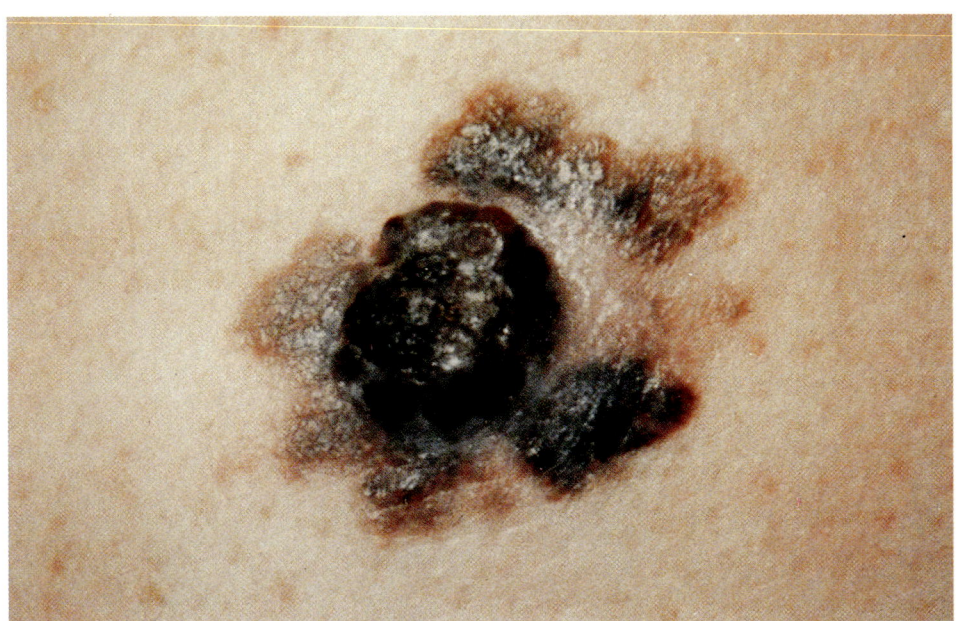

Figure 21-10 *Superficial spreading melanoma, vertical growth phase. In addition to the striking notching of borders and complexity of color, there is a central dome-shaped blue-black nodule with central keratotic surface.* (Courtesy Alfred W. Kopf, M.D., with permission.)

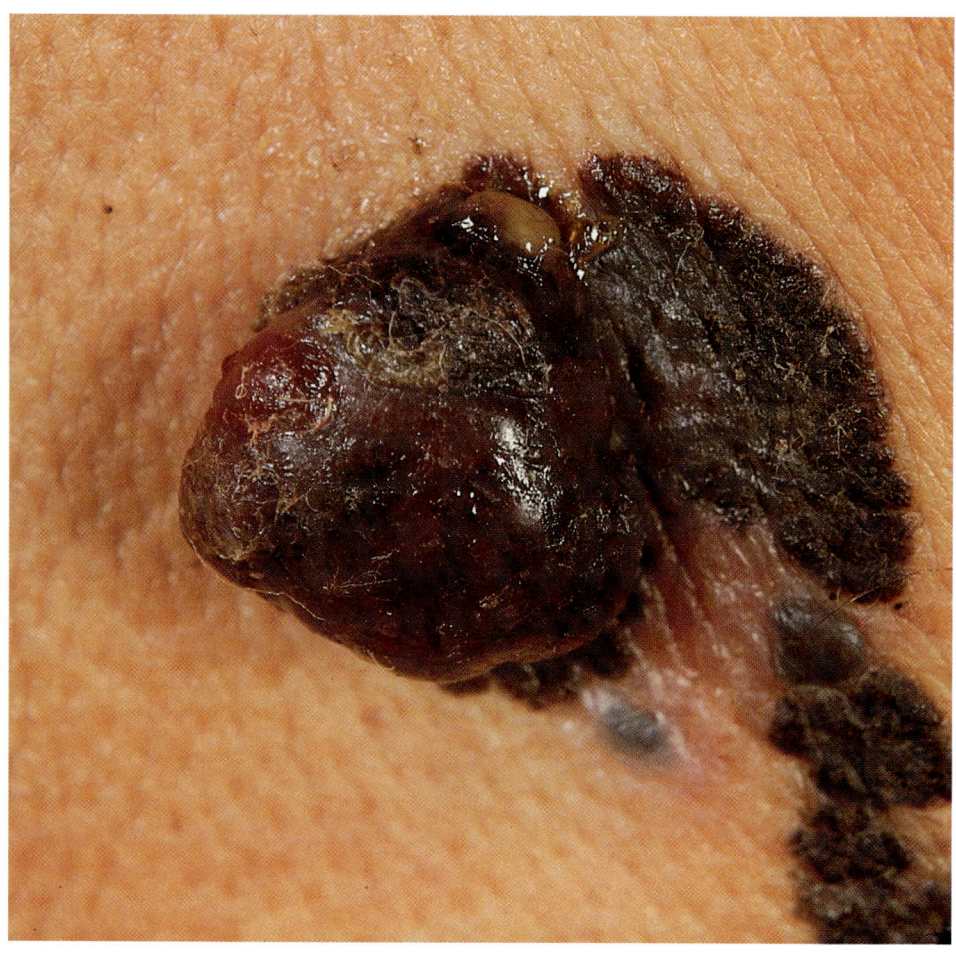

Figure 21-11 *Superficial spreading melanoma, vertical growth phase. The lesion is notable for a large eccentric, ulcerated nodule with colors ranging from pink-brown to blue-black.*

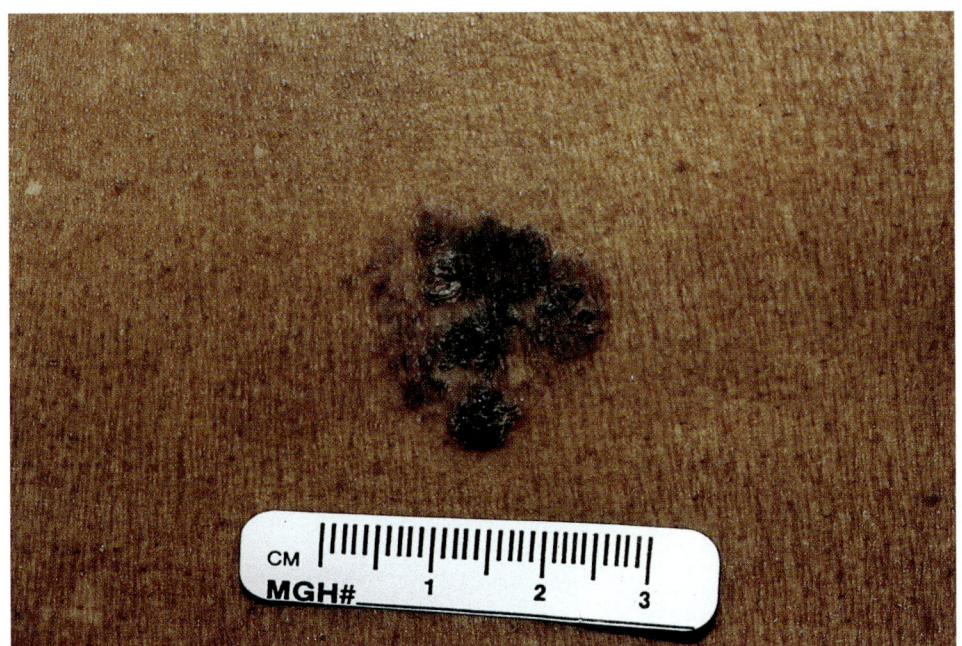

Figure 21-12 *Pigmented Bowen's disease. This lesion, which measures approximately 2.5 cm in diameter, shows strikingly irregular borders and variegation of pigmentation. Also note the scalloping of borders. This lesion was noted on the trunk of an elderly African-American patient and was highly suspicious for melanoma.*

22. Nodular Melanoma

Nodular melanoma (NM) is a primary form of cutaneous melanoma that by definition develops without any residual or detectable radial growth phase. Although NM shares many characteristics in common with superficial spreading melanoma (SSM), NM may develop on any epithelial surface and may represent rapid tumor progression from any intraepidermal component, whether pagetoid or lentiginous.

EPIDEMIOLOGY AND ETIOLOGY

NM occurs with equal incidence in both sexes and is diagnosed at a slightly older age than SSM, i.e., 40 to 50 years. NM is associated with rapid onset, e.g., from 4 months to 2 years, and generally has the same distribution pattern as SSM. Remnants of melanocytic nevi are noted less commonly in association with NM (e.g., 6 percent) than with SSM (42 percent in one series).

CLINICAL FEATURES

NM is a raised papule or nodule which less commonly may be sessile or polypoid (Figs. 22–1 to 22–6). Surface ulceration is frequently present (see Figs. 22-3 and 22-5). Colors range from blue-black to amelanotic (Figs. 22-1 to 22-6). This form of melanoma is notable for well-defined borders and symmetry, in contrast to other melanomas with a radial growth phase. The size ranges from 0.4 to 3.0 cm or larger.

HISTOPATHOLOGIC FEATURES

NM is characterized by a cohesive cellular nodule or plaque expanding the papillary dermis, with elevated polypoid, dome-shaped, or sessile morphology. The tumor is most commonly composed of epithelioid melanoma cells. Although an intraepidermal component may overlie the invasive tumor, this component generally does not extend laterally beyond the dermal nodule. More advanced tumors may invade the reticular dermis and subcutaneous fat.

DIFFERENTIAL DIAGNOSIS

The differential diagnosis includes primarily vascular lesions—pyogenic granuloma, angiokeratoma, the sclerosing hemangioma variant of dermatofibroma, Kaposi's sarcoma, metastatic melanoma, Spitz nevus, pigmented spindle-cell nevus, blue nevus, appendage tumors such as eccrine poroma (Fig. 22–7), and pigmented basal cell carcinoma. The striking symmetry and obvious vascular character of many angiomatous lesions allow for clinical distinction from NM in many instances (Fig. 22-8). However, histopathologic examination is necessary to rule out NM. Distinction of NM from metastatic melanoma may be impossible without detailed clinical information. In many instances cutaneous lesions of metastatic melanoma are smaller than primary NM.

ADDITIONAL READINGS
(See Chapter 23.)

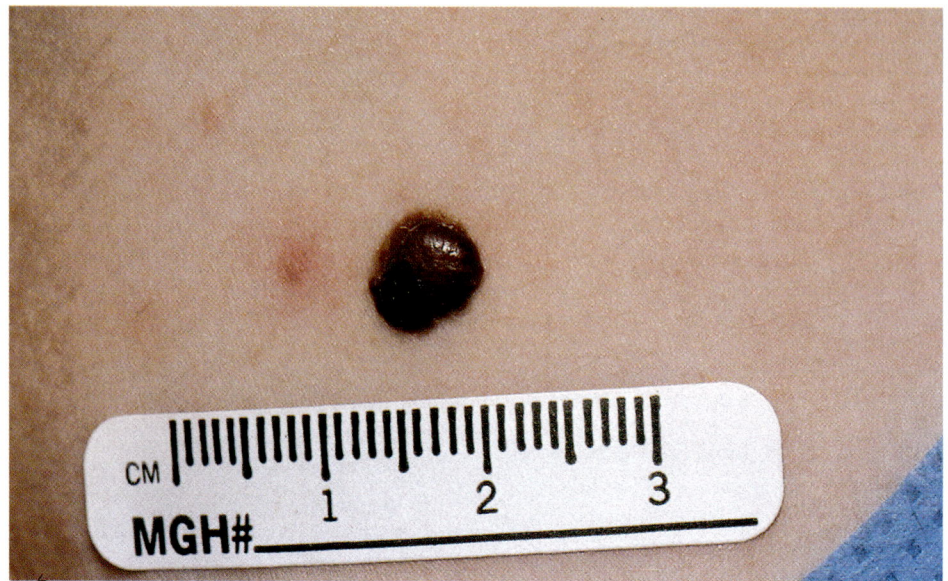

Figure 22-1 *Small nodular melanoma. This melanoma measures approximately 8 mm in greatest diameter and exhibits a reddish-brown to dark brown color.*

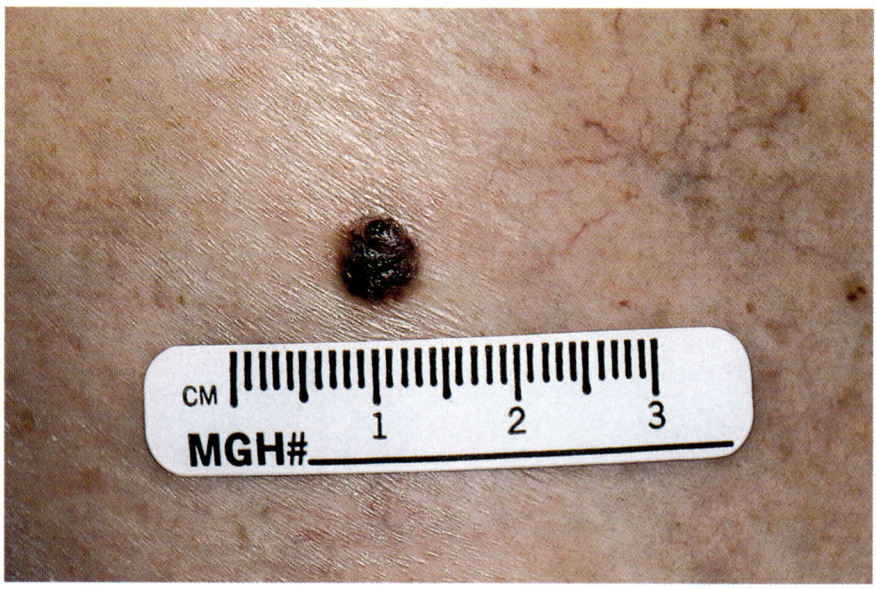

Figure 22-2 *Small nodular melanoma. This lesion is well defined and fairly symmetric but shows prominent variation in the pigmentary pattern.*

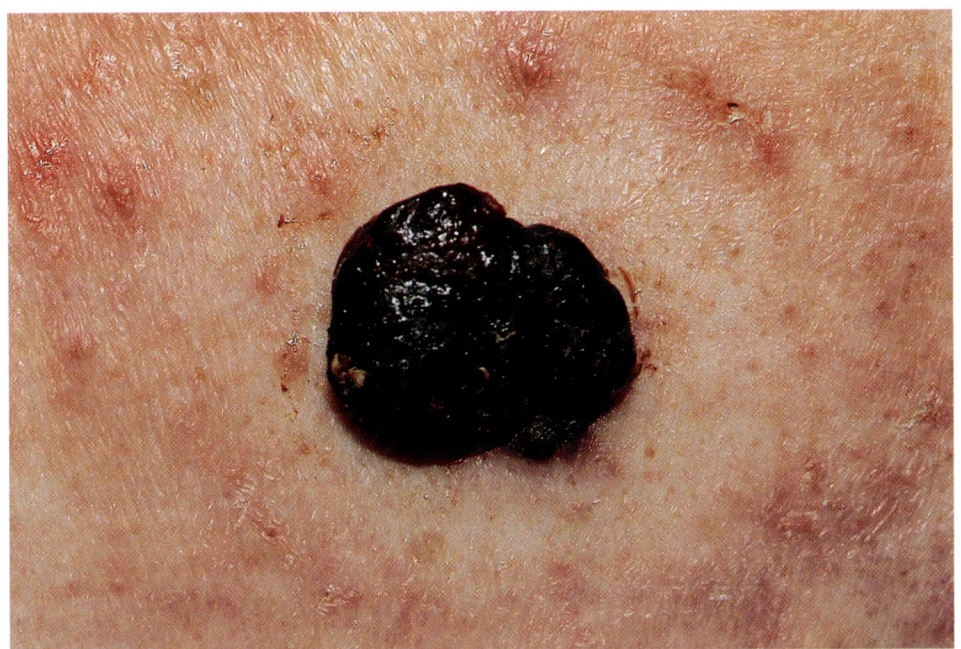

Figure 22-3 *Nodular melanoma. This melanoma is well defined but exhibits asymmetry, a pedunculated configuration, and black color. The surface is ulcerated with a hemorrhagic eschar.*

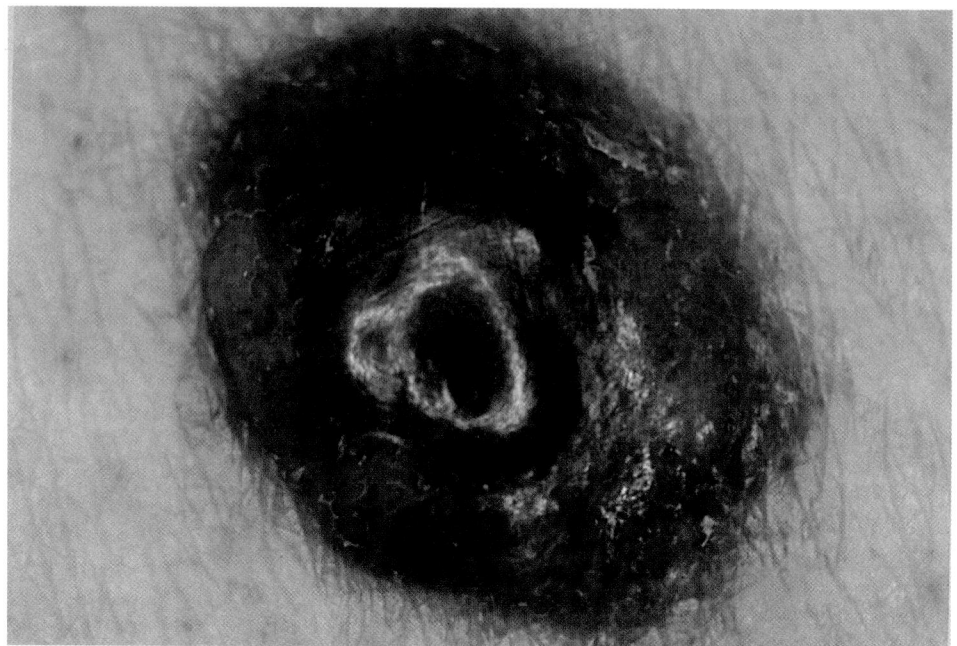

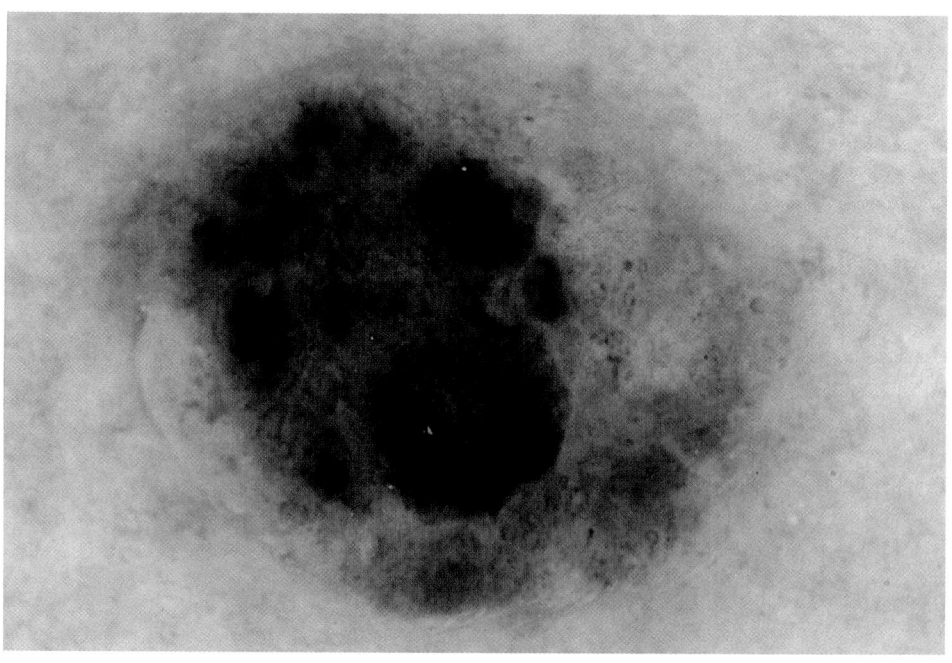

Figure 22-4

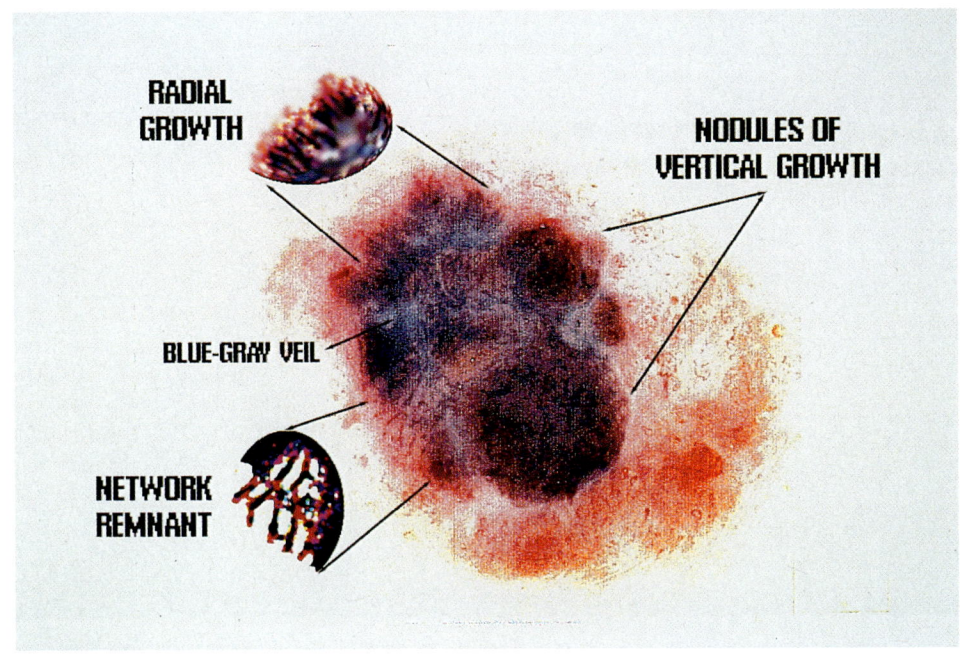

c

Figure 22-4 Nodular melanoma, 2.92 mm depth. Nodular pattern. Note elevated nodules with obliteration of skin markings. Maximum diameter 11 mm. (b, c) Global features: nodular pattern (multiple, irregular regions of dense pigment concentration that correspond to raised areas in the clinical surface view) and remnant of obliterated network pattern (arrow). Local features: whitish veil (milky way)/blue-gray veil (b), telangiectasia [3 o'clock position (b)], radial streaming [arrow (c)]. (a) Digital clinical surface view (without oil); (b) digital epiluminescence microscopic subsurface view (with oil); and (c) pigment pattern enhancement of epiluminescence microscopic subsurface view. (c) (Digital enhancement of subsurface morphology): Computer enhancement with diagramatic inserts demonstrates three important clinical histomorphologic features. (i) Remnant of pigment network which demonstrates that this lesion has a very high probability of being melanocytic (rather than a nonmelanocytic lesion mimicking melanoma), (ii) subtle features of the radial growth phase of melanoma, i.e., subtle linear projections at the periphery often called radial streaming, and (iii) large, dark nodules that are raised in the clinical view (a), with irregular borders, that appear to be virtually obliterating the pigment network. (Reprinted with permission from RO Kenet et al: Clinical diagnosis of pigmented lesions using digital epiluminescence microscopy: Grading protocol and atlas. *Arch Dermatol* 129:157, 1993.)

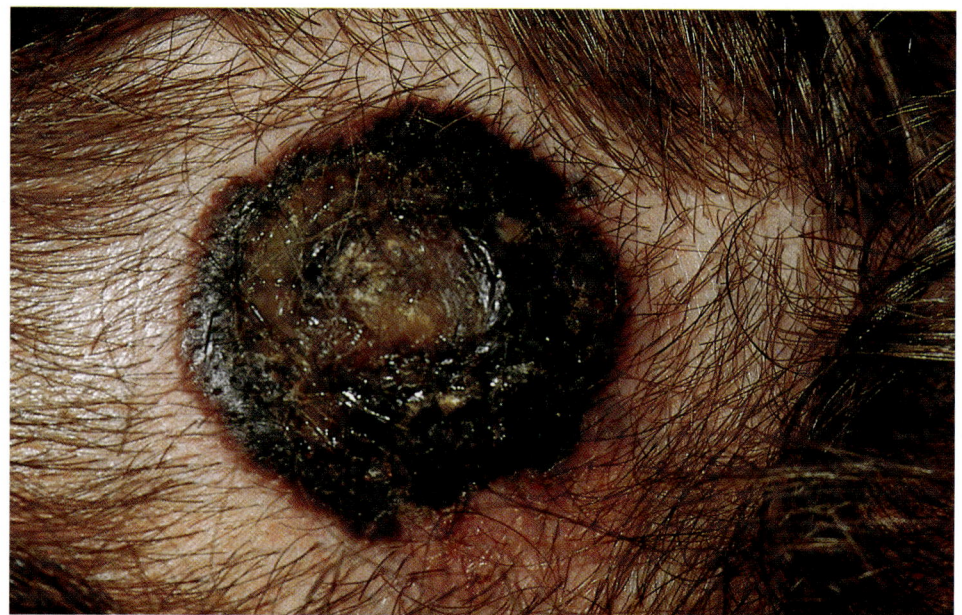

Figure 22-5 *Nodular melanoma. This melanoma from the scalp is remarkable for a dome-shaped morphology, almost uniformly black color, and central ulceration.*

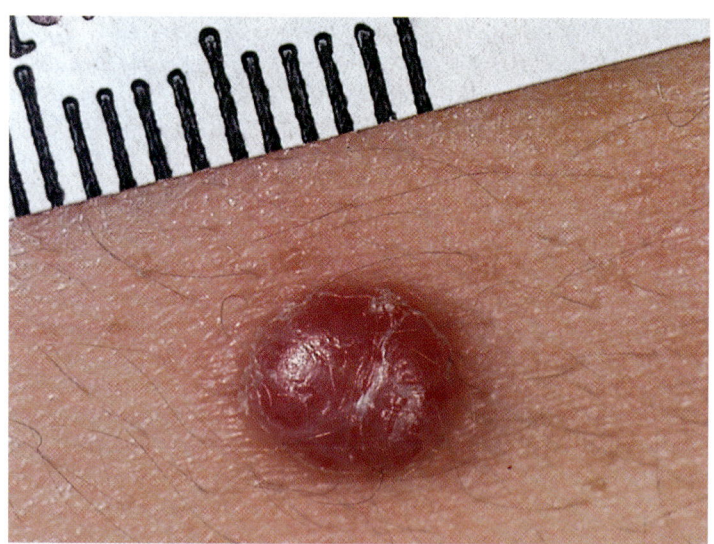

Figure 22-6 *Nodular melanoma, amelanotic type. This melanoma has a dusky red color. Because of the complete absence of pigmentation, these lesions are exceedingly difficult to diagnose clinically.*

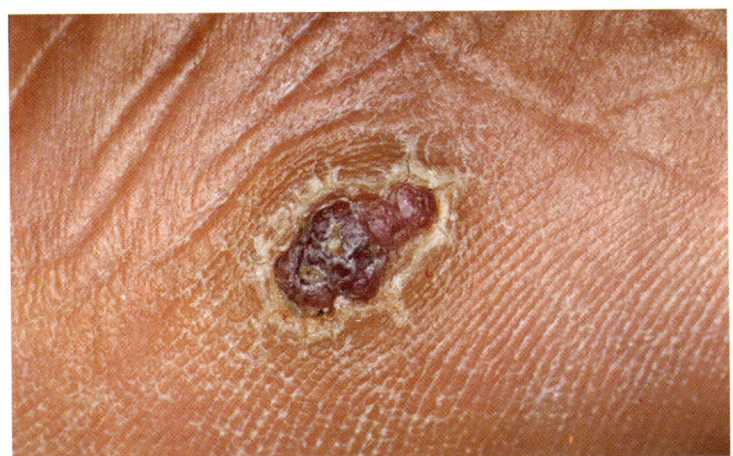

Figure 22-7 *Eccrine poroma. This well-demarcated nodule on the sole is suspicious for nodular melanoma. The lesion is notable for a reddish-blue translucent color and is indistinguishable from amelanotic nodular melanoma.* (From TB Fitzpatrick et al (eds): *Dermatology in General Medicine,* 4th ed. New York, McGraw-Hill, 1993, p 878, with permission.)

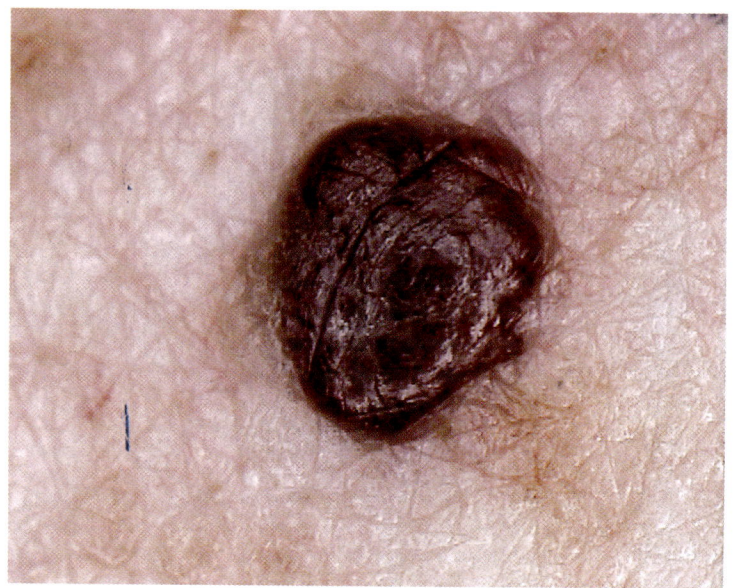

A

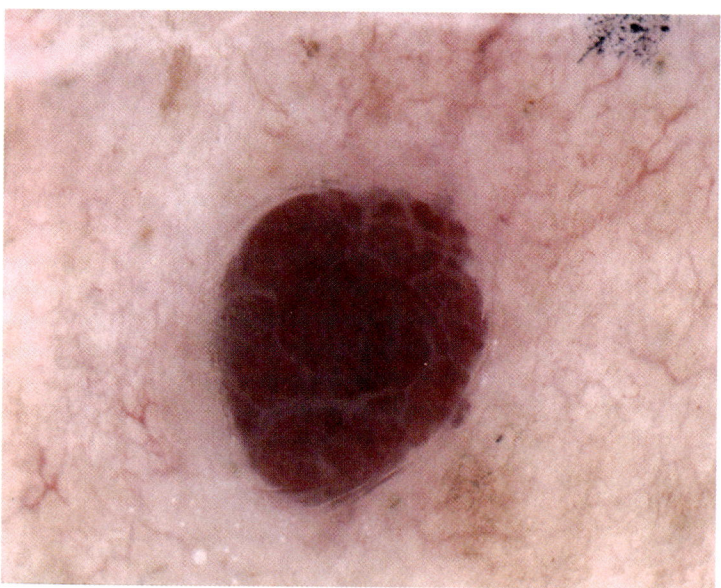

B

Figure 22-8

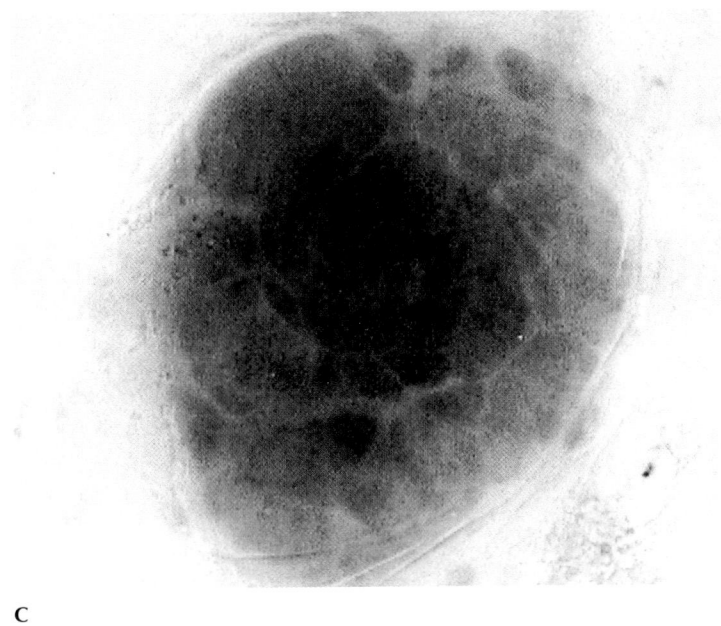

c

Figure 22-8 *Hemangioma. (a) Red elevated lesion that is relatively symmetric and with smooth borders. (b) No brown pigment is visible, just a typical "saccular pattern" consisting of a cluster of smooth bordered red sacs. (c) Enhancement helps confirm that there is no region with a pigment network remnant as in Figure 22-4, thus confirming that this is a nonmelanocytic lesion.*

23. Acral Lentiginous Melanoma

Acral lentiginous melanoma (ALM) is an uncommon form of melanoma in Caucasian populations but is the most common type of melanoma in Asian and black populations. ALM involves the palms, soles, and nail apparatus of digits as well as mucosae.

Synonyms: palmar-plantar-subungual-mucosal melanoma, lentigo maligna melanoma of the sole

EPIDEMIOLOGY AND ETIOLOGY

Men are affected more commonly than women (ratio 3:1), and ALM is generally diagnosed at a late stage in older individuals, e.g., 60 to 65 years of age. While melanoma is less common in black and Asian populations (about 1/7 to 1/20 the incidence in white populations), ALM accounts for about 50 to 70 percent of the melanomas in these races. The duration before diagnosis is difficult to ascertain but ranges from 1 to 10 years.

Little is known concerning the etiology of ALM. Sunlight would seem to have little, if any, role in its pathogenesis compared with other types of melanoma. Lentiginous precursor lesions (particularly in African blacks) have been implicated in the development of ALM. Although frequently mentioned, there is no convincing evidence that trauma is an important risk factor for ALM.

CLINICAL FEATURES

The coloration is less varied than that seen with SSM; in flat areas, dark brown predominates with blue and black (Fig. 23-1). In raised areas (plaques), brown-black or blue-black predominates. Depigmented and gray areas indicative of regression are also noted (Figs. 23-2 and 23-3). Borders may show marked irregularity and notching (use of the Wood's lamp is necessary to determine the full extent of the borders). The size ranges from 0.9 to 12.0 cm or greater. Advanced tumors exhibit raised papules or nodules that are blue, black, or amelanotic and often ulcerated (Figs. 23-4 to 23-6).

Subungual melanoma and melanomas involving the nail apparatus (periungual sites) most often involve the thumb or great toe. Pigmented longitudinal bands >0.6 cm in width are suspicious for melanoma (Table 23-1 and Fig. 23-7). Often the entire nail is pigmented, and there may be color variation, nail deformity, shedding, and focal ulceration (Figs. 23-8 and 23-9). Extension of pigmentation onto the periungual skin is termed *Hutchinson's sign* and should raise suspicion for subungual melanoma (see Figs. 23-7 and 23-8).

HISTOPATHOLOGIC FEATURES

The radial growth phase is notable for a lentiginous proliferation of often highly pleomorphic melanocytes within a hyperplastic epidermis. The invasive tumor

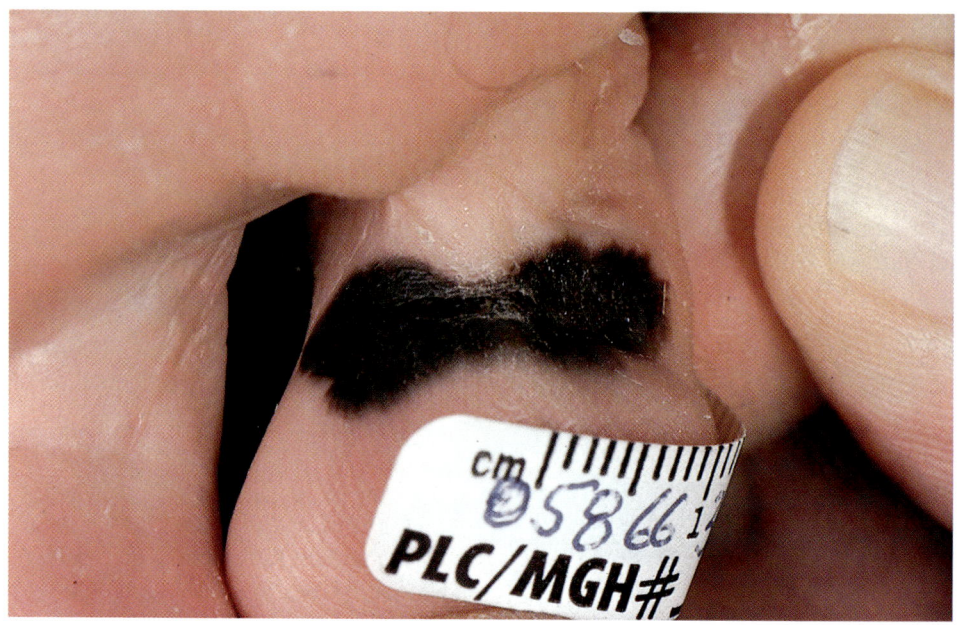

Figure 23-1 *Acral lentiginous melanoma, radial growth phase. This interdigital lesion is entirely macular and remarkable for a jet-black color. Note the irregularity and notching of the borders.*

most commonly contains spindle cells and, as with other lentiginous melanomas, may exhibit desmoplasia and neurotropism.

DIFFERENTIAL DIAGNOSIS

ALM must be distinguished from melanocytic nevi and lentiginous proliferations on acral skin, verrucae, vascular lesions (pyogenic granuloma, Kaposi's sarcoma), trauma-related hemorrhage (talon noir), and appendage tumors such as eccrine poroma. ALM tends to show larger size (>0.6 cm), greater irregularity of borders, and greater complexity of color than do benign melanocytic lesions. Ulcerated, nodular, and amelanotic lesions generally require biopsy for diagnosis.

Subungual melanomas may be confused with lentigines and nevi of the nail bed, trauma-related hemorrhage (very common) or dystrophy, verrucae, squamous cell carcinoma, pyogenic granuloma, and fungal infection. Melanonychia striata (pigmented bands) involving the nail bed are often multiple, present in persons of color, have uniform color, and are <0.6 cm in width. Biopsy is essential to rule out melanoma.

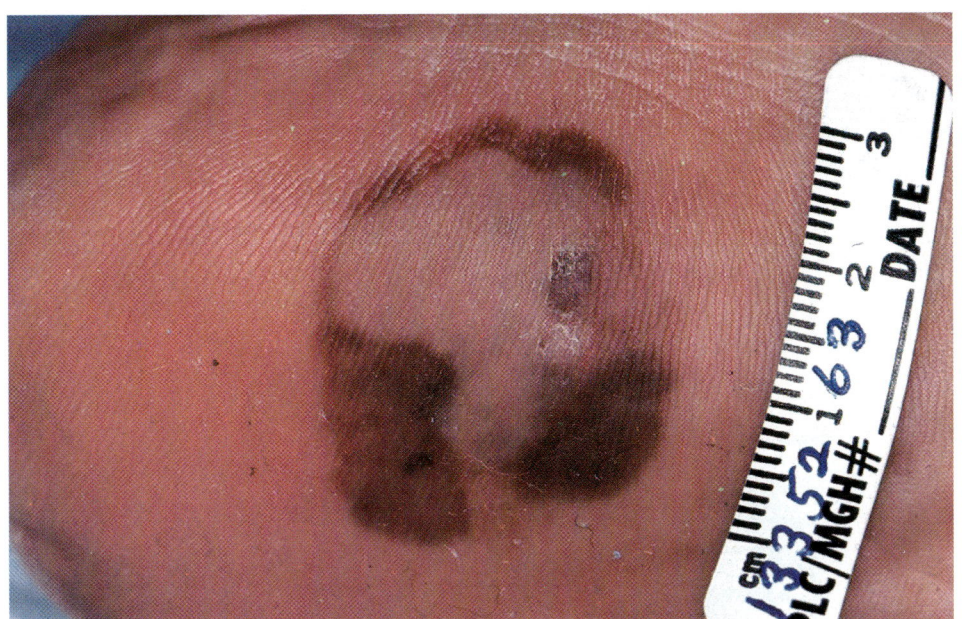

Figure 23-2 *Acral lentiginous melanoma, radial growth phase. The lesion is almost completely macular and exhibits marked irregularity of color. A large, confluent central area has a bluish-gray appearance, possibly indicating regression.* (From TB Fitzpatrick et al (eds.): *Dermatology in General Medicine*, 4th ed. New York, McGraw-Hill, 1993, p 1095, with permission.)

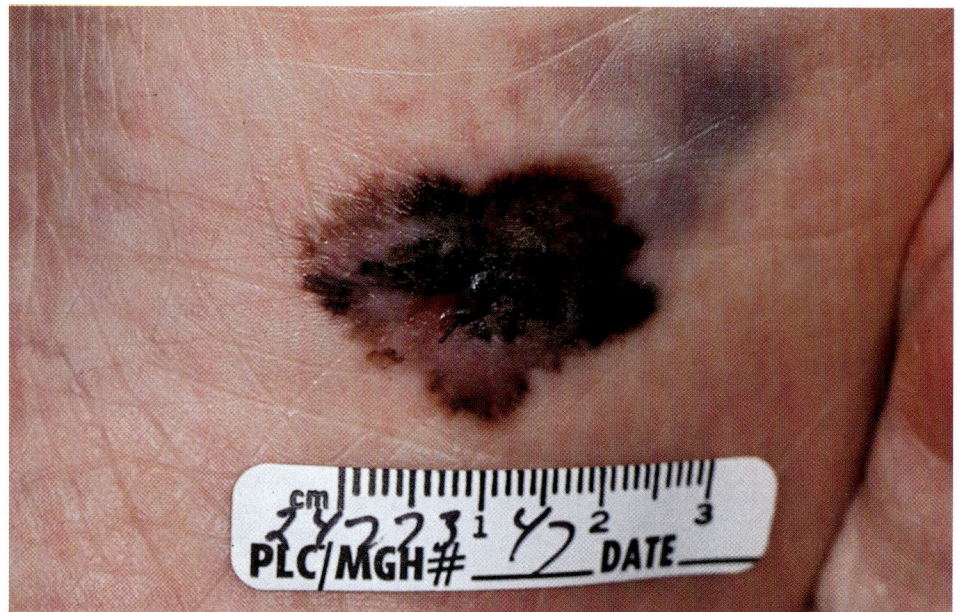

Figure 23-3 *Acral lentiginous melanoma. This melanoma exhibits prominent asymmetry, notching of borders, and complex variation in color. The areas of gray, blue, and pink indicate the presence of regression.*

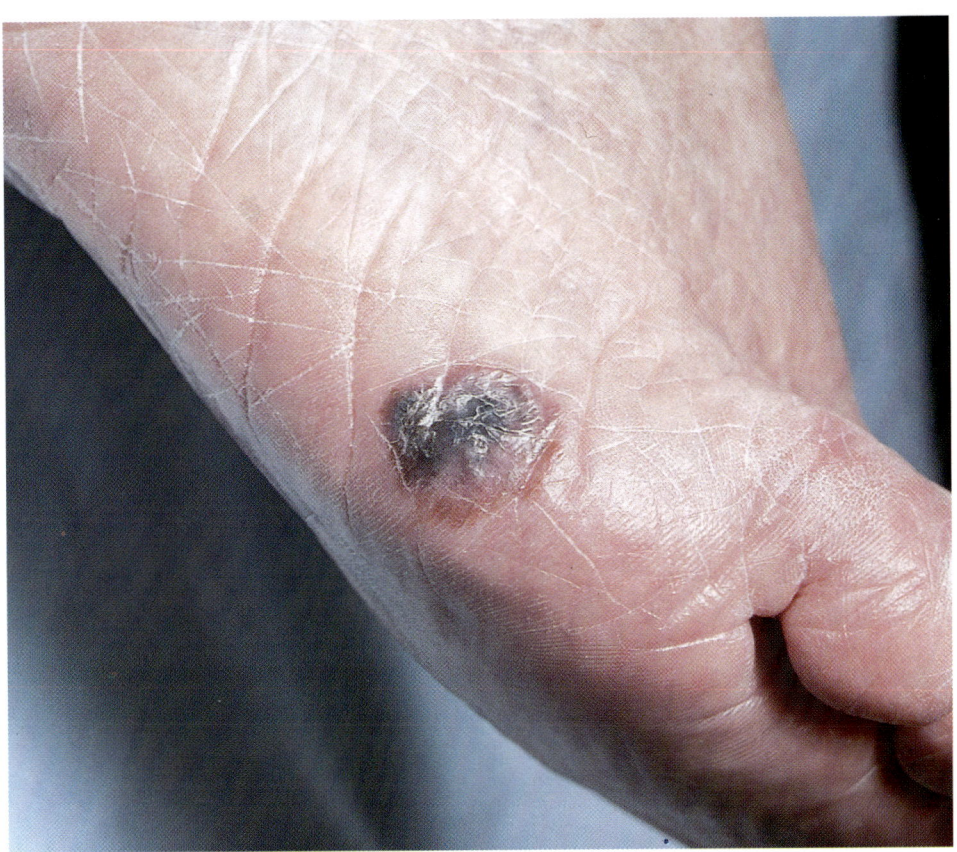

Figure 23-4 *Acral lentiginous melanoma. This well-circumscribed melanoma on the lateral aspect of the foot has a somewhat translucent appearance with the colors pink, gray, and blue.*

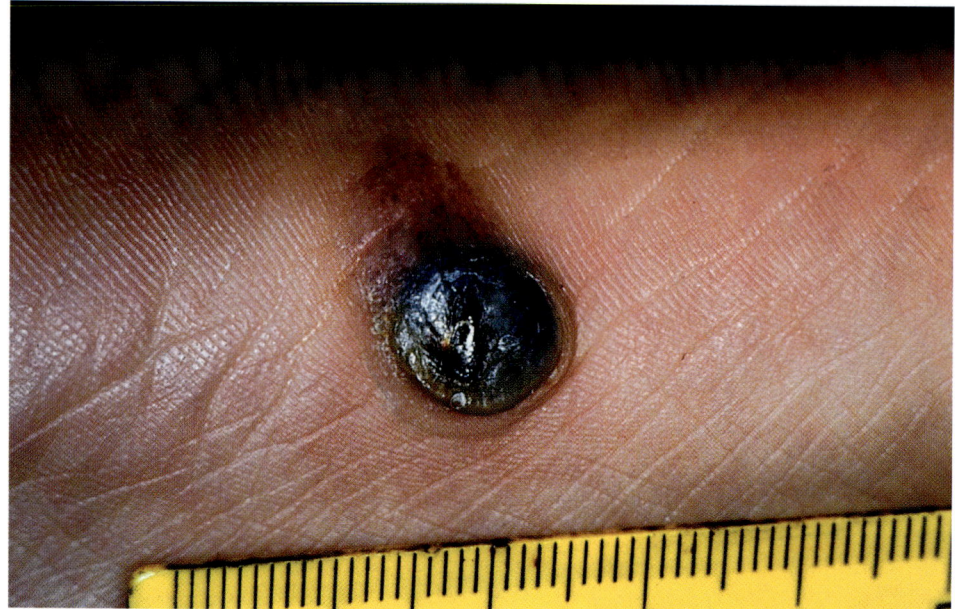

Figure 23-5 *Acral lentiginous melanoma, vertical growth phase. The presence of an eccentric blue-black nodule superimposed on a relatively flat brown area is consistent with the development of a vertical growth phase component.*

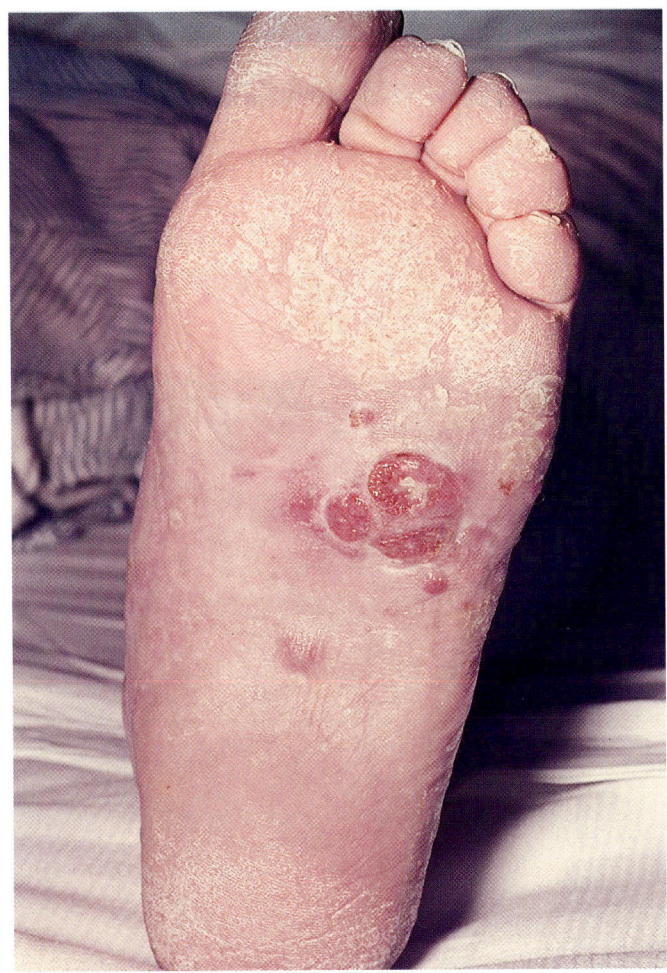

Figure 23-6 *Acral lentiginous melanoma, amelanotic type. The central nodular lesion on the sole is notable for three ulcerated nodular components. The surrounding skin shows smaller papules consistent with satellite lesions.*

Table 23-1 Clinical Features Suggesting Early Subungual Melanoma

Development of melanonychia striata in adulthood
Pigmented band >6 mm in width or involving entire nail plate
Variation in pigmented band
Hutchinson's sign (pigmentation of periungual skin)
Any degree of nail deformity

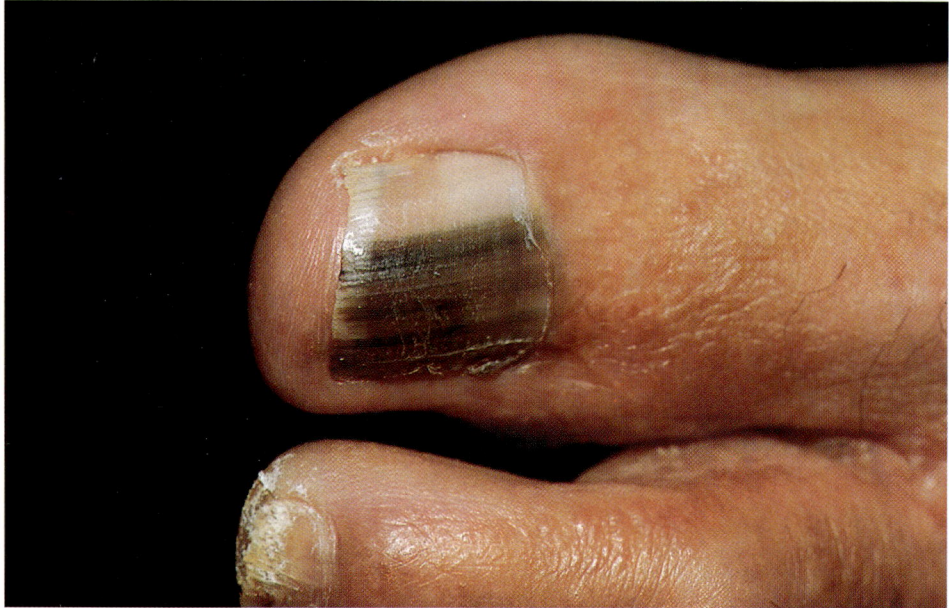

Figure 23-7 *Melanonychia striata. This toenail displays a broad, variegated pigmented band. The colors within this band vary from light brown to black. The lesion is also notable for the spread of pigmentation onto the immediately adjacent periungual skin (Hutchinson's sign). Biopsy of this lesion revealed an atypical lentiginous melanocytic proliferation, consistent with early acral lentiginous melanoma in situ.*

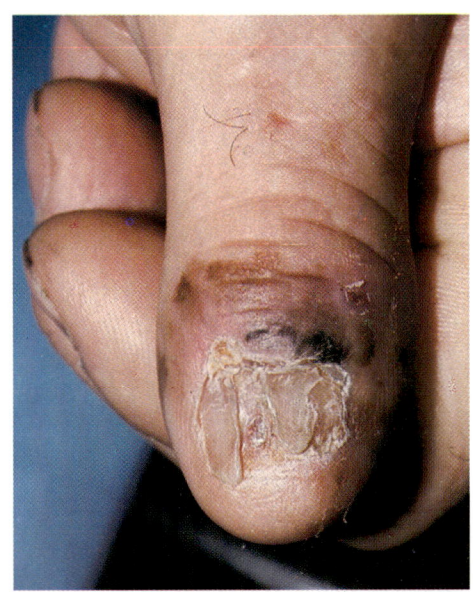

Figure 23-8 *Subungual melanoma with extensive involvement of periungual skin (Hutchinson's sign). There is dystrophy and loss of the nail plate secondary to the tumor.* (From TB Fitzpatrick et al (eds): *Dermatology in General Medicine,* 4th ed. New York, McGraw-Hill, 1993, p 1095, with permission.)

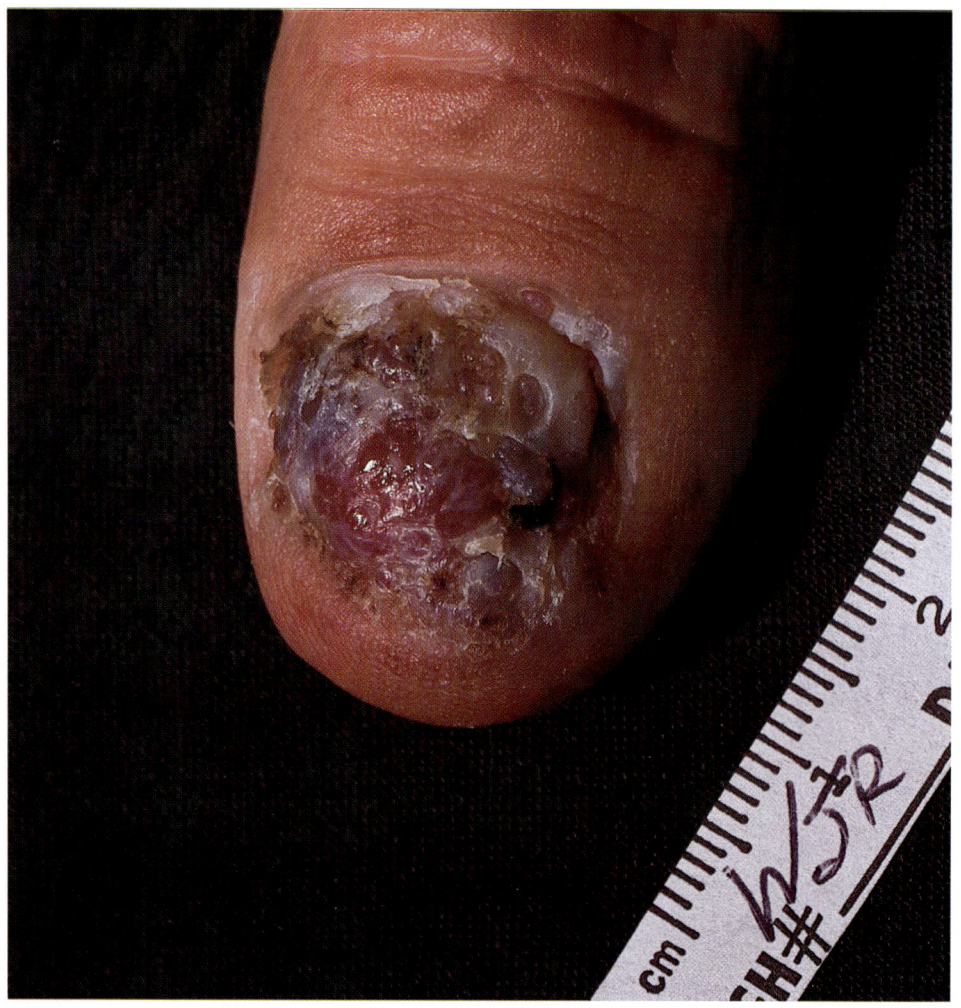

Figure 23-9 *Subungual melanoma, advanced stage. The nail has been shed, and there is an ulcerated tumor occupying the nail bed. The melanoma is remarkable for an ulcerated surface and highly irregular coloration.*

ADDITIONAL READINGS

Ackerman AB: Malignant melanoma: A unifying concept. *Human Pathol* **71**:591, 1980.

Barnhill RL, Mihm MC Jr: The histopathology of cutaneous malignant melanoma. *Semin Diagnost Pathol* **10**:47, 1993.

Clark WH Jr. et al: Model predicting survival in stage I melanoma based on tumor progression. *J Natl Cancer Inst* **81**:1893, 1989

Clark WH Jr. et al: The histogenesis and biologic behavior of primary human malignant melanomas of the skin. *Cancer Res* **29**:705, 1969

Gruber SB et al: Nevomelanocytic proliferations in association with cutaneous malignant melanoma: A multivariate analysis. *J Am Acad Dermatol* **21**:773, 1989

Ho VC, Sober AJ: Therapy for cutaneous melanoma: An update. *J Am Acad Dermatol* **22**:159, 1990

Holman CDJ et al: Relationship of cutaneous malignant melanoma to individual sunlight-exposure habits. *J Natl Cancer Inst* **76**:403, 1986

Koh HK: Cutaneous melanoma. *N Engl J Med* **325**:171, 1991

Koh HK et al: Lentigo maligna melanoma has no better prognosis than other types of melanoma. *J Clin Oncol* **2**:994, 1984

MacKie RM et al: Personal risk-factor chart for cutaneous melanoma. *Lancet* **2**:487, 1989

Mihm MC Jr et al: The clinical diagnosis, classification and histogenetic concepts of the early stages of cutaneous malignant melanomas. *N Engl J Med* **284**:1078, 1971

National Cancer Institute: *Cancer Statistics Review 1973–1987* (NIH Publication No. 90-2789). Bethesda, Md, Department of Health and Human Services, 1990

Rhodes AR et al: Risk factors for cutaneous melanoma. *JAMA* **258**:3146, 1987

Saida T et al: Clinical guidelines for the early detection of plantar malignant melanoma. *J Am Acad Dermatol* **23**:37, 1990

Saida T, Ohshima Y: Clinical and histopathologic characteristics of early lesions of subungual malignant melanoma. *Cancer* **63**:556, 1989

Sober AJ et al: Early recognition of cutaneous melanoma. *JAMA* **242**:2795, 1979

24. Desmoplastic Melanoma

This is an uncommon variant of melanoma primarily defined histologically by a desmoplastic stromal response and usually presenting as a firm nodule in sun-damaged skin.
Synonyms: desmoplastic-neurotropic melanoma

EPIDEMIOLOGY

Desmoplastic melanoma is uncommon, as judged by the number of cases reported thus far in the English-language literature (<400 cases). The tumor most commonly arises in elderly individuals (average age 60 years) and in association with lentigo maligna melanoma.

ETIOLOGY

The tumor is believed to result from collagen synthesis by functionally altered melanocytes in the connective-tissue stroma.

CLINICAL FEATURES

The tumor often presents as an indurated papule, nodule, or plaque on sun-exposed skin with or without pigmentation; it is often skin-colored (Figs. 24-1 to 24-4). Its size ranges from <1 to ≥2 cm in greatest diameter. If lentigo maligna is present, it is as an associated macular, hyperpigmented lesion that usually displays irregular borders and a variegated pigment pattern (see Fig 24-3) (see also Chap. 20). Desmoplastic melanoma is often first diagnosed as a recurrent lesion because of failure to recognize the tumor at its initial presentation and because firm nodules recurring at the site of previous surgery are a common manifestation of desmoplastic melanoma.

HISTOPATHOLOGIC FEATURES

The tumor is characterized by a fibrous nodule occupying the dermis and often extending into subcutaneous fat. Its constituent cells are pleomorphic spindle cells disposed singly or in organized fascicles. In most instances, the cells do not contain melanin. The tumor frequently also exhibits neural differentiation or neurotropism (infiltration of preexisting nerve structures) or both. Examination of the epidermis, particularly in initially presenting tumors, often will reveal lentigo maligna.

DIFFERENTIAL DIAGNOSIS

If pigmentation is present, the differential diagnosis may include clinically atypical (dysplastic) nevi, blue nevus, desmoplastic or sclerosing forms of Spitz nevus, solar lentigo, and seborrheic keratosis. Because desmoplastic melanoma occurs commonly in association with lentigo maligna, the clinical features of lentigo maligna may facilitate recognition of desmoplastic melanoma (see Chap. 20). If no pigmentation is present, clinical diagnosis

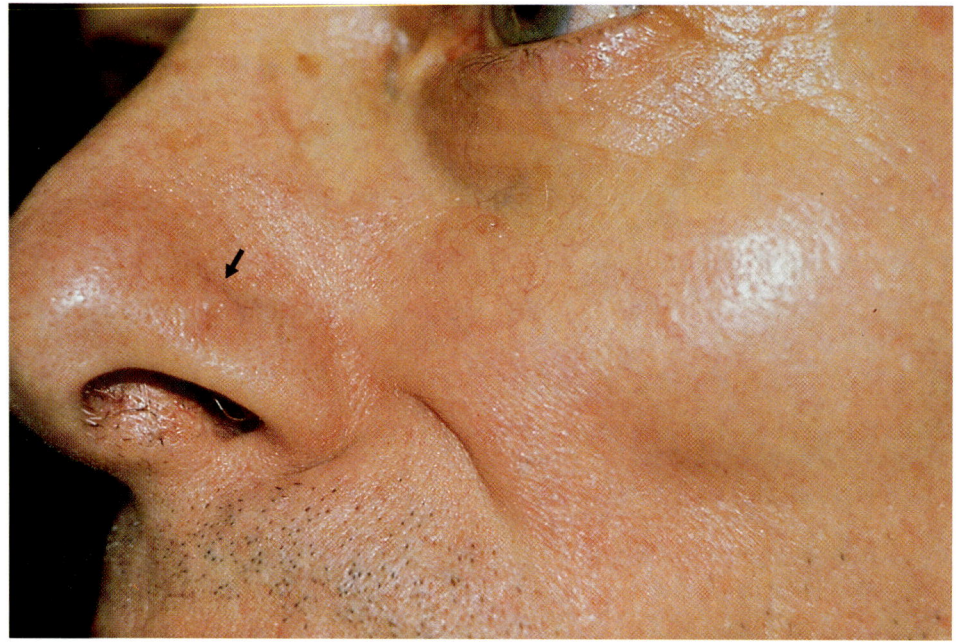

Figure 24-1 *Desmoplastic melanoma. The lesion is a relatively small, flesh-colored papule located on the midportion of the distal nose. This tumor exemplifies the great difficulty in diagnosing many desmoplastic melanomas. Fortunately, this tumor was rather early in its development, which would probably result in a favorable prognosis.*

is exceedingly difficult and must rely on a high index of suspicion. Any persistent indurated papule, nodule, or plaque on sun-exposed skin should be evaluated for biopsy. Desmoplastic melanoma might be confused with a wide variety of lesions, such as scar, keloid, dermatofibroma, fibromatosis, amelanotic blue nevus, desmoplastic Spitz nevus, and many other flesh-colored tumors. Biopsy is necessary for establishing a diagnosis.

BIOLOGIC COURSE

Desmoplastic melanoma and its closely related variant, neurotropic melanoma, are usually thick lesions at diagnosis, often reaching 4 to 5 mm or greater in Breslow depth and anatomic level IV or V. Because of the thickness of desmoplastic melanoma at presentation, the frequent initial failure to diagnose the tumor, and inadequate excision, these tumors recur at a high rate (generally reported in the vicinity of 50 percent and ranging from 25 to 82 percent of cases). Tumors with prominent neurotropism are prone to the highest rates of recurrence. Neurotropic tumors often infiltrate cranial nerves and may extend into the central nervous system. Desmoplastic melanoma is thus often associated with multiple recurrences that may eventuate in distant metastases.

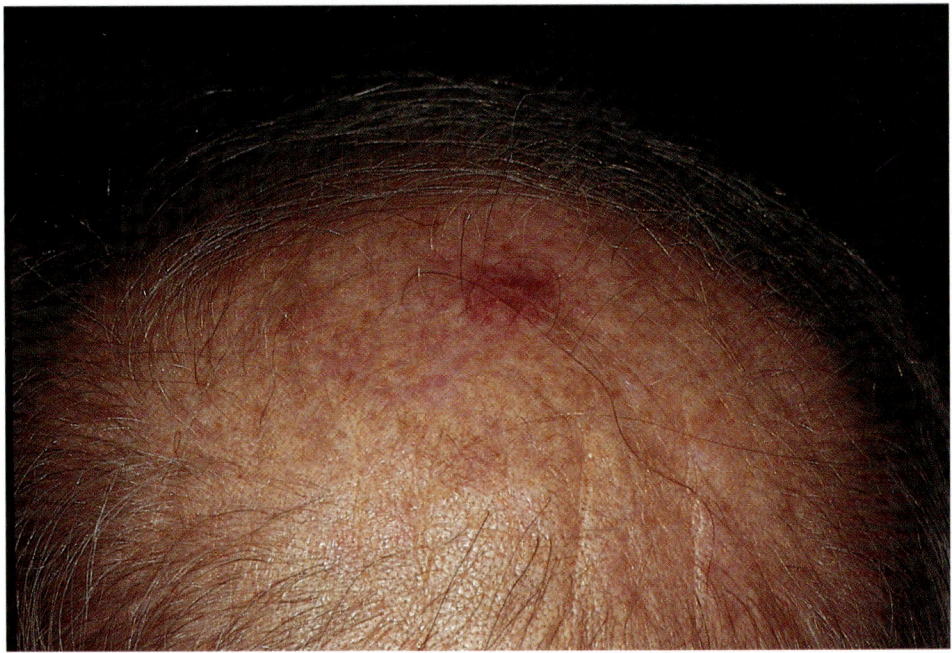

Figure 24-2 *Desmoplastic melanoma. This elderly patient presented with a raised, firm, but ill-defined nodule involving the vertex of the scalp. There was some associated subtle pigmentation overlying this nodule.*

Regional lymph node metastases are probably less common than in conventional melanoma. Overall, the rates of distant metastases and survival have not been clearly established because of the rarity of the tumor and the lack of long-term follow-up in sufficient numbers of patients. It is possible that desmoplastic melanoma has a more indolent course than conventional melanomas.

MANAGEMENT

As with other forms of melanoma, diagnosis as early as possible affords the best chance for adequate surgery and control of the disease. Unusual fibrous tumors in sun-exposed skin should always be suspect for desmoplastic melanoma. Such tumors should be evaluated by immunohistochemistry and possibly by electron microscopy and, if necessary, reviewed by a reference pathologist. Initial surgery is aimed at complete removal for diagnosis. Definitive surgery for thick desmoplastic melanomas should include margins of 2 to 3 cm. It is mandatory that the surgical margins be carefully evaluated for involvement by the tumor and particularly for neurotropism. If nerve involvement is present, further resection is usually indicated in an attempt to extirpate the entire tumor.

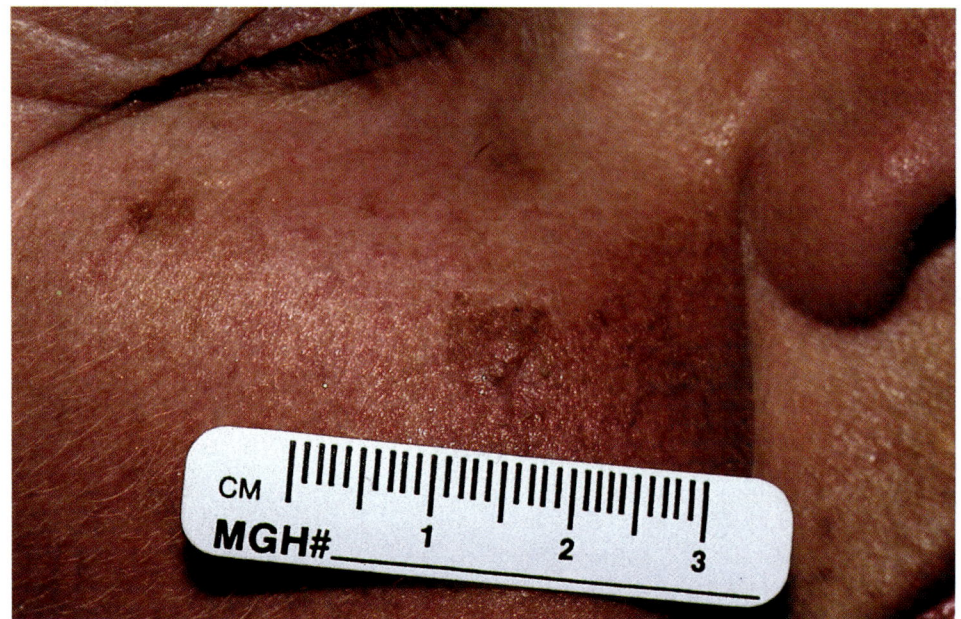

Figure 24-3 *Early desmoplastic melanoma arising in association with lentigo maligna melanoma. There is an asymmetric, variably pigmented lesion on the cheek consistent with lentigo maligna.*

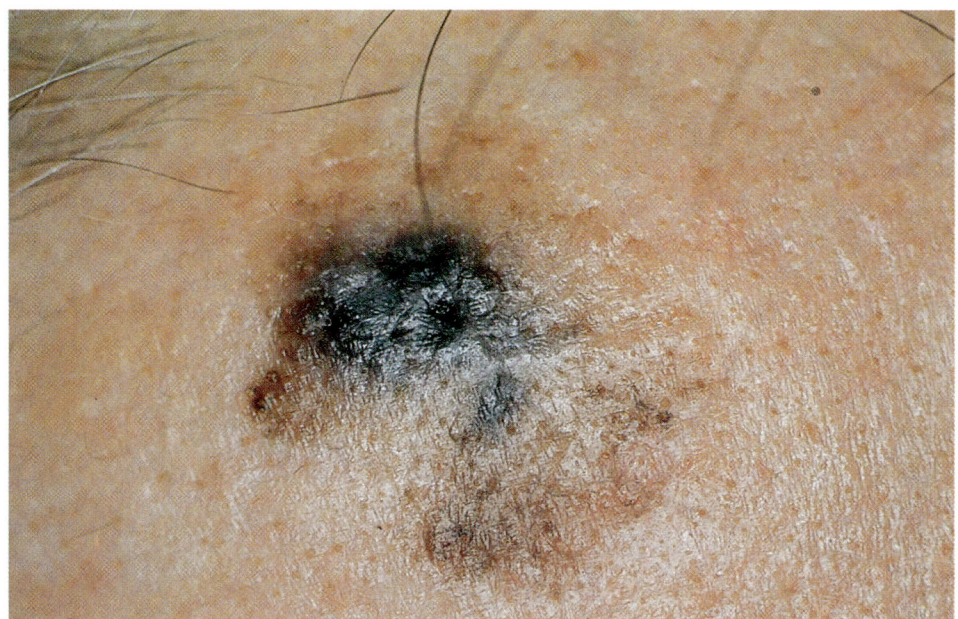

Figure 24-4 *Desmoplastic melanoma developing on the forehead of a young woman. This lesion is notable for striking asymmetry, irregularity of borders, and complexity of color. Although this lesion exhibited all the features of conventional melanoma, desmoplastic melanoma was noted in the dermal component of the tumor.*

ADDITIONAL READINGS

Beenken S et al: Desmoplastic melanoma: Histologic correlation with behavior and treatment. *Arch Otolaryngol Head Neck Surg* **115**:374, 1989

Bruijn J et al: Desmoplastic melanoma. *Histopathology* **20**:197, 1992

Conley J et al: Desmoplastic malignant melanoma (a rare variant of spindle cell melanoma). *Cancer* **28**:914, 1971

Egbert B et al: Desmoplastic malignant melanoma: A clinicohistopathologic study of 25 cases. *Cancer* **62**:2033, 1988

From L et al: Origin of the desmoplasia in desmoplastic malignant melanoma. *Hum Pathol* **14**:1072, 1983

Jain S, Allen PW: Desmoplastic malignant melanoma and its variants: A study of 45 cases. *Am J Surg Pathol* **13**:358, 1989

Reed RJ, Leonard DD: Neurotropic melanoma: A variant of desmoplastic melanoma. *Am J Surg Pathol* **3**:301, 1979

Reiman HM et al: Desmoplastic melanoma of the head and neck. *Cancer* **60**:2269, 1987

Smithers BM et al: Desmoplastic, neural transforming and neurotropic melanoma: A review of 45 cases. *Aust NZ J Surg* **60**:967, 1990

Walsh NMG et al: Desmoplastic malignant melanoma: A clinicopathologic study of 14 cases. *Arch Pathol Lab Med* **112**:922, 1988

Warner TFCS et al: Immunocytochemistry of neurotropic melanoma. *Cancer* **53**:254, 1984

25. Mucocutaneous Melanoma

Mucocutaneous melanomas occurring on the mucosae of conjunctivae, nasal cavity, oral cavity, vulvovaginal area, urogenital tract, anorectal area, or esophagus.

Synonym: mucous membrane melanoma

EPIDEMIOLOGY

Melanomas at these sites are uncommon, accounting for approximately 3 to 4 percent of all melanomas, and do not appear to be increasing in incidence, in contrast with cutaneous melanoma. Mucosal melanomas comprise a higher percentage of total melanomas in Asians, blacks, and persons of color in contrast to Caucasians of light complexion. Between 40 and 50 percent of mucosal melanomas occur on the mucosae of the head and neck, of which 55 percent are in the nasal cavity, 40 percent in the oral cavity, and the remaining 5 percent in the proximal esophagus, larynx, and pharynx. Approximately 400 cases of vulvar melanoma have been reported, representing about 10 percent of cancers at that site. Their site distribution is as follows: mucosa of labia minora, 80 percent; labia majora, 13 percent; and clitoris, 7 percent. Because more than 75 percent of vulvar melanomas extend to the vagina, it is usually difficult to ascertain the precise site of origin. Less than 150 cases of vaginal melanoma are recorded in the literature.

Esophageal melanomas are even less common. Of malignant tumors of the anorectum, melanoma accounts for 0.5 to 1 percent. Tumors at this site occur with equal frequency in men and women. The mean age of occurrence is 58 years.

ETIOLOGY

As with cutaneous melanoma, mucosal melanomas are thought to arise principally from a proliferation of intraepithelial melanocytes. Certain mucocutaneous melanomas may develop from cutaneous melanocytes extending onto mucosal surfaces. Some mucosal melanomas may originate from mucous membrane nevi or melanocytic dysplasias, but almost no information is available to address this issue.

CLINICAL FEATURES

Early diagnosis of these lesions is difficult because they develop at sites not routinely inspected, and consequently, mucosal melanomas are often detected because of prominent symptoms or signs, such as pain, bleeding, obstruction, and tumoral masses, that vary according to the mucosal site involved (Figs. 25-1 to 25-3). Epistaxis and obstruction are typical for nasal tumors. Oral lesions present with pigmented, sometimes friable masses, and pain is very often noted. Vulvar melanomas are usually characterized by pain

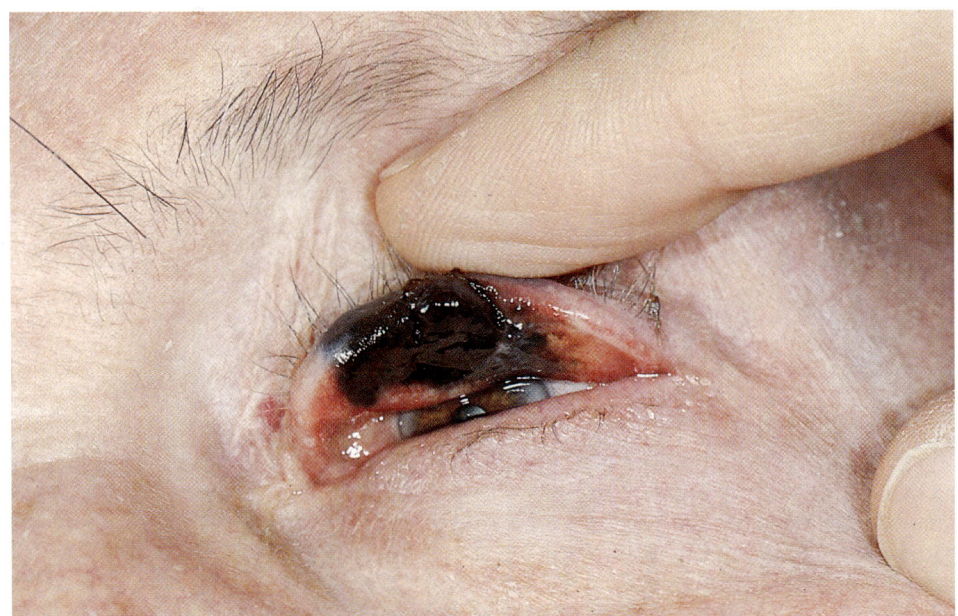

Figure 25-1 *Conjunctival melanoma. An advanced, jet-black melanoma involves the upper eyelid of this patient. The surrounding palpebral conjunctival surface exhibits a variegated grayish-blue color. Such a lesion would be associated with a very poor prognosis.*

and bleeding. Vaginal melanomas often present with bleeding and/or a malodorous discharge. Rectal bleeding, a painful mass, or a change in bowel habits is typical for anorectal melanoma.

HISTOPATHOLOGY

Mucosal melanomas may develop with or without a radial or horizontal growth phase. If such an intraepithelial component is present, it is usually lentiginous, i.e., composed of mainly basilar melanoma cells. The invasive tumors consist of spindle cells most commonly but also epithelioid cells and small nevus-like cells or any combination of the latter cell types. Mucosal melanomas are also prone to desmoplastic and neurotropic invasive components.

BIOLOGIC BEHAVIOR

Insufficient numbers of cases preclude a detailed evaluation of prognostic factors. Late presentation is associated with relatively poor survival. The 5-year survival rates range from 10 to 25 percent for head and neck melanomas. Two series have reported 5-year survival rates of 35 to 45 percent in these locations. For vulvar sites, a 56 percent 5-year survival has been noted in patients without nodal involvement. For patients with nodal disease, the 5-year survival rate was 15 percent. Five-year survival for anorectal melanoma

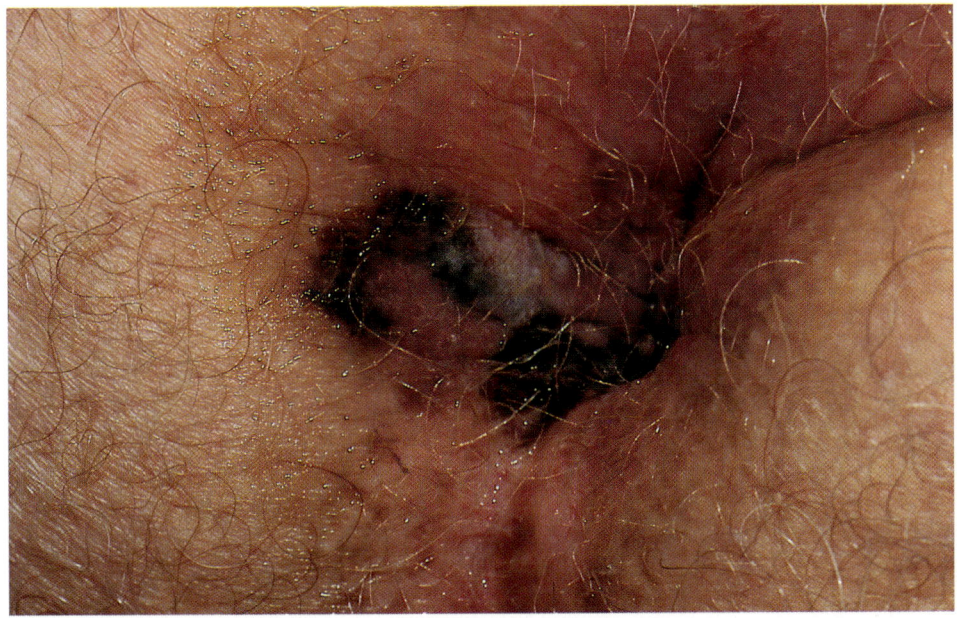

Figure 25-2 *Anorectal melanoma. This lesion demonstrates prominent asymmetry and variegation of color. There are grayish-blue foci which are most likely indicative of regression.*

ranges from 5 to 10 percent. In a series of 36 patients from Memorial Sloan-Kettering Cancer Center, New York, 4 patients survived 5 years; 3 of the latter patients had primary tumors less than 2 mm in thickness.

DIFFERENTIAL DIAGNOSIS

Melanosis (benign) of the oral cavity is common in blacks but, in contrast to melanoma, is usually bilateral and symmetric. Melanocytic nevi occur uncommonly on oral mucosal surfaces. Biopsy may be needed to distinguish such oral nevi from melanoma. Vascular lesions (angiomas, venous lakes), lentigines, and dental-amalgam tattoos also must be distinguished from melanoma. Genital lentiginosis must be differentiated from melanoma at vulvar and penile sites (see Chap. 7). In the anorectal area, hemorrhoids may enter into the differential diagnosis of melanoma.

MANAGEMENT

Sufficiently wide surgical excision is the treatment of choice for primary mucosal melanoma. Since most of these tumors present at an advanced point in their natural history, metastases often have preceded detection of the primary lesion. Radical surgery with one or more nodal basins electively dissected has not been shown to improve survival.

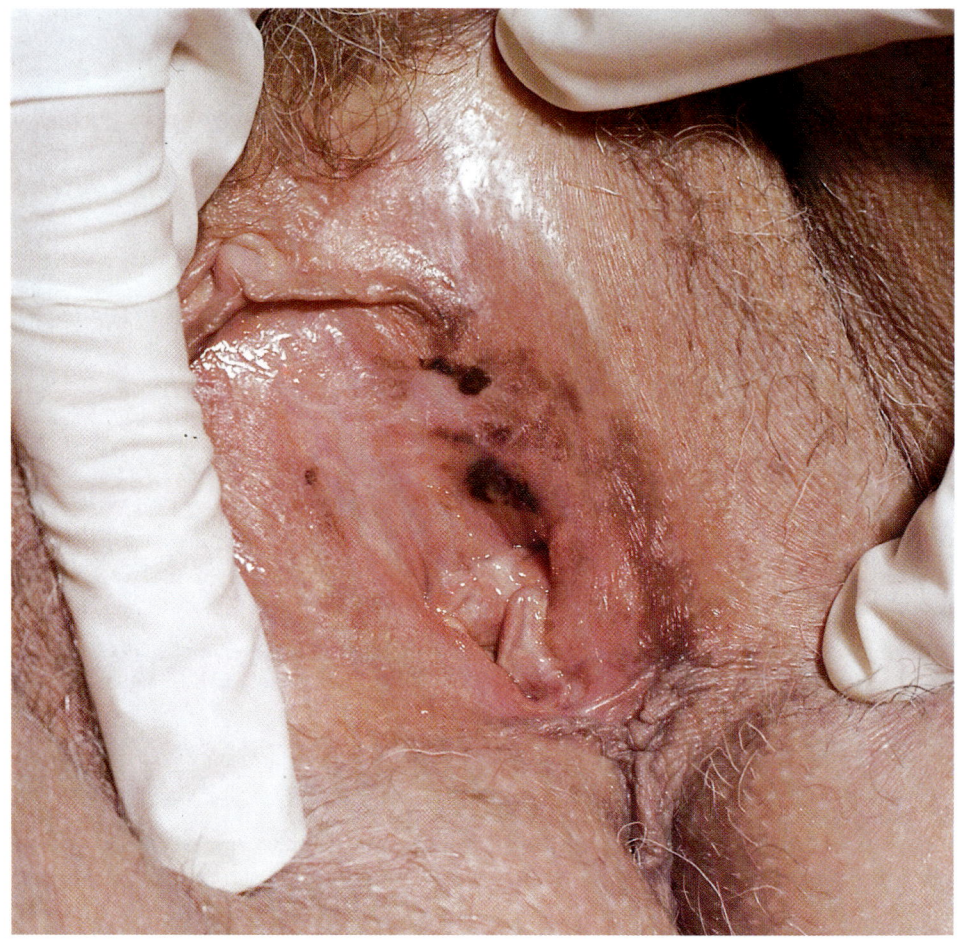

Figure 25-3 *Vulvar melanoma. This lesion is notable for poorly defined margins, striking asymmetry, and highly complex variegated pigmentary pattern. There are irregular blue-black foci that are separated by epithelium of normal color, slight hyperpigmentation, and areas of hypopigmentation.*

ADDITIONAL READINGS

Barnhill RL et al: Genital lentiginosis: A clinical and histopathologic study. *J Am Acad Dermatol* **22**(3):453, 1990

Berthelsen A et al: Melanomas of the mucosa in the oral cavity and the upper respiratory passages. *Cancer* **54**:907, 1984

Brand E et al: Vulvovaginal melanoma: Report of seven cases and literature review. *Gynecol Oncol* **33**:54, 1989

Chung AF et al: Malignant melanoma of the vulva: A report of 44 cases. *Obstet Gynecol* **45**:638, 1975

Frank W et al: Anorectal melanoma—A case report and brief review of the literature. *J Dermatol Surg Oncol* **18**:333, 1992

Shah JP et al: Mucosal melanomas of the head and neck. *Am J Surg* **134**:531, 1977

Stern SJ, Guillamondegui O: Mucosal melanoma of the head and neck. *Head Neck Surg* **13**:22, 1991

Wanebo HJ et al: Anorectal melanoma. *Cancer* **47**:1891, 1981

26. Unusual Presentations of Melanoma, Including Metastatic Melanoma

DOCUMENTATION OF EVOLUTION OF MELANOMA WITH SERIAL PHOTOGRAPHY

Cutaneous malignant melanoma is most often diagnosed because of atypical clinical features and/or a history of recent change, i.e., enlargement in area or elevation, changes in color, pruritus, bleeding, etc., often in a long-standing pigmented lesion. Despite this familiar history from patients, the actual evolution of such gross morphologic changes has rarely been recorded photographically (Fig. 26-1).

MALIGNANT MELANOMA DEVELOPING IN A CONGENITAL NEVUS SPILUS

Nevus spilus was described in Chap. 13. Although there are insufficient data to specifically define the melanoma risk of such lesions, well-documented cases of melanoma arising in association with nevus spilus have been reported (Fig. 26-2). Clinical details are not available for all the latter cases described, but some of the nevi spili have been large or giant variants; a number also have been congenital and have exhibited a background of melanocytic atypia.

MALIGNANT MELANOMA WITH PROMINENT HALO PHENOMENON

The development of a hypopigmented halo in association with primary or metastatic melanoma, analogous to halo nevus, is well recognized but rare. In contrast to halo nevus, the halo developing with melanoma is usually asymmetric and irregular in appearance. Often the development of such hypo- or depigmentation is a manifestation of tumor regression, and there may be partial or complete regression of the melanoma, whether primary or metastatic. The end stage of such regression may consist of circumscribed hypo- or depigmentation, indistinguishable from vitiligo.

Halo nevi (see Chap. 12) are much more common and may be seen in association with patients who have cutaneous melanoma at another site. Since halo melanomas are so rare, the prognostic implications of these lesions cannot be reliably ascertained. In the image shown in Fig. 26-3, the halo cutaneous melanoma developed in a 30-year-old woman. The pigmented lesion had been slowly enlarging for about 7 years. The patient had no evidence of halo nevi elsewhere. Removal of the lesion confirmed the presence of malignant melanoma, level IV, 1.5 mm in thickness. Five years later, during a pregnancy, the patient developed metastases.

CUTANEOUS MELANOSIS ASSOCIATED WITH ADVANCED MELANOMA

Generalized diffuse darkening of the skin (melanosis) may occur as an unusual complication of advanced melanoma. The skin appears slate-gray or bluish without alter-

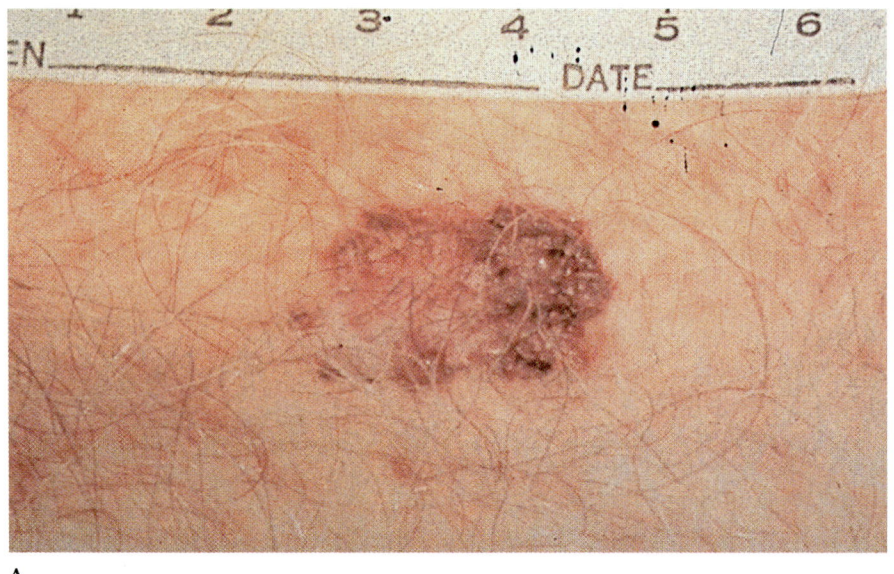

A

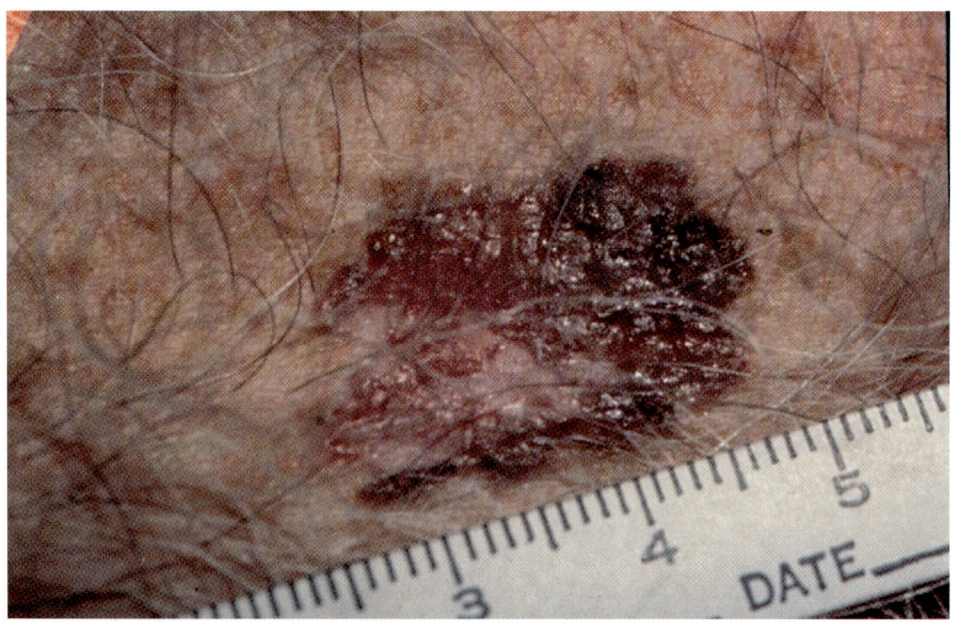

B

Figure 26-1

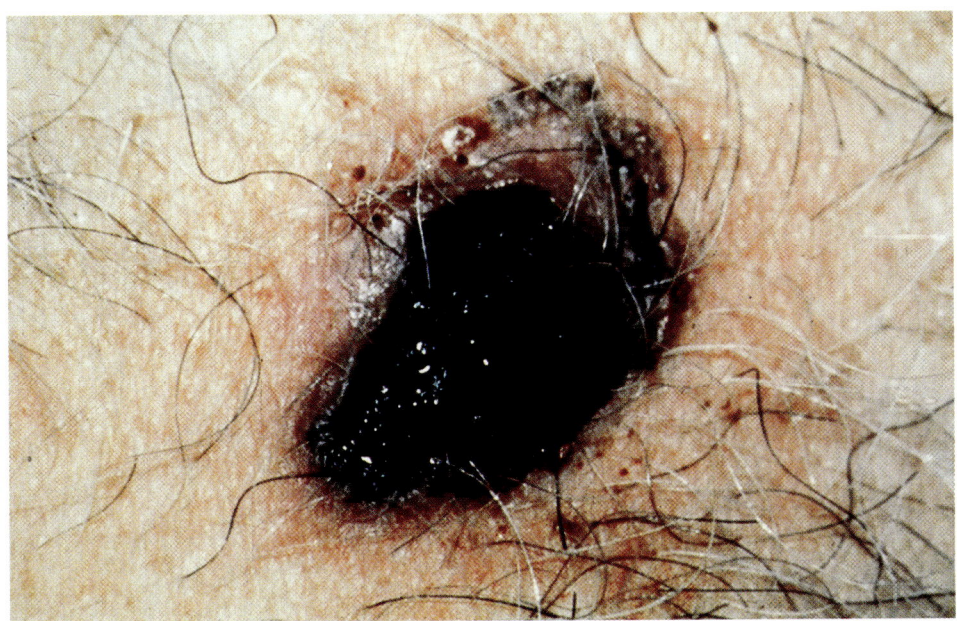

C

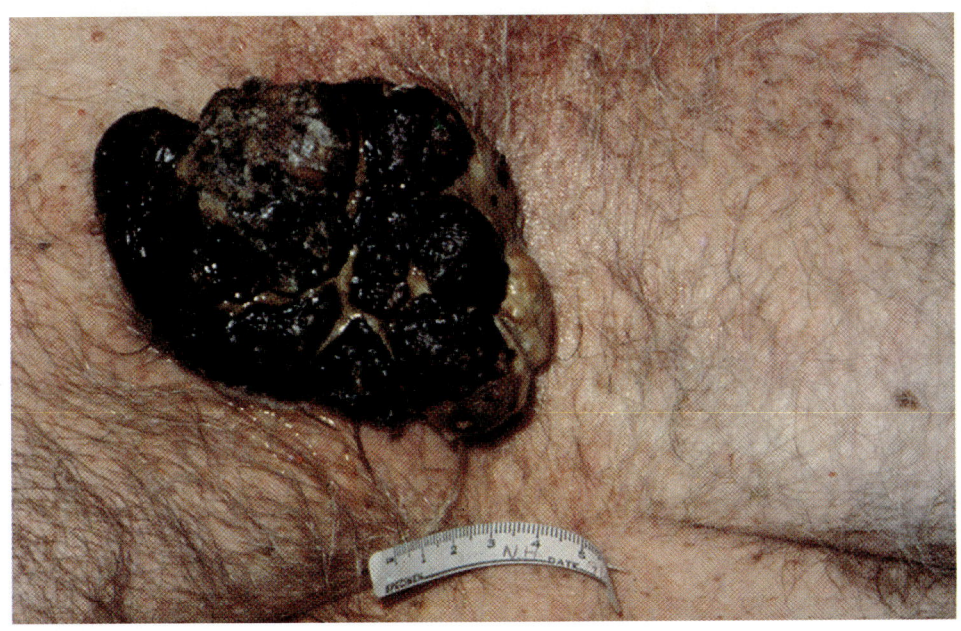

D

26 UNUSUAL PRESENTATIONS OF MELANOMA

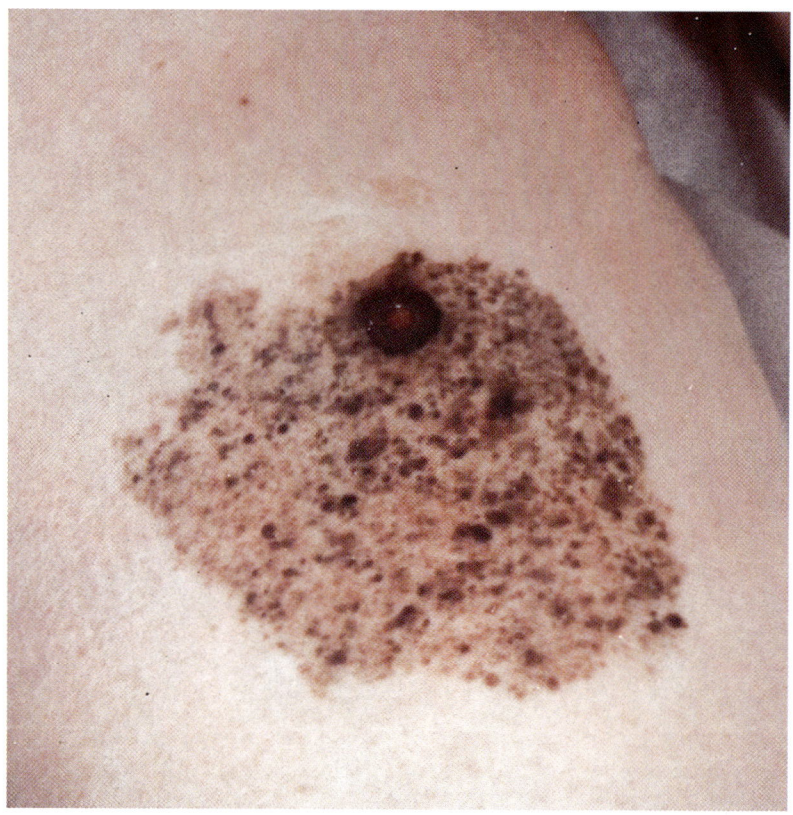

Figure 26-2 *Malignant melanoma arising in congenital nevus spilus. A 79-year-old woman had a congenital nevus spilus on the medial aspect of her right calf. The lesion measured 75 × 80 mm and had a typical speckled appearance. A blue-black nodule, 10 mm in diameter, was noted near the superior pole. Histopathologic examination revealed invasive melanoma in contiguity with the nevus spilus. The melanoma measured 0.8 mm in thickness, anatomic level III. The patient died of other causes 5 years later without evidence of recurrent melanoma. (Courtesy of Arthur R. Rhodes, M.D.)*

Figure 26-1 (See pages 212 and 213) *Evolution of superficial spreading melanoma over a 7-year period. (a) This lesion was first seen in 1983. The lesion measures approximately 2 cm in greatest diameter and exhibits asymmetry, irregularity of borders, and a variegated pigment pattern. A biopsy at this time confirmed a diagnosis of melanoma. (b) The lesion 4 years later in 1987. The lesion demonstrates unequivocal clinical features of melanoma at this time. The lesion measures approximately 2.5 cm in greatest length. Also note the striking notching and complexity of color. There are grayish-blue foci consistent with regression. (c) The lesion 3 years later. Most of the lesion consists of a raised, blue-black nodule. (d) There has been striking growth of the tumor by the time the patient presented 7 months later with metastatic melanoma. By this time, the tumor had a pedunculated, irregular surface with ulceration. (Courtesy of HC Maguire, Jr., M.D.)*

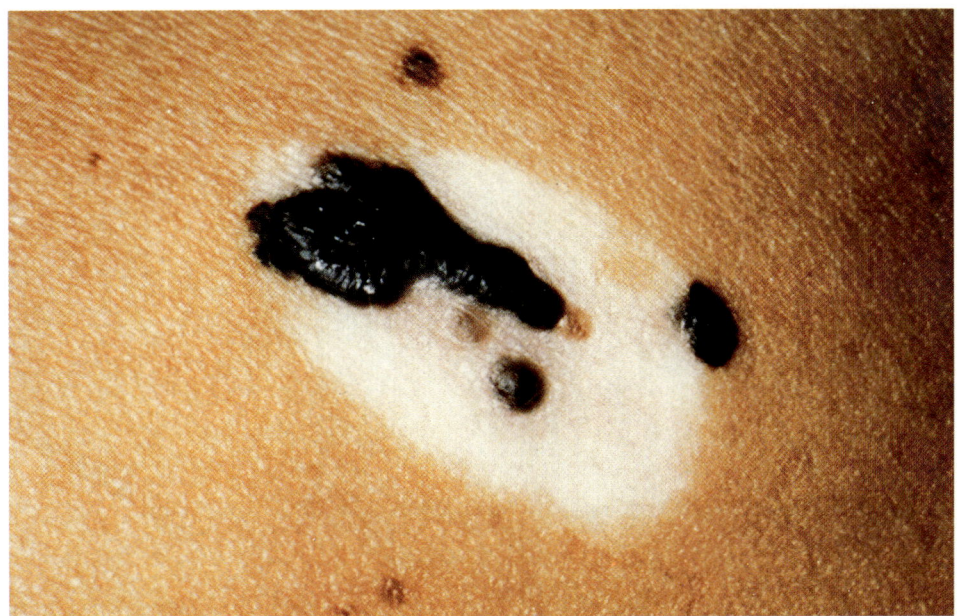

Figure 26-3 *Halo melanoma. Note the striking asymmetry of the lesion, irregular raised black foci present within and at periphery of the depigmented halo.* (Courtesy of TP Habif, MD: *Clinical Dermatology: A Color Guide to Diagnosis and Therapy*, 2nd ed. St. Louis, CV Mosby, 1990, p.571, with permission.)

ation in texture (Fig. 26-4) and is accompanied by melanuria (excretion of dark urine). All patients reported thus far have had disseminated metastatic disease, and the onset of melanosis has usually developed near the end of the patient's course. Explanations for the skin discoloration include (1) tyrosine intermediates deposited in the skin are oxidized to melanin, (2) diffuse single-cell metastases to the skin, and (3) circulating melanosomes which are carried to the skin are phagocytosed by macrophages.

MELANOMA-ASSOCIATED LEUKODERMA

Melanoma-associated leukoderma (MAL) is reported to occur in approximately 1 to 20 percent of melanoma patients. This phenomenon develops distant from the primary melanoma and is characterized by diffuse, often widespread mottled macular hypo- or depigmentation resembling vitiligo. In many instances, the trunk is initially affected (Fig. 26-5), followed by the extremities in a symmetric or asymmetric

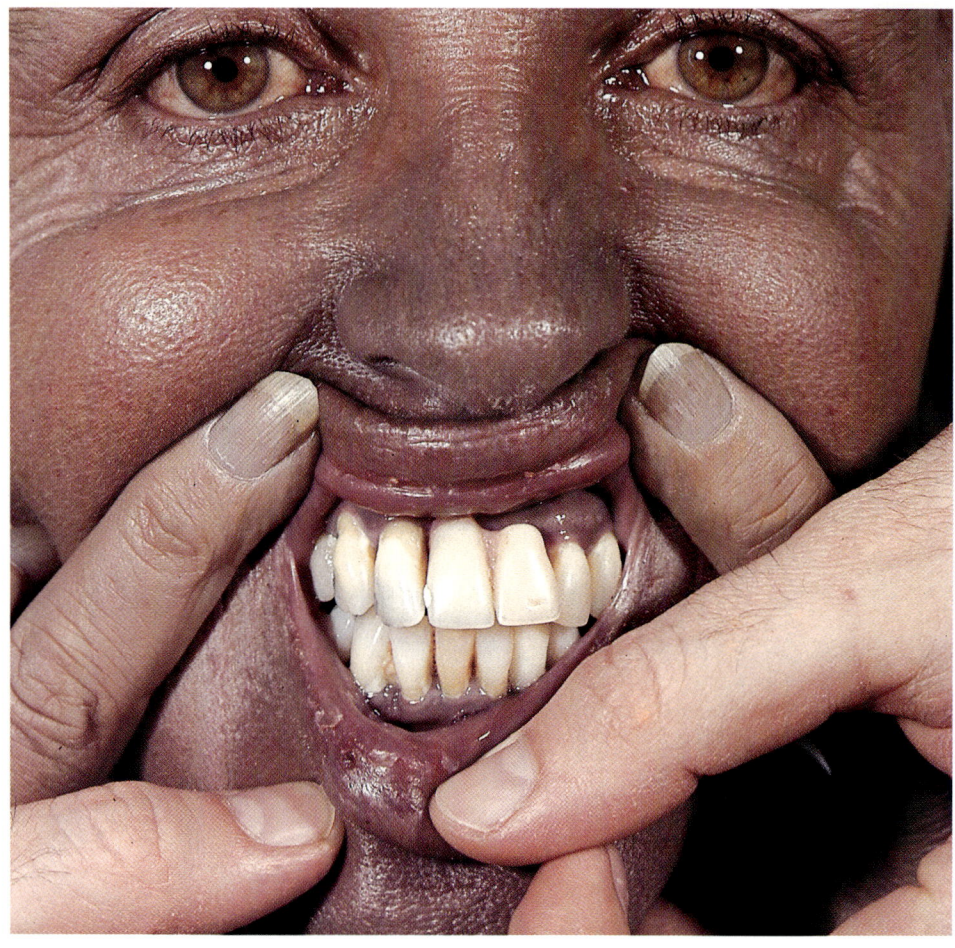

Figure 26-4 *Diffuse melanosis associated with disseminated melanoma. The skin and mucous membranes of this patient are notable for a diffuse, bluish-gray color. The texture of the skin is unchanged.*

pattern. The onset of this leukoderma is often coincident with the development of melanoma or may follow the tumor by months to as long as 5 years. Two cases have been reported to precede the diagnosis of primary melanoma. Most patients have been more than 40 years of age and have had concomitant lymph node and/or visceral metastases.

Melanoma-associated leukoderma is most likely associated with an immunologic host response against tumor and has been reported as a favorable prognostic feature. A number of authors have observed prolonged survival of melanoma patients exhibiting MAL. It should be emphasized that sufficient numbers of patients, long-term follow-up, and rigorous statistical

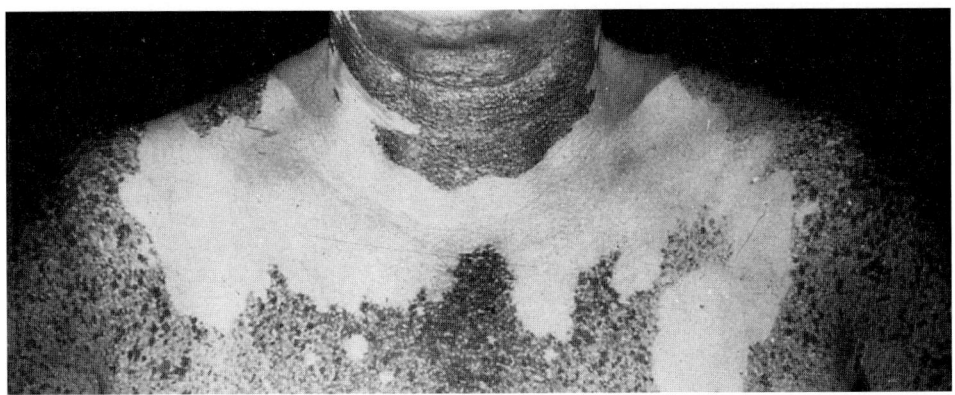

Figure 26-5 *Melanoma-associated leukoderma. This hypomelanosis may resemble vitiligo clinically and may be characterized by absence of melanocytes. It may be associated with a favorable prognosis.* (From TB Fitzpatrick et al (eds): *Dermatology in General Medicine*, 4th ed. New York, McGraw-Hill, 1993, p 957, with permission.)

analysis are needed to confirm the favorable prognostic effect of MAL.

RECURRENT AND METASTATIC MELANOMA INVOLVING SKIN AND SUBCUTANEOUS TISSUE

Malignant melanoma recurs with some frequency at the original site of excision and is primarily related to original tumor thickness rather than the margins of excision (Figs. 26-6 and 26-7). For example, melanomas >4.0 mm in thickness have a local recurrence rate of 13 percent with 5-year follow-up.

The skin and subcutaneous tissue are very common sites of regional and distant metastases from cutaneous melanoma. Local or regional metastases, defined as melanoma recurring between the primary site of excision and the regional lymph nodes, have been termed *satellite* and *in-transit metastases*. Multiple cutaneous metastases occurring near the original primary site have been described as *satellitosis*. These various lesions often present as papules or nodules with or without pigmentation (Fig. 26-8). They are often small (<0.5 mm) and commonly exhibit a pink or bluish color. Larger lesions are frequently ulcerated. Extensive involvement of a single extremity, most commonly a lower extremity, results in a distinctive clinical presentation that has been depicted as *chronic limb melanoma* (Fig. 26-9). Subcutaneous metastases usually present as painless firm nodules with or without a bluish appearance.

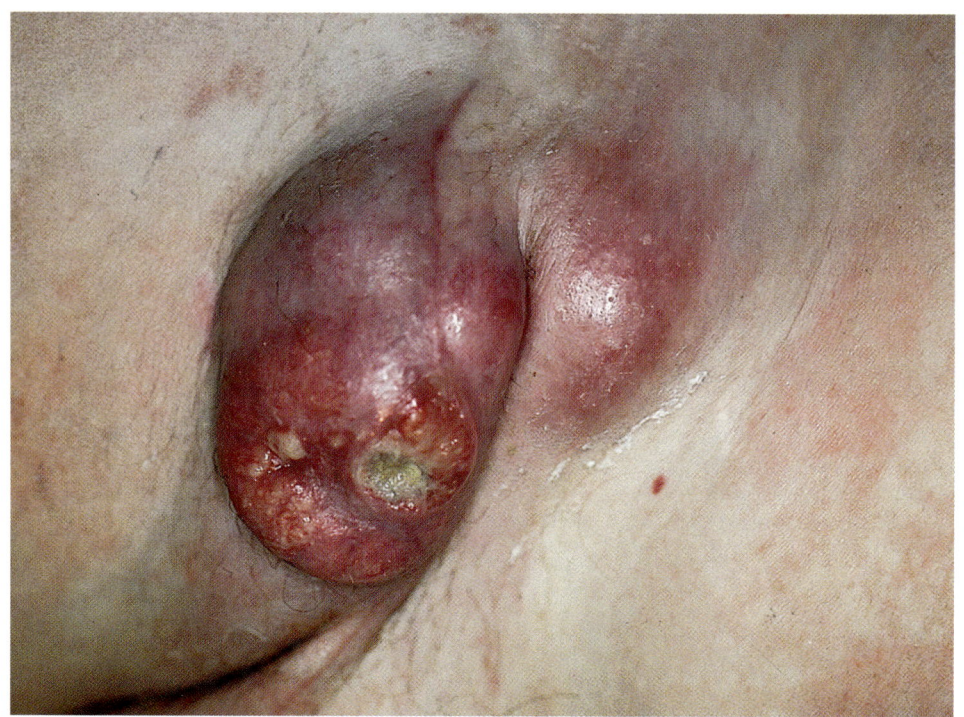

Figure 26-6 *Recurrent melanoma. There is a large, bluish-red, lobulated and ulcerated tumor that has recurred at the site of previous excision of a primary melanoma.*

Figure 26-8 (See opposite page) *Metastatic melanoma with unknown primary. (a) This pyogenic granuloma-like lesion has been present for 2 months; no primary was identified. (b) Enlargement of lesion.* (From TB Fitzpatrick et al (eds): *Dermatology in General Medicine,* 4th ed. New York, McGraw-Hill, 1993, p 1099, with permission.)

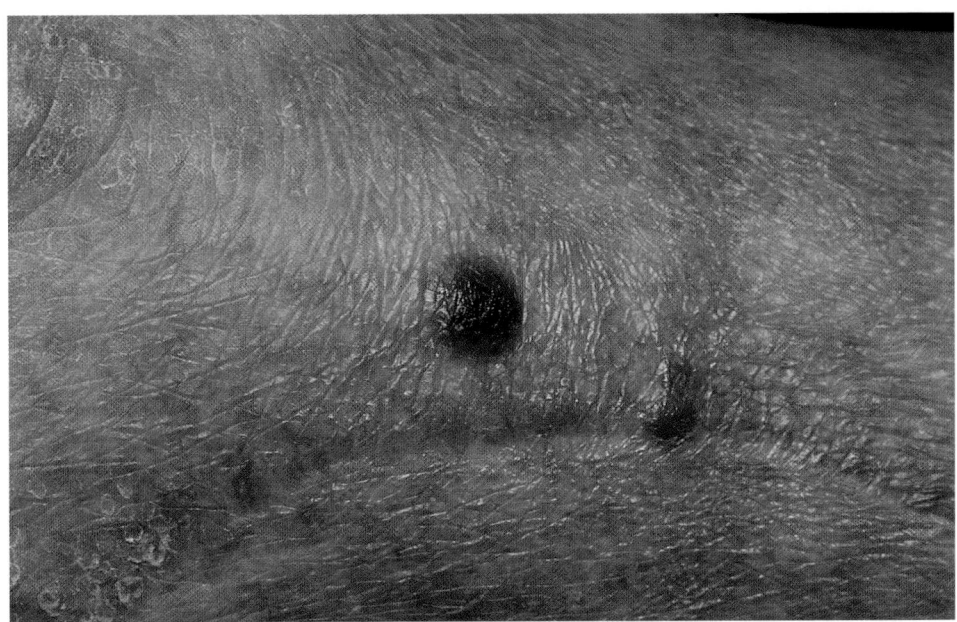

Figure 26-7 *Two papules are noted in or near the scar from a previous melanoma excision. The larger papule exhibits a dark brown color.*

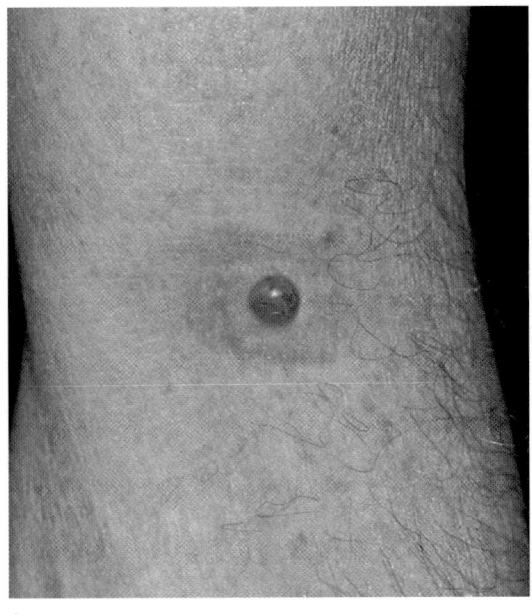

A

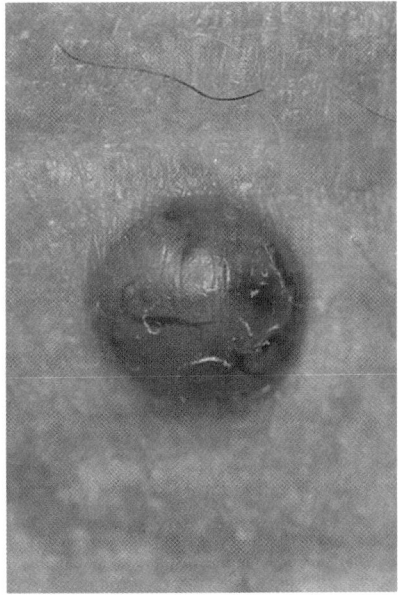

B

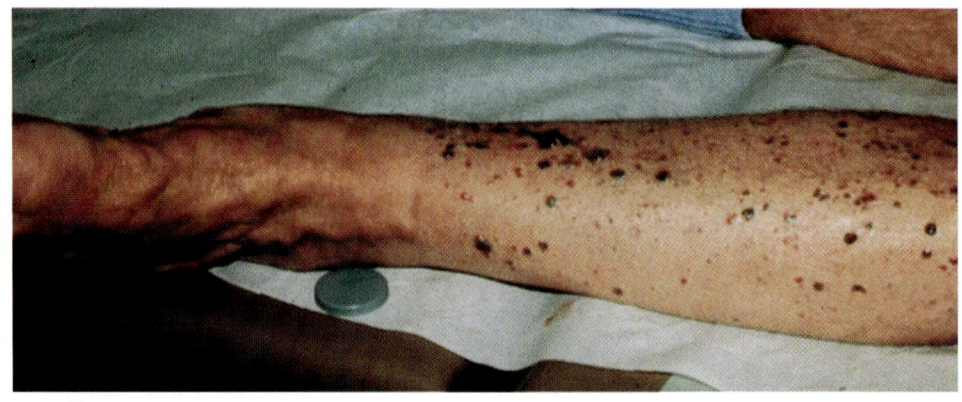

Figure 26-9 *Metastatic melanoma of the lower extremity. The lower extremity of this patient is notable for numerous darkly pigmented papules of metastatic melanoma. These metastases were confined to the lower extremity, which was the site of the patient's primary melanoma. This phenomenon has been termed* chronic limb melanoma *and is an uncommon but characteristic presentation of some lower extremity melanomas. Some patients may survive for a number of years with metastatic melanoma localized to a lower extremity.*

ADDITIONAL READINGS

Ackerman AB: Disagreements with the current classification of malignant melanomas. *Am J Surg Pathol* **6**(8):733, 1982

Adrian RM et al: Diffuse melanosis secondary to metastatic melanoma: Light and electron microscopic findings. *J Am Acad Dermatol* **5**:308, 1981

Ames FC et al: Local recurrences and their management, in *Cutaneous Melanoma,* 2d ed, edited by CM Balch et al. Philadelphia, Lippincott, 1992, pp 287–294

Balabanov K et al: Malignant melanoma and vitiligo. *Dermatologica* **139**:211, 1969

Balch CM, Houghton AN: Diagnosis of metastatic melanoma at distant sites, in *Cutaneous Melanoma,* 2d ed, edited by CM Balch et al. Philadelphia, Lippincott, 1992, pp 439–467 and 485–497

Bolognia JL: Fatal melanoma arising in a zosteriform speckled lentiginous nevus (letter). *Arch Dermatol* **127**:1240, 1991

Gebhart W, Kokoschka EM: Generalized diffuse melanosis secondary to malignant melanoma, in *Pathology of Malignant Melanoma,* edited by AB Ackerman. New York, Masson, 1981, pp 243–249

Goodall P et al: Malignant melanoma with melanosis and melanuria, and with pigmented monocytes and tumour cells in the blood: Autoradiographic demonstration of tyrosinase in malignant cells from peritoneal fluid. *Br J Surg* **48**:549, 1960

Guillot B et al: Malignant melanoma occurring on a "naevus on naevus" (letter). *Br J Dermatol* **124**:610, 1991

Koh HK et al: Malignant melanoma and vitiligo-like leukoderma: An electron microscopic study. *J Am Acad Dermatol* **9**:690, 1983

Konrad K, Wolff K: Pathogenesis of diffuse melanosis secondary to malignant melanoma. *Br J Dermatol* **91**:635, 1974

Kopf AW: Broad spectrum of leukoderma acquisitum centrifugum. *Arch Dermatol* **92**:14, 1965

Kurban RS et al: Occurrence of melanoma in "dysplastic" nevus spilus: Report of case and analysis by flow cytometry. *J Cutan Pathol* **19**:423, 1992

Lerner AB, Moellmann G: Two rare manifestations of melanomas: Generalized cutaneous melanosis and rapid solar induction of showers of small pigmented lesions. A critical review of the literature and presentation of two additional cases. *Acta Dermatol Venereol (Stockh)* **73**:241, 1993

Lerner AB, Nordlund JJ: Should vitiligo be introduced in patients after resection of primary melanoma? (editorial). *Arch Dermatol* **113**:421, 1977

Rhodes AR, Mihm MC Jr: Origin of cutaneous melanoma in a congenital dysplastic nevus spilus. *Arch Dermatol* **126**:500, 1990

Schuler G et al: Diffuse melanosis in metastatic melanoma: Further evidence for disseminated single cell metastases in the skin. *J Am Acad Dermatol* **3**:363, 1980

Schwartz BK et al: Pregnancy and hormonal influences on malignant melanoma. *J Dermatol Surg Oncol* **13**:276, 1987

Silberberg I et al: Diffuse melanosis in malignant melanoma: Report of a case and of studies by light and electron microscopy. *Arch Dermatol* **97**:671, 1968

Singletary SE, Balch CM: Recurrent regional metastases and their management, in *Cutaneous Melanoma,* 2d ed, edited by CM Balch et al. Philadelphia, Lippincott, 1992, pp 427–435

Sohn N et al: Generalized melanosis secondary to malignant melanoma: Report of a case with serum and tissue tyrosinase studies. *Cancer* **24**:897, 1969

Spremulli EN et al: Nude mouse model of the melanosis syndrome. *J Natl Cancer Inst* **71**:933, 1983

Section V

Nonmelanocytic Pigmented Lesions Entering Into The Differential Diagnosis of Melanoma

27. Seborrheic Keratosis

Seborrheic keratosis is a highly prevalent benign epidermal proliferation that is characterized by a well-demarcated, often pigmented, keratotic, or verrucous appearance.

Synonyms: seborrheic wart, seborrheic verruca

EPIDEMIOLOGY

This tumor is very common in individuals beyond the age of 30 years and increases in frequency with age. The lesion is most commonly observed on the trunk and in the head and neck areas. A slightly greater prevalence in men has been reported. There is also evidence supporting an autosomal dominant mode of inheritance.

ETIOLOGY

Little is known concerning the cause of seborrheic keratoses. As mentioned earlier, a genetic predisposition to the lesions is likely.

CLINICAL FEATURES

This lesion characteristically exhibits a well-defined, slightly elevated, waxy, "stuck-on" or greasy appearance (Figs. 27-1 to 27-3). The surface may be finely stippled in early lesions or typically warty and keratotic. The size varies from a few millimeters to 6.0 cm or larger. Examination with a hand lens often will disclose small keratotic cysts. The color varies from flesh colored to tan, light brown, brown, gray, or black. Variegation of color is sometimes also noted. In general, the lesions are round or oval in shape. Seborrheic keratoses most commonly are present as multiple symmetric lesions and in some instances may be profuse.

HISTOPATHOLOGY

The lesions are characterized by papillomatous epidermal hyperplasia of monotonous, slightly basaloid keratinocytes. Delicate, laminated hyperorthokeratosis and pseudo-horn cysts are observed.

BIOLOGIC COURSE

In general, the lesions gradually enlarge or remain stable indefinitely.

DIFFERENTIAL DIAGNOSIS

The relatively flat varieties of incipient seborrheic keratosis enter into the differential diagnosis of solar lentigo, pigmented actinic keratosis, and lentigo maligna. Careful inspection of these incipient forms of seborrheic keratosis usually discloses a slightly keratotic or verrucous surface topography and presence of horn cysts, which allow discrimination from the preceding three entities. Fully developed seborrheic keratoses with typical warty surfaces may be confused with verruca, epidermal nevus, and—of particular importance—an unusual verruca-like presentation of malignant melanoma. The lat-

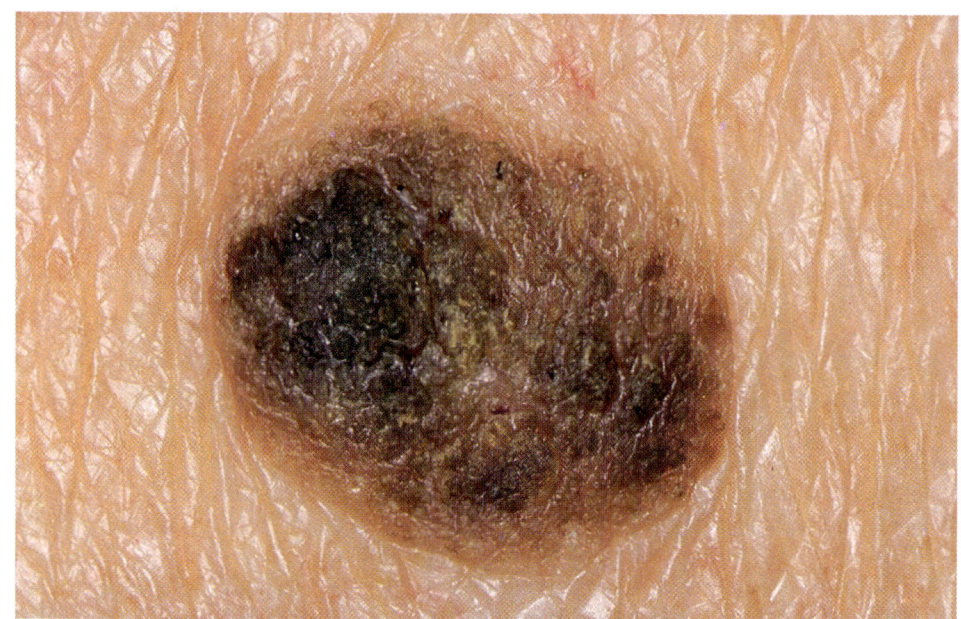

Figure 27-1 *Seborrheic keratosis. This lesion is slightly asymmetric but has a characteristic "stuck-on" appearance and well-defined margins. The surface is also somewhat keratotic, and the lesion exhibits colors of tan and brown.* (From TB Fitzpatrick et al (eds.): *Dermatology in General Medicine*, 4th ed. New York, McGraw-Hill, 1993, p 856, with permission.)

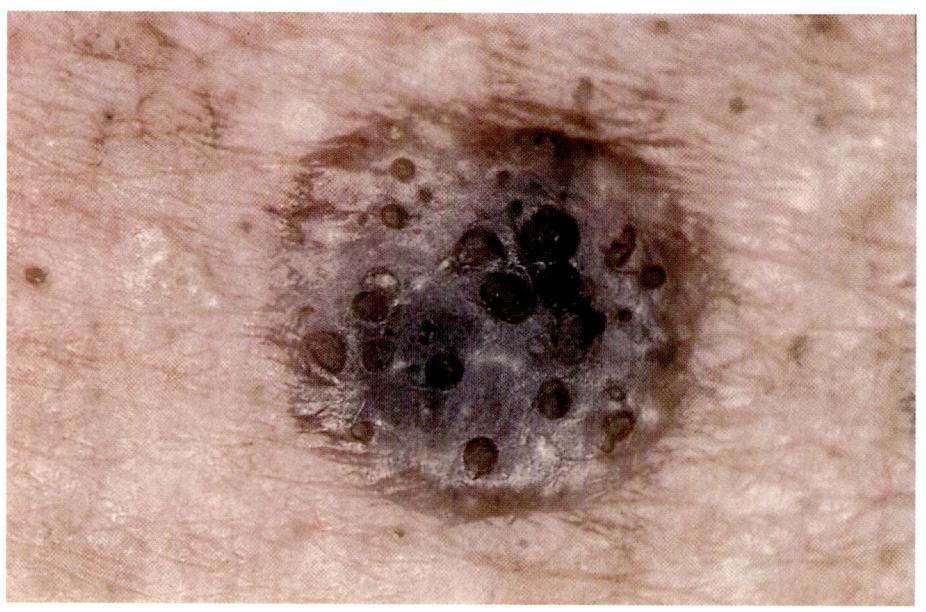

A

Figure 27-2

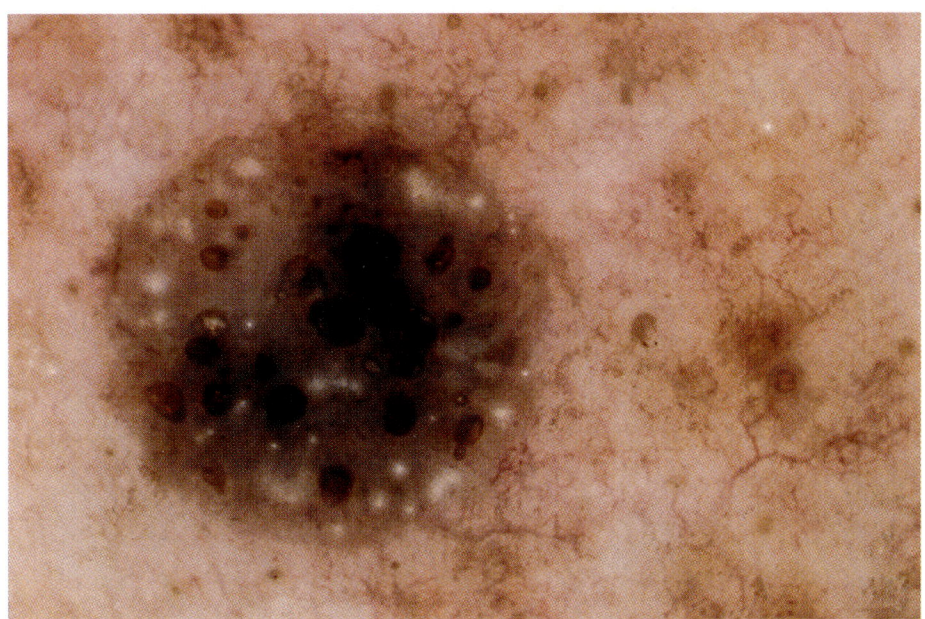

B

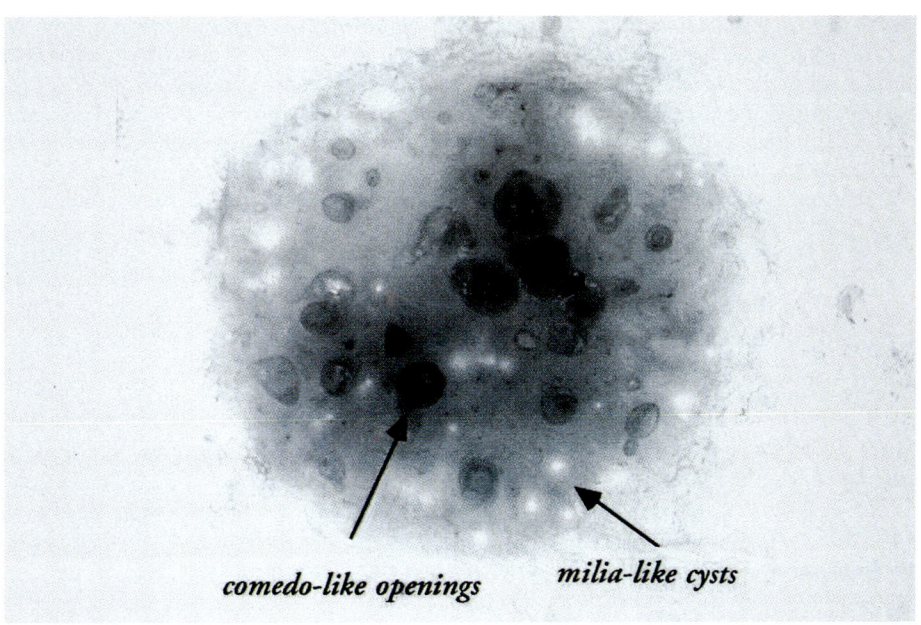

C

Figure 27-2 *(cont.)*

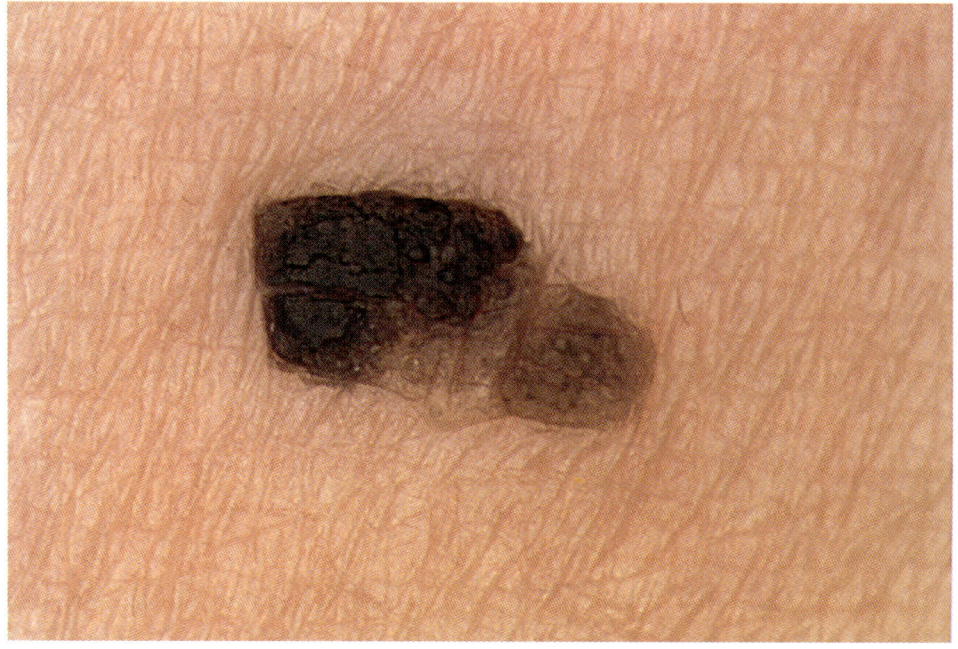

A

Figure 27-3 *Pigmented seborrheic keratosis. (a) (Clinical surface view without oil): Small vary dark lesion with surface typical of a seborrheic keratosis. (b) (Subsurface gross tissue architecture, ELM with oil): There are a few milia-like cysts that suggest that this is a seborrheic keratosis; however, there are no multiple comedo-like openings that would be more specific for a seborrheic keratosis. Note that there is a small region with a pigment network in the upper left corner of the lesion; this represents the exception to the rule that a pigment network has a high specificity for melanocytic lesions. (c) pigment pattern enhancement of epiluminescence microscopic subsurface view.*

Figure 27-2 (See pages 226 and 227) *Seborrheic keratosis. Comedo-like openings and milia-like cysts. (a) Multiple comedo-like openings. Maximum diameter 7 mm. (b, c) Local features: multiple comedo-like openings and milia-like cysts (arrows). (a) Digital clinical surface view (without oil); (b) digital epiluminescence microscopic subsurface view (with oil); and (c) pigment pattern enhancement of epiluminescence microscopic subsurface view.* (Reprinted with permission from RO Kenet et al: Clinical diagnosis of pigmented lesions using digital epiluminescence microscopy: Grading protocol and atlas. *Arch Dermatol* 129:157, 1993.)

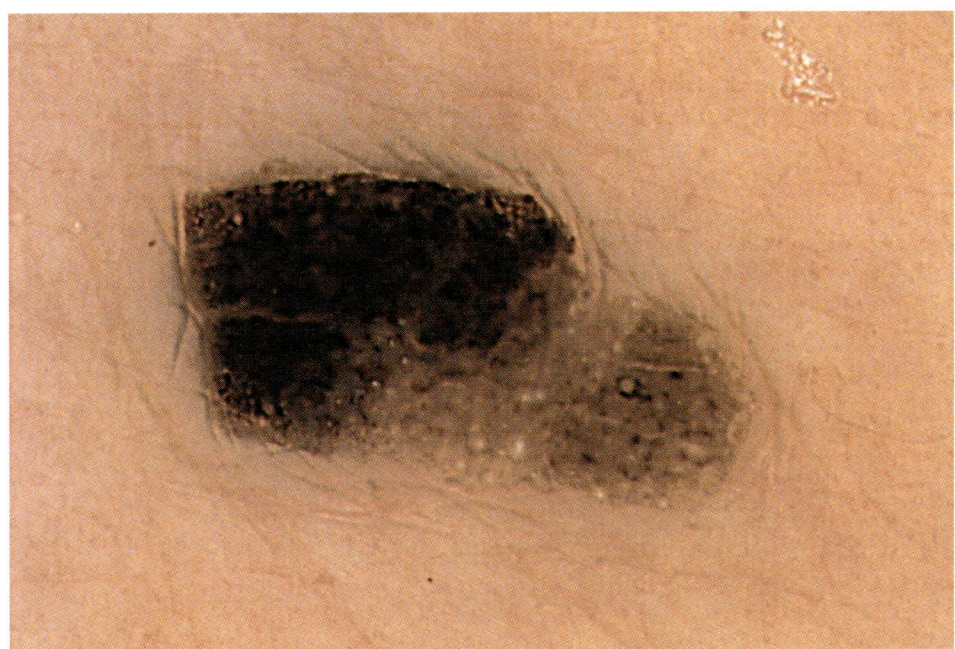

B

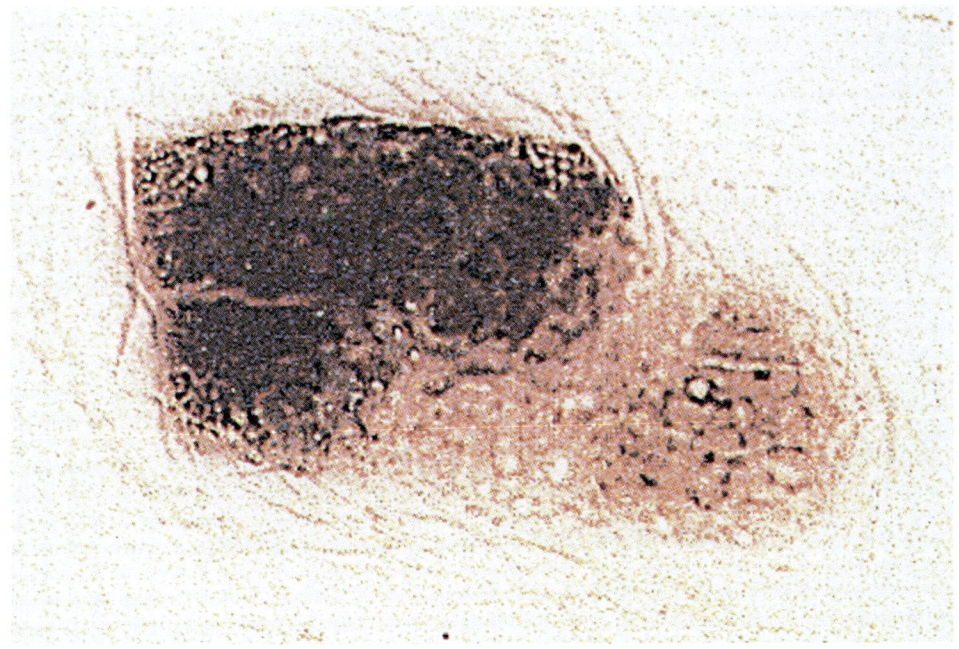

C

Figure 27-3 *(cont.)*

ter entity was originally described by Clark in his classification of melanoma but was subsequently dropped. The usual gross morphologic features of seborrheic keratosis, namely, well-demarcated borders, typical "stuck-on" appearance, and presence of horn cysts, should allow distinction from melanoma. However, in some instances, this may be impossible without histopathologic examination.

MANAGEMENT

Typical seborrheic keratoses do not require treatment. If removal is desired, it can be accomplished by cryotherapy, curettage, or electrodesiccation. In any lesion that is atypical, histologic evaluation is required.

ADDITIONAL READINGS

Freudenthal W: Verruca senilis und keratoma senile. *Arch Dermatol Syphilol* **152**:505, 1926

Sanderson KV: The structure of seborrheic keratoses. *Br J Dermatol* **80**:588, 1968

28. Pyogenic Granuloma

The pyogenic granuloma is a vascular proliferation with rapid onset, protuberant shape, and bright red or dusky color.

Synonyms: granuloma telangiectaticum, lobular capillary hemangioma

EPIDEMIOLOGY

These lesions most commonly affect individuals less than 30 years of age. Men and women are equally affected.

ETIOLOGY

The sudden appearance of pyogenic granuloma has suggested external injury or trauma as a principal factor in the etiology of these lesions.

CLINICAL FEATURES

These lesions characteristically present as reddish polypoid nodules with an often eroded or crusted surface (Fig. 28-1). The color may vary from bright red to dusky to brown-black. In general, these lesions are isolated and <1.5 cm in greatest diameter. Pyogenic granulomas most commonly involve the lips, digits, trunk, and mucosal surfaces.

HISTOPATHOLOGY

Histologic examination usually shows a raised tumor with often ulcerated surface and containing well-defined vascular lobules separated by fibrous septa. An epidermal collarette is characteristically present at the base of the tumor.

BIOLOGIC COURSE

These lesions usually persist or gradually involute with fibrosis.

DIFFERENTIAL DIAGNOSIS

The differential diagnosis primarily includes nodular malignant melanoma (particularly with an amelanotic presentation), basal cell carcinoma, squamous cell carcinoma, appendageal tumors such as eccrine poroma, Kaposi's sarcoma, and bacillary angiomatosis. Distinction from malignant melanoma may be impossible without histopathologic examination. However, the small size of the lesion, rapid development, typical location, and usually young age of the patient as a rule favor pyogenic granuloma.

MANAGEMENT

Usually, removal by excision or a shave biopsy technique is accomplished for histologic examination.

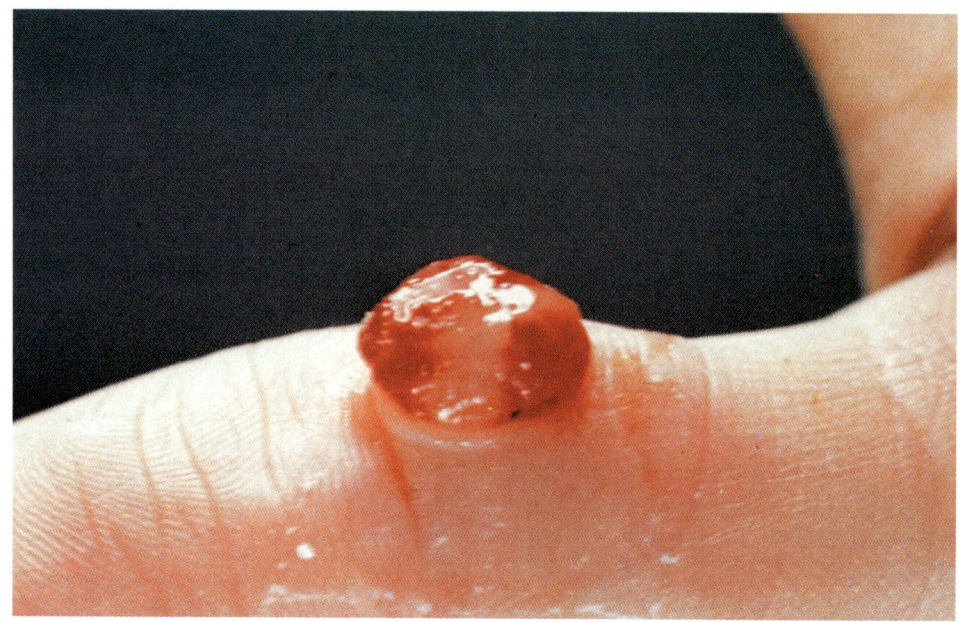

Figure 28-1 *Pyogenic granuloma. An ulcerated, glistening, reddish papule is surrounded by a collarette. The differential diagnosis includes amelanotic nodular melanoma.* (From TB Fitzpatrick et al (eds): *Dermatology in General Medicine,* 4th ed. New York, McGraw-Hill, 1993, p 1232, with permission.)

ADDITIONAL READING

Wolf JE Jr, Hubler WR Jr: Origin and evolution of pyogenic granuloma (editorial). *Arch Dermatol* **110**:958, 1974

29. Sclerosing Hemangioma Variant of Fibrous Histiocytoma

The sclerosing hemangioma is a variant of dermatofibroma that is generally characterized by a firm, raised, vascular appearance and is often located on the extremities.

Synonym: dermatofibroma

EPIDEMIOLOGY

These lesions may affect individuals of any age and have a somewhat greater incidence in women versus men.

ETIOLOGY

A response to external trauma, as from an arthropod bite, is suspected.

CLINICAL FINDINGS

These lesions usually present as solitary, raised, firm papules or nodules usually <1 to 2 cm in diameter (Fig. 29-1). The surface is often smooth but may exhibit scaling or slight keratotic texture. The color may be red, brown, or blue. Although these proliferations may occur in virtually any location, they are noted most commonly on the lower extremities, followed by the upper extremities and trunk.

HISTOPATHOLOGY

Histologic evaluation usually reveals a fairly well circumscribed dermal tumor composed of varying admixtures of ectatic vascular channels and a diffuse proliferation of spindle-shaped or histiocyte-like cells or both. Varying degrees of hemorrhage, hemosiderin deposition, and fibrosis are also present.

BIOLOGIC COURSE

The lesions tend to persist indefinitely.

DIFFERENTIAL DIAGNOSIS

The differential diagnosis primarily involves nodular malignant melanoma, blue nevus, and vascular proliferations such as Kaposi's sarcoma or bacillary angiomatosis. Histologic examination may be indispensable for discrimination of sclerosing hemangioma from malignant melanoma. However, the overall symmetry, firm texture, and striking vascular character may more strongly suggest sclerosing hemangioma.

MANAGEMENT

Excision is often needed for diagnosis as well as for appropriate treatment of the lesion.

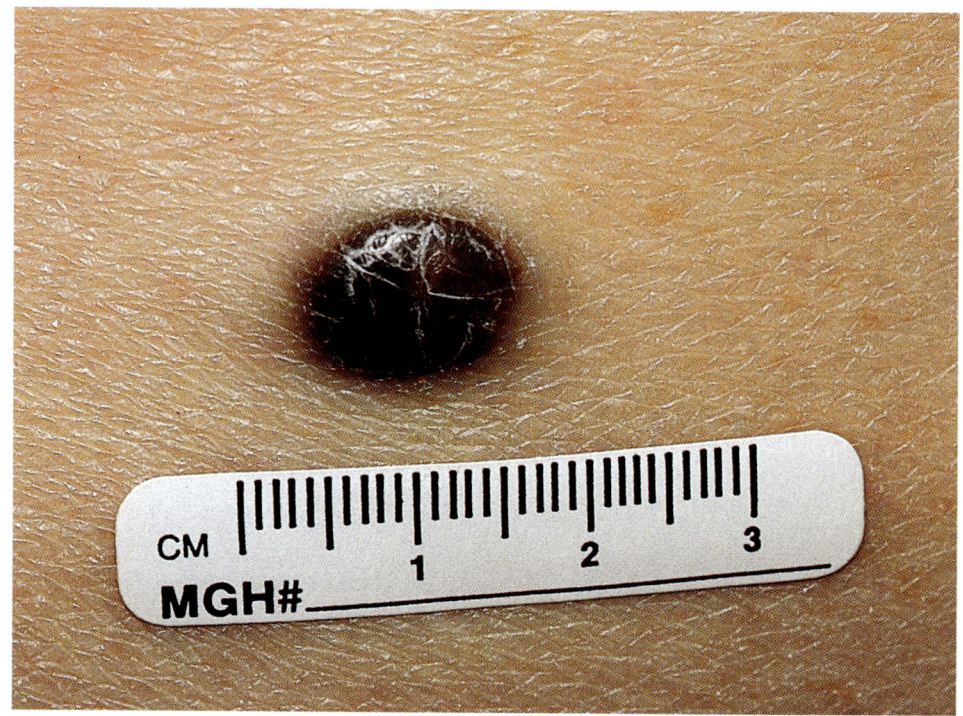

Figure 29-1 *Sclerosing hemangioma, variant of fibrous histiocytoma. This dome-shaped nodule is notable for striking symmetry and well-defined borders. The lesion also exhibits a dark brown, dusky color.*

ADDITIONAL READINGS

Hairston MA Jr, Reed RJ: Aneurysmal sclerosing hemangioma of skin. *Arch Dermatol* **93**:439, 1965

Vilanova JR, Flint A: The morphological variations of fibrous histiocytoma. *J Cutan Pathol* **1**:155, 1974

30. Angiokeratoma

Angiokeratoma is a circumscribed, raised, usually blue-black vascular lesion often present on the extremities.

Synonyms: angiokeratoma corporis circumscriptum, angiokeratoma of Mibelli

EPIDEMIOLOGY

Angiokeratoma corporis circumscriptum is an uncommon vascular malformation, usually present at birth and usually on the lower extremities. The angiokeratoma of Mibelli is usually noted in adolescent females, commonly affecting both lower and upper extremities.

ETIOLOGY

No information is available concerning the causes of these lesions.

CLINICAL FEATURES

The lesions usually present as raised plaques measuring up to 3 cm in diameter and associated with a characteristic red-blue-black color (Figs. 30-1 to 30-3). A keratotic or scaling surface also may be present. Lesions are most commonly located on the extremities and may involve digits, elbows, or knees.

HISTOPATHOLOGY

The characteristic histologic findings consist of markedly dilated, thin-walled vascular channels in the papillary dermis that are enveloped by closely apposed hyperplastic epidermis. Extravasation of erythrocytes and thrombosis are also common features.

BIOLOGIC COURSE

The lesions may exhibit gradual enlargement.

DIFFERENTIAL DIAGNOSIS

The principal process to be excluded is malignant melanoma. Histopathologic examination is often mandatory to exclude melanoma.

MANAGEMENT

Complete excision for diagnosis will be required in many instances.

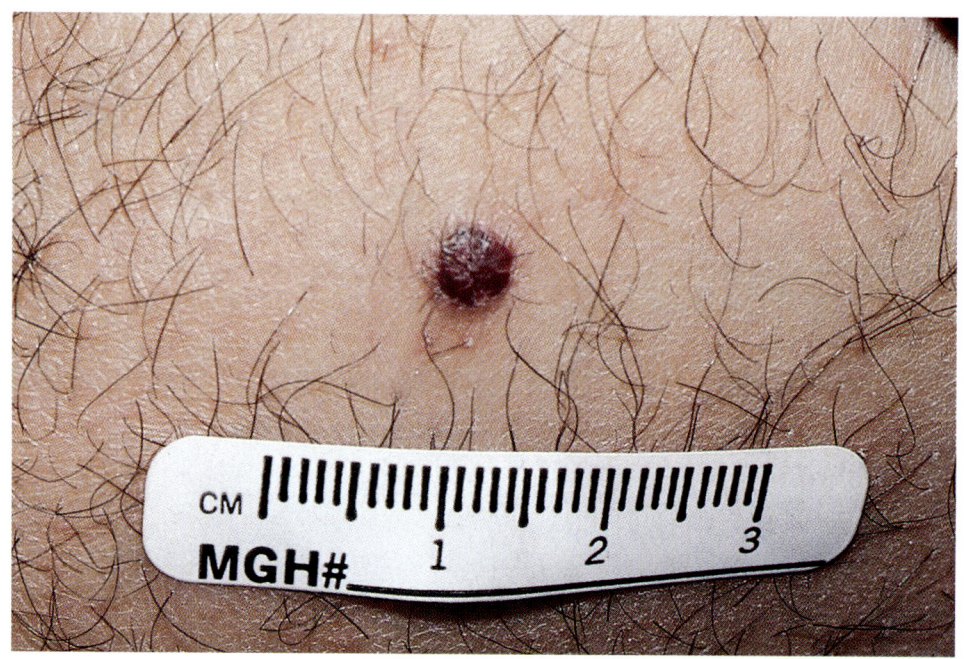

Figure 30-1 *Angiokeratoma. This raised reddish-blue nodule measures approximately 4 mm in diameter. Such a lesion is difficult to distinguish from nodular melanoma.*

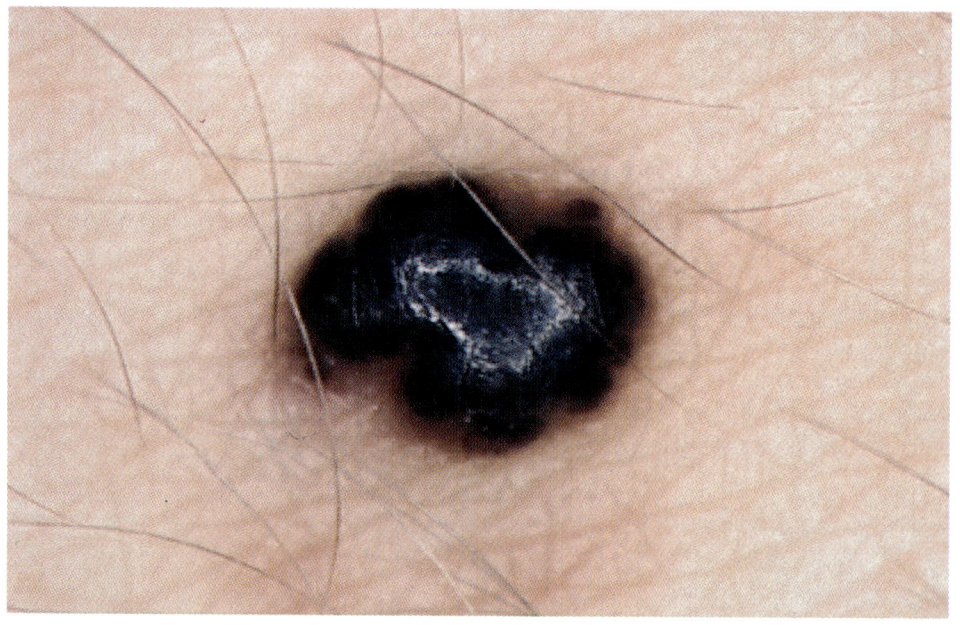

A

Figure 30-2

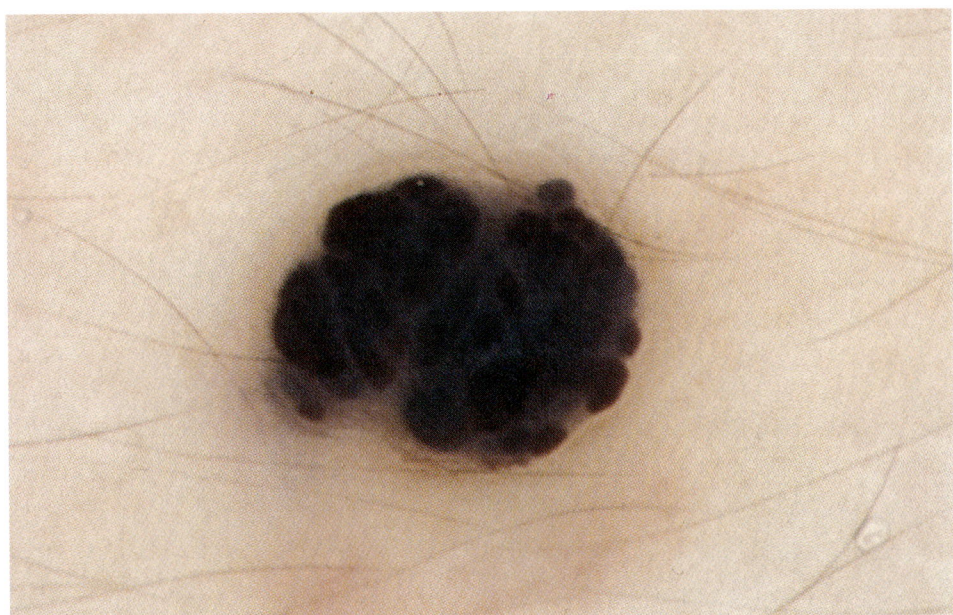

B

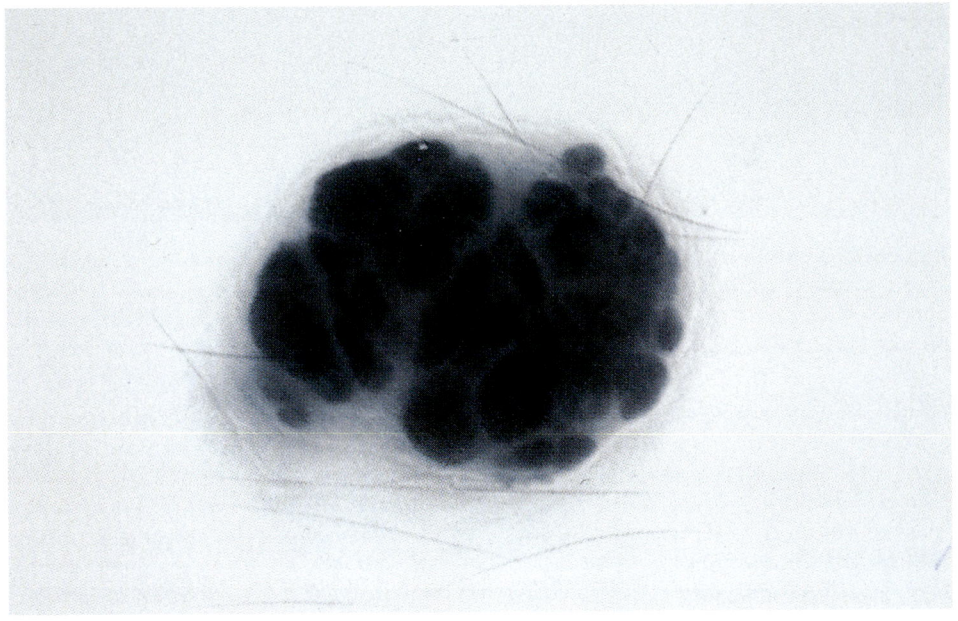

C

Figure 30-2 *(cont.)*

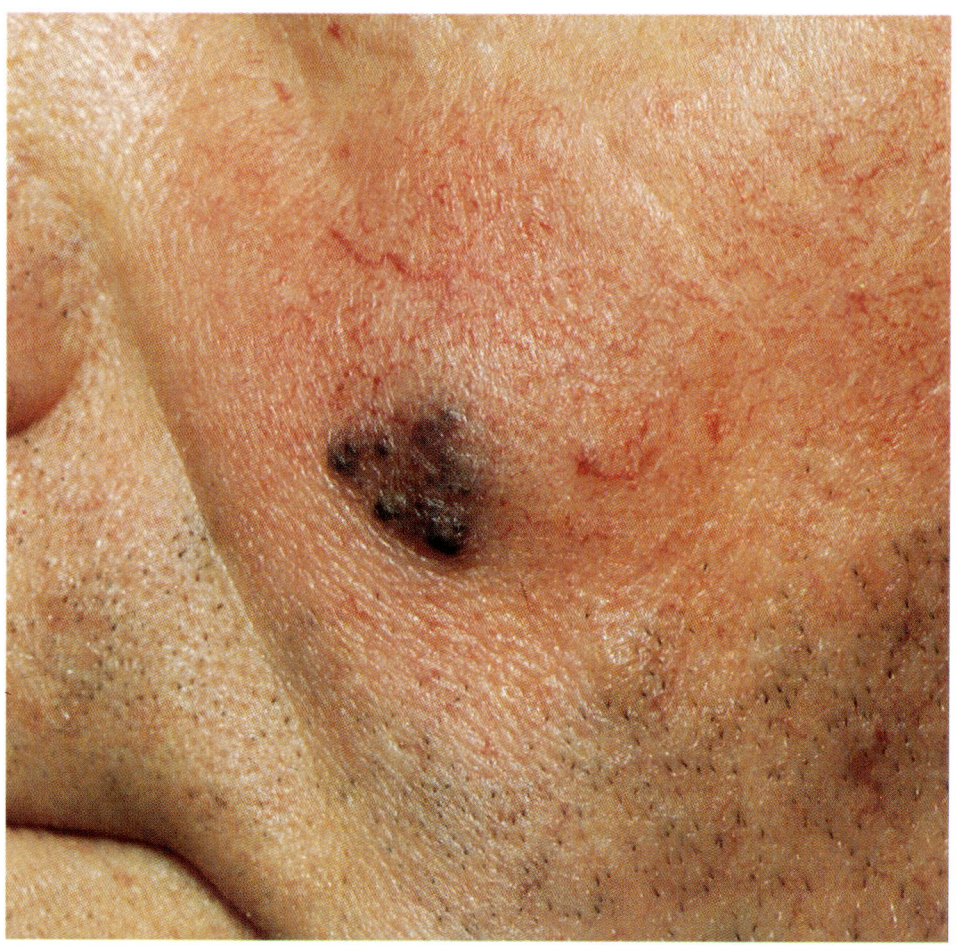

Figure 30-3 *Venous lake. This irregular nodule on the cheek demonstrates a cobblestone, purplish-red appearance and is indistinguishable from melanoma.* (From TB Fitzpatrick et al: *Color Atlas and Synopsis of Clinical Dermatology*, 2nd ed. New York, McGraw-Hill, 1992, p 167 with permission.)

Figure 30-2 (See pages 236 and 237) *Thrombosed hemangioma. Saccular pattern. (a) Dark, elevated lesion with obliteration of skin markings and scalloped borders. Compare with nodular melanoma in Fig. 22-3a. Maximum diameter 3.5 mm. (b, c) Global features: saccular pattern (cluster of smooth-bordered, purplish, nearly black sacculi without any trace of a pigment network). Local features: smooth blue-gray veil. (a) Digital clinical surface view (without oil); (b) digital epiluminescence microscopic subsurface view (with oil); and (c) pigment pattern enhancement of epiluminescence microscopic subsurface view.* (Reprinted with permission from RO Kenet et al: Clinical diagnosis of pigmented lesions using digital epiluminescence microscopy: Grading protocol and atlas. *Arch Dermatol* 129:164, 1993.)

ADDITIONAL READINGS

Bruce DH: Angiokeratoma circumscriptum and angiokeratoma scroti. *Arch Dermatol* **81**:388, 1968

Haye KR, Rebello DJA: Angiokeratoma of Mibelli. *Acta Derm Venereol (Stockh)* **41**:56, 1961

Hayen DO: Thrombosed angiokeratoma simulating malignant melanoma. *Arch Dermatol* **93**:358, 1966

31. Pigmented Basal Cell Carcinoma

Pigmented basal cell carcinoma is a heavily melaninized variant of basal cell carcinoma that may be clinically indistinguishable from melanoma.

Synonym: basal cell epithelioma

EPIDEMIOLOGY

Basal cell carcinomas are the most common form of skin cancer and generally affect individuals over the age of 40 years. Pigmented basal cell carcinomas occur more commonly in persons with skin phototypes IV or V.

CLINICAL FEATURES

These lesions usually present as dark brown, blue, or black papules or nodules with frequent erosion or ulceration. The overall size ranges from 2 to 3 mm to 3 cm. A translucent quality is commonly present, even in the darkly pigmented types. A papular border may provide a clue to the correct diagnosis (Figs. 31-1 and 31-2).

HISTOPATHOLOGY

The tumor is characterized by lobules of basaloid cells associated with melanin pigment that may be present either in the tumor lobules, in the tumor stroma, or both.

DIFFERENTIAL DIAGNOSIS

Pigmented basal cell carcinoma must be distinguished primarily from superficial spreading or nodular malignant melanoma. Complete removal for histologic examination is usually necessary for definitive diagnosis.

MANAGEMENT

For small lesions, excision. For large lesions, a diagnostic biopsy and then treatment with cryosurgery or electrocautery.

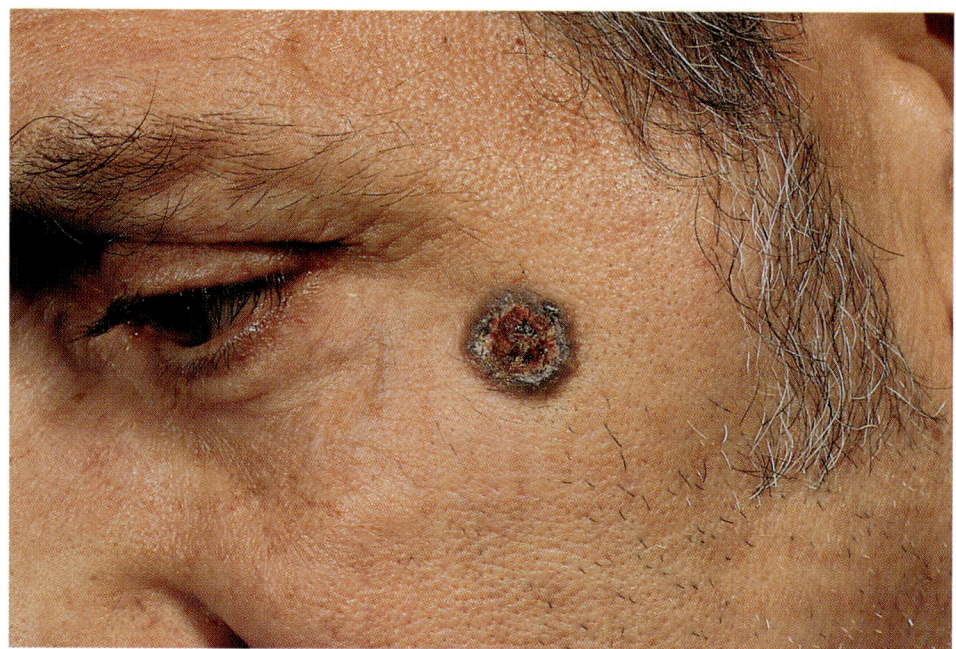

Figure 31-1 *Pigmented basal cell carcinoma. This well-circumscribed, bluish-black nodule demonstrates central ulceration. Such a lesion may be impossible to differentiate from melanoma without histologic examination.*

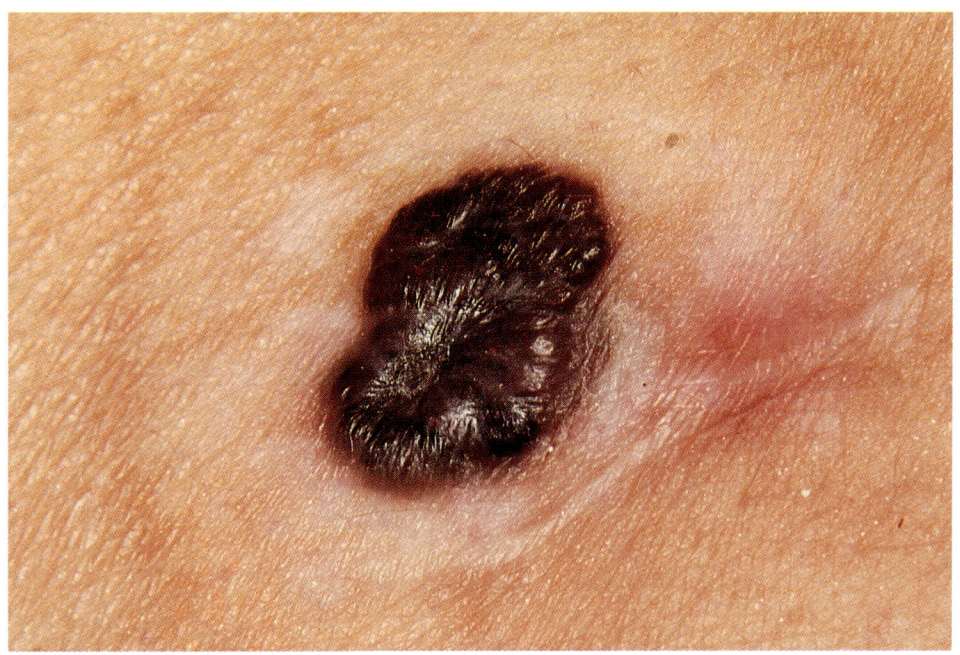

Figure 31-2 *Pigmented basal cell carcinoma. This lobular blue-black tumor is also indistinguishable from nodular melanoma.*

ADDITIONAL READINGS

Bleehen SS: Pigmented basal cell epithelioma: Light and electron microscopic studies on tumors and cell cultures. *Br J Dermatol* **93**:361, 1975

Fellner, MJ, Katz JM: Pigmented basal cell cancer masquerading as superficial spreading malignant melanoma. *Arch Dermatol* **113**:946, 1976

Index

ABCDE system for melanoma recognition, 11, 12
Actinic keratosis:
  dysplastic nevi vs., 127
  lentigo maligna vs., 158, 161
  solar lentigo vs., 48
Albright's syndrome, 35–36
Angiokeratoma, 235–38
  clinical features, 235–38
  epidemiology, 235
  histopathology, 235
  nodular melanoma vs., 236, 238
Anorectal melanoma, 206, 207
Antibodies, melanoma, halo nevus and, 95
Atypical nevus. *See also* Dysplastic nevus.
  melanoma risk and, 7, 8
Auflickmikroskopie. *See* Epiluminescence.

Basal cell carcinoma, pigmented, 241–43
  clinical features, 241–43
  differential diagnosis and management, 241
  epidemiology, 241
  histopathology, 241
Bathing-trunk nevus. *See* Congenital melanocytic nevus.
Becker's melanosis, 39–41
  associated abnormalities, 41
  biologic behavior and prognosis, 41
  clinical features, 39–41
  differential diagnosis, 41

Becker's melanosis (*cont.*):
  epidemiology and etiology, 39
  histologic features, 41
  management, 41
Benign pigmented lesions, 29–106
B-K mole. *See* Dysplastic nevus.
Black-ray, 12–13
Bloom's syndrome, 35
Blue nevus, 75–81
  biologic behavior and prognosis, 79
  cellular, 75, 77, 80, 81
  clinical features, 75–76
  combined, 75–76, 79
  common, 75–79
  differential diagnosis, 80–81
  epidemiology and etiology, 75
  halo, 98–99
  histologic features, 76–79
  malignant, 76
  management, 81
  Ota's nevus vs., 73
  plaque-type, 75, 79
Border characteristics, 10–11
Bowen's disease, 175

Café au lait macules, 33–36
  associated diseases, 34–36
  Becker's melanosis vs., 41
  clinical and histologic features, 33
  differential diagnosis, 36
  epidemiology and etiology, 33
  management, 36
  melanocytic nevi vs., 86
  nevus spilus and, 102
  Ota's nevus vs., 73

Capillary hemangioma, lobular, 231
Carcinoma, basal cell, pigmented, 241–43
 clinical features, 241–43
 differential diagnosis and management, 241
 epidemiology, 241
 histopathology, 241
Cardiocutaneous syndrome, 56
Cardiomyopathic lentiginosis, 56
Carney's syndrome. See Ephelides.
Centrofacial lentiginosis, 62
Chronic limb melanoma, 217, 220
Clark's nevus. See Dysplastic nevus.
Coloration of lesion, 11–12
Comedo-like opening of seborrheic keratosis, 228
Compound nevus, 83
 clinical features, 84, 86–89
 differential diagnosis, 86
 dysplastic, 125, 129, 131
 "fried-egg," 124, 125
 halo around, 97, 98
 of nail bed, 92
Congenital melanocytic nevus, 135–42
 biologic behavior, 138–39
 clinical features, 135–37
 differential diagnosis, 139–40
 epidemiology and etiology, 135
 giant, 136, 139–41
 histopathologic features, 137–38
 management, 140–41
 melanoma and, 138–42
 nodules, 136, 139, 142
 satellite, 136, 141
Conjunctiva:
 melanoma of, 206
 melanosis of, 54
Cost containment, ELM and, 21–23
Cronkhite-Canada syndrome, 62
Cysts, of seborrheic keratosis:
 horn, 225, 230
 milia-like, 228

Depigmentation:
 halo nevus, 95
 melanoma and, 215–17
Dermal melanocyte hamartoma, 72
Dermal melanocytoma. See Blue nevus.
Dermal melanocytosis, 72
 congenital. See Mongolian spot.
Dermal nevus, 83
 clinical features, 84, 90–91
Dermatofibroma, 233
Dermoscopy. See Epiluminescence microscopy.
Desmoplastic melanoma. See Melanoma, desmoplastic.
Diagnosis, 3–13
 ELM enhancement of, 18
 nonmelanocytic pigmented lesions and, 223–43
 remote, telemedicine and, 25
Dubreuilh's melanosis. See Melanoma, lentigo maligna.
Dysplastic nevus, 123–33
 actinic keratosis vs., 127
 biologic behavior, 127
 clinical features, 9, 124–26
 compound, 125, 129, 131
 differential diagnosis, 127
 epidemiology, 123–24
 etiology, 124
 extensive numbers of, 125, 126
 follow-up and photography, 130
 "fried-egg," 124, 125
 halo nevi vs., 98
 histopathologic features, 126–27
 junctional, 126
 management, 127–30
 melanocytic nevi vs., 87
 recurrent, 110
 melanoma risk and, 7, 8
 melanoma vs., superficial spreading, 171
 seborrheic keratosis vs., 127
 variegated, 124, 131–33

Eccrine poroma, 183
ELM. *See* Epiluminescence microscopy.
Ephelides, 29–32
   biologic behavior and prognosis, 29–30
   CALM vs., 36
   clinical and histologic features, 29
   differential diagnosis, 30–31
   epidemiology and etiology, 29
   management, 31
   melanocytic nevi vs., 86
   solar lentigines vs., 48, 50
Epidermal nevus:
   Becker's melanosis vs., 41
   CALM vs., 36
Epiluminescence microscopy (ELM), 15–25
   definition, 15
   diagnosis enhanced by, 18
   grading protocol for, 20–21
   network pattern of pigment and, 15–18
   risk stratification by, 19–24
      for cost containment, 21–24
      for melanoma screening, 19–21
   steps in assessment by, 18–19
   telemedicine and, 24
Epithelioid-cell nevus. *See* Spindle- and epithelioid-cell nevus.
Epithelioma, basal cell, 241–43
Eschar, nodular melanoma, 179
Examination of skin, 6
   sidelighting, 12
   Wood's lamp, 12–13
Eye:
   melanoma of, 206
   Ota's nevus and, 70, 71

Family history, 6
FAMM mole. *See* Dysplastic nevus.
Fibrous dysplasia, polyostotic, 35, 36
Fibrous histiocytoma, sclerosing hemangioma and, 233–34

Freckles. *See* Ephelides.
   Hutchinson's. *See* Melanoma, lentigo maligna.
   senile. *See* Solar lentigo.
"Fried-egg" compound nevus, 124, 125

Garment nevus. *See* Congenital melanocytic nevus.
Genital lentiginosis, 53–54. *See also* Lentigo simplex.
Giant hairy nevus. *See* Congenital melanocytic nevus.
Giant pigmented nevus. *See* Congenital melanocytic nevus.
Granuloma:
   pyogenic, 231–32
   telangiectaticum, 231
Growth:
   radial. *See* Radial growth.
   vertical. *See* Vertical growth phase.

Hairiness, Becker's melanosis and, 39
Hairy nevus, giant. *See* Congenital melanocytic nevus.
Halo melanoma, 211, 215
Halo nevus, 95–99
   biologic behavior, 96–99
   clinical features, 96
   congenital vs. acquired, 98
   differential diagnosis, 98–99
   epidemiology, 95
   etiology, 95–96
   histopathology, 96
   management, 99
   melanoma vs., 211
Hamartoma:
   Becker's pigmentary. *See* Becker's melanosis.
   dermal melanocyte, 72
Hemangioma, 184–85
   lobular capillary, 231
   sclerosing, 233
   thrombosed, 238

Histiocytoma, fibrous, sclerosing hemangioma and, 233–34
Histomorphology, 15
History, 3–6
　family, 6
Horn cysts, seborrheic keratosis and, 225, 230
Hutchinson's melanotic freckle. See Melanoma, lentigo maligna.
Hutchinson's sign, 187, 194, 195
Hypermelanotic lentigo, 43
Hypertrichosis, Becker's melanosis and, 39
Hypopigmentation, melanoma and, 215–17

Immune response, halo nevi and, 95
Incident-light microscopy. See Epiluminescence microscopy.
"Ink spot" lentigo, 43
Intradermal nevi. See Dermal nevus.
Ito's nevus, 72

Jadassohn-Tièche nevus. See Blue nevus.
Junctional nevus, 83
　clinical features, 84, 85
　differential diagnosis, 86
　dysplastic, 126

Keratosis:
　actinic. See Actinic keratosis.
　seborrheic. See Seborrheic keratosis.

LAMB syndrome, 62
　vulvar lentigines and, 62
Laugier-Hunzider syndrome, 62
Lentigines. See Lentigo.
Lentiginosis, 53
　cardiomyopathic, 56
　centrofacial, 62

Lentiginosis (*cont.*):
　eruptive, 62
　generalized, 54, 56
　genital, 53–54. See also Lentigo simplex.
　inherited patterned, 62
　localized, 62
　partial unilateral, 62
　perigenitoaxillaris, 62
　segmental, 105
　syndrome of, 56
Lentiginous nevus, speckled. See Nevus spilus.
Lentigo:
　ephelides vs., 30–31
　generalized, 54, 56
　hypermelanotic, 43
　"ink spot," 43
　labial (lip), 53, 56, 61
　maligna, 153–61
　　clinical features, 153
　　desmoplastic melanoma and, 199, 202
　　differential diagnosis, 158
　　epidemiology and etiology, 153
　　melanoma. See Melanoma, lentigo maligna.
　　Ota's nevus vs., 73
　　solar lentigo vs., 48
　melanoma vs., 188
　multiple, 56–57
　penile, 54, 58
　PUVA-induced, 47
　senilis. See Solar lentigo.
　simplex, 53–62
　　associated syndromes, 56–57, 62
　　biologic behavior and prognosis, 56
　　clinical features, 54
　　differential diagnosis, 57–59
　　epidemiology, 53–54
　　etiology, 54
　　histologic features, 54–55
　　management and follow-up, 59

Lentigo (cont.):
  simplex (cont.):
    melanocytic nevus vs., 58, 86
    melanoma vs., 58–59
    solar lentigo vs., 58
    sunburn, 43, 44
    vulvar, 57, 59
LEOPARD syndrome, 56–57, 60
Leukoderma:
  acquisitum centrifugum. See Halo nevus.
  melanoma-associated, 215–17
Limb melanoma, chronic, 217, 220
Lip, lentigo of, 53, 56, 61
Liver spot. See Solar lentigo.
Lobular capillary hemangioma, 231

Macules, 11
  café au lait. See Café au lait macules.
  melanotic, 53
Melanoblasts, nevi and, 83
Melanocytes:
  blue nevus and, 76–77
  in CALM, 33
  in ephelides, 29
  Mongolian spot and, 66
  Ota's nevus and, 71–72
  solar lentigo and, 43, 46
Melanocytic lesions:
  benign, 29–106
  cost-containment for, risk stratification and, 24
  diagnosis, 3–13
  hyperplastic, 53. See also Lentigo simplex.
  morphologic assessment, 6–13
  network pattern in, 15–21
  nevi. See Nevus, melanocytic; also specific nevi.
Melanocytoma, dermal. See also Blue nevus.

Melanocytosis:
  dermal, 72
    acquired, 73
    congenital. See Mongolian spot.
  oculodermal. See Ota's nevus.
Melanoma:
  ABCDE system for, 11, 12
  acral lentiginous, 187–96
    amelanotic type, 193
    clinical features, 187
    differential diagnosis, 188
    epidemiology and etiology, 187
    histopathologic features, 187–88
    radial growth phase, 187–89
    regression, 189, 190
    ulceration, 193, 196
    variegation of color, 190, 191, 194
    vertical growth phase, 192
  anorectal, 206, 207
  antibodies to, halo nevus and, 95
  blue nevus and, 76, 80
  changes associated with, 5, 6
  chronic limb, 217, 220
  classification of, 146
  clinical characteristics, 9
  congenital melanocytic nevus and, 138–42
  conjunctival, 206
  desmoplastic, 199–204
    biologic course, 200–01
    clinical/histopathologic features, 199
    differential diagnosis, 199–200
    epidemiology and etiology, 199
    management, 201
    metastases, 200–01
  diagnostic guidelines, 3
  dysplastic nevi and, 123–25, 127, 129, 133
  epidemiology, 145–46
  halo, 211, 215
  halo nevus vs., 98
  history-taking guide, 149
  in situ, 146, 163

Index 249

Melanoma (cont.):
  lentigo maligna, 153–61
    biologic course, 158
    clinical features, 153
    desmoplastic melanoma and, 202
    differential diagnosis, 158
    epidemiology and etiology, 153
    histopathologic features, 153
    radial growth phase, 153, 158, 159
    regression phenomenon, 154–56
    of sole. See acral lentiginous subentry above.
    variegation of color, 153, 154, 156, 158–60
    vertical growth phase, 153, 160
  lentigo simplex vs., 58–59
  leukoderma associated with, 215–17
  management, 148–50
  melanocytic nevus and, 85
  melanosis associated with, 211, 215, 216
  metastases from, 146, 217
    chronic limb melanoma, 217, 220
    desmoplastic, 200–201
  mucocutaneous, 205–9
    biologic behavior, 206–7
    clinical features, 205–6
    differential diagnosis, 207
    epidemiology and etiology, 205
    histopathology, 206
    management, 207
  natural history, 146–47
  neurotropic, 199, 200. See also desmoplastic subentry above.
  nevus spilus and, 102, 211, 214
  nodular, 177–85
    amelanotic, 182
    pyogenic granuloma vs., 232
    angiokeratoma vs., 236, 238
    carcinoma vs., basal cell, 242, 243
    clinical/histopathologic features, 177
    differential diagnosis, 177
    epidemiology and etiology, 177
    ulceration, 179, 182

Melanoma (cont.):
  nonmelanocytic pigmented lesions vs., 223–43
  oral, 205
    differential diagnosis, 207
    lentigo simplex and, 53
  pagetoid spread of, 166
  periungual, 187, 194–95
  photographic recording of evolution of, 211, 212–14
  physical examination guide, 150
  precursors, 121–42
  prevention, 150
  pseudopods, 169, 170
  pyogenic lesion, 218
  radial growth of, 146
    acral lentiginous melanoma, 187–89
    lentigo maligna melanoma, 153, 158, 159
  recurrent, 217–19
    recurrent melanocytic nevus vs., 110
    scar and, 219
    ulcerated, 218
  risk factors for, 4
    algorithm for, 145
    atypical (dysplastic) nevi and, 7, 8
    checklist for, 4
    general assessment of, 6–8
    numbers of nevi and, 7, 9
    stratification of, 5
    ELM and, 19–21
  satellites of, 146
  spindle- and epithelioid-cell nevus and, 115, 118
  Spitz's juvenile. See Spindle- and epithelioid-cell nevus.
  staging, 148
  subungual, 194–96
    differential diagnosis, 188
  sunlight and, 150
  superficial spreading, 163–75
    clinical features, 166

Melanoma (*cont.*):
  superficial spreading (*cont.*):
    differential diagnosis, 171
    epidemiology and etiology, 163–66
    evolution of, 212–14
    histopathologic features, 166–71
    radial growth phase, 166–71
    variegation in color of, 163, 165–67, 172–74
    vertical growth phase, 166, 172–74
  surgical guidelines for, 149, 151
  survival probabilities and, 147
  ulceration, 217, 218
    acral lentiginous melanoma, 193, 196
    nodular melanoma, 179, 182
  unusual presentation of, 211–20
  vertical growth of, 146
    acral lentiginous melanoma, 192
    lentigo maligna melanoma, 153, 160
    superficial spreading melanoma, 166, 172–74
  vulvar, 205, 208
Melanonychia striata, 188, 194
Melanosis, 53
  Becker's (nevoid). *See* Becker's melanosis.
  bulbi, congenital. *See* Ota's nevus.
  Dubreuilh's. *See* Melanoma, lentigo maligna.
  Hutchinson's. *See* Melanoma, lentigo maligna.
  melanoma with, 211, 215, 216
  oculi, progressive, *See* Ota's nevus.
Melanosomes, solar lentigo and, 43, 46
Melanuria, 215
Melasma:
  CALM vs., 36
  Ota's nevus vs., 73
Metastases, 146, 217
  chronic limb, 217, 220

Metastases (*cont.*):
  desmoplastic, 200–201
  in-transit, 217
  satellite, 217
Mibelli's angiokeratoma, 235
Microscopy, epiluminescence, 15–25
Milia-like cysts of seborrheic keratosis, 228
Mole. *See* Nevus, melanocytic, acquired.
  B-K. *See* Dysplastic nevi.
  FAMM. *See* Dysplastic nevi.
Mongolian spot, 65–67
  biologic behavior and prognosis, 67
  clinical features, 65–66
  differential diagnosis, 67
  epidemiology and etiology, 65
  histologic features, 66
  management, 67
  nevus of Ota and, 66, 67, 73
  Wood's lamp examination, 66
Morphologic assessment, 6–13
Mucosa:
  melanoma of. *See* Melanoma, mucocutaneous.
  melanotic macules of. *See* Lentigo simplex.
Mucocutaneous melanoma. *See* Melanoma, mucocutaneous.

Nail bed, melanocytic nevi of, 84, 92
Nails, melanoma of, 187, 188, 194–96
Network, pigment, 15–21
  lentigo maligna melanoma and, 154, 156
  superficial spreading melanoma, 165, 170
Neurofibromatosis, CALM and, 33, 34
Neuronevus, blue. *See* Blue nevus.
Neurotropic melanoma, 199, 200. *See also* Melanoma, desmoplastic.
Nevocellular nevus. *See* Nevus, melanocytic, acquired.

Nevomelanocytic nevus, congenital. *See* Congenital melanocytic nevus.
Nevus (nevi):
  with architectural disorder and cytologic atypia. *See* Dysplastic nevus.
  atypical. *See* Dysplastic nevus.
  bathing-trunk. *See* Congenital melanocytic nevus.
  Becker's. *See* Becker's melanosis.
  blue. *See* Blue nevus.
  Clark's. *See* Dysplastic nevus.
  compound. *See* Compound nevus.
  dermal. *See* Dermal nevus.
  dysplastic. *See* Dysplastic nevus.
  epithelioid-cell. *See* Spindle- and epithelioid-cell nevus.
  fuscocaeruleus acromiodeltoideus, 72
  fuscocaeruleus ophthalmomaxillaris. *See* Ota's nevus.
  fuscocaeruleus zygomaticus, 72–73
  garment. *See* Congenital melanocytic nevus.
  genital, 53. *See also* Lentigo simplex.
  giant hairy. *See* Congenital melanocytic nevus.
  giant pigmented. *See* Congenital melanocytic nevus.
  halo. *See* Halo nevus.
  intradermal. *See* Dermal nevus.
  of Ito, 72
  junctional. *See* Junctional nevus.
  melanocytic. *See also specific nevi.*
    acquired, 9, 83–92
      biologic behavior, 85
      clinical features, 84
      differential diagnosis, 85–87
      epidemiology, 83
      etiology, 83–84
      histologic features, 84
      management, 87
    acral lentiginous melanoma vs., 188

Nevus (nevi) (*cont.*):
  melanocytic (*cont.*):
    Becker's melanosis vs., 41
    CALM vs., 36
    congenital. *See* Congenital melanocytic nevus.
    dysplastic. *See* Dysplastic nevus.
    halo nevus and, 96
    lentigo simplex vs., 58
    of nail bed, 84, 92
    recurrent, 109–10
      clinical and histologic features, 109
      differential diagnosis, 110
      epidemiology and etiology, 109
      management, 110
  nevocellular. *See* Nevus, melanocytic, acquired.
  nevomelanocytic, 75–76
    congenital. *See* Congenital melanocytic nevus.
    epithelioid cell-spindle cell. *See* Spindle- and epithelioid-cell nevus.
  of Ota. *See* Ota's nevus.
  phenotype for, 6–7, 9
  pigmentosus et pilosus. *See* Congenital melanocytic nevus.
  spilus, 101–3
    biologic behavior, 101–2
    clinical features, epidemiology, etiology, and histopathology, 101
    differential diagnosis, 102
    management, 102
    melanoma arising in, 211, 214
    Ota's nevus vs., 73
    segmental lentiginosis vs., 105
  spindle-cell. *See* Spindle- and epithelioid-cell nevus.
    pigmented. *See* Spindle-cell nevus, pigmented.
  Spitz. *See also* Spindle- and epithelioid-cell nevus.

Nevus (nevi) (*cont.*):
　Spitz (*cont.*):
　　malignant, 115
　　pigmented variant of. *See* Spindle-cell nevus, pigmented.
　Sun's, 72–73
　Sutton's. *See* Halo nevus.
　tardive, congenital, 135
Nodular melanoma. *See* Melanoma, nodular.
Nonmelanocytic pigmented lesions in differential diagnosis of melanoma, 223–43

Oculodermal melanocytosis. *See* Ota's nevus.
Oil-immersion microscopy, 15–25
Old age spot. *See* Solar lentigo.
Oral melanoma, 205
　differential diagnosis, 207
　lentigo simplex and, 53
Ota's nevus, 69–73
　associated abnormalities, 72–73
　biologic behavior and prognosis, 72
　clinical features, 69–71
　differential diagnosis, 73
　epidemiology and etiology, 69
　histologic features, 71–72
　management and follow-up, 73
　Mongolian spot and, 66, 67

Pagetoid spread of melanoma, 166
Palmar melanoma. *See* Melanoma, acral lentiginous.
Papules, 11
Penile lentigo, 54, 58
Perinevoid vitiligo. *See* Halo nevus.
Periungual melanoma, 187, 194–95
Peutz-Jeghers syndrome, 57, 61
Phenotype, nevus, 6–7, 9
Photography:
　atypical nevi and, 130

Photography (*cont.*):
　serial, of melanoma evolution, 211, 212–14
Phototype, 10
Phyophotodermatitis, CALM vs., 36
Pigment network, 15–21. *See also* Network, pigment.
Plantar melanoma. *See* Melanoma, acral lentiginous.
Polyostotic fibrous dysplasia, 35, 36
Poroma, eccrine, 183
Postinflammatory hyperpigmentation, CALM vs., 36
Pseudomelanoma. *See* Nevus, melanocytic, recurrent.
Pseudopods, melanoma, 169, 170
Psoralen, ultraviolet A plus, lentigo and, 47
Pulmonic stenosis, lentigines induced by, 47
PUVA, lentigines induced by, 47
Pyogenic granuloma, 231–32
　clinical/histopathologic features, 231, 232
　differential diagnosis, 231
　epidemiology and etiology, 231
　management, 231
Pyogenic melanoma, 218

Radial growth, 19, 21
　acral lentiginous melanoma, 187–89
　lentigo maligna melanoma, 153, 158, 159
　streaming, 181
　superficial spreading melanoma, 166–71
Rectal melanoma, 206, 207
Recurrent melanocytic nevus. *See* Nevus, melanocytic, recurrent.
Reed's pigmented spindle-cell tumor. *See* Spindle-cell nevus, pigmented.

Risk factors (for melanoma), 4
  algorithm for, 145
  atypical (dysplastic) nevi and, 7, 8
  checklist for, 4
  general assessment of, 6–8
  numbers of nevi and, 7, 9
  stratification of, 5
    ELM and, 19–21

Satellitosis, 217
Scar, melanoma recurrence and, 219
Sclerosing hemangioma, 233–34
  clinical findings, 233, 234
  differential diagnosis, 233
  epidemiology and etiology, 233
  histopathology, 233
  management, 233
Sclerosis, tuberous, 35
Screening, risk stratification for, 19–21
Seborrheic keratosis, 225–30
  clinical/histopathologic features, 225
  color variation of, 226
  comedo-like openings of, 228
  differential diagnosis, 225, 230
  dysplastic nevi vs., 127
  epidemiology and etiology, 225
  management, 230
  melanocytic nevi vs., 86
  melanoma vs., superficial, 171
  milia-like cysts of, 228
  pigment network of, 228
  "stuck-on" appearance of, 226
SECN. *See* Spindle- and epithelioid-cell nevus.
Segmental lentiginosis, 105
Senile freckle. *See* Solar lentigo.
Sidelighting, 12
Silver-Russell syndrome, 35
Size of lesion, 10
Solar lentigo, 43–50
  associated diseases, 47–48
  biologic behavior and prognosis, 46
  CALM vs., 31, 36

Solar lentigo, (*cont.*):
  clinical features, 43
  differential diagnosis, 48
  ephelides vs., 48, 50
  epidemiology and etiology, 43
  histologic features, 43–46
  lentigo simplex vs., 58
  management, 49
  xeroderma pigmentosum and, 48, 49
Sole, lentigo maligna melanoma of. *See* Melanoma, acral lentiginous.
Speckled lentiginous nevus. *See* Nevus spilus.
Spindle cell(s):
  blue nevi and, 77, 79
  desmoplastic melanoma and, 199
Spindle-cell nevus, pigmented (PSCN), 117–19
  biologic behavior, 118
  clinical features, 117
  differential diagnosis, 118–19
  epidemiology and etiology, 117
  histopathology, 117–18
  management, 119
Spindle- and epithelioid-cell nevus (SECN), 113–16
  agminated (grouped), 16
  biologic course, 114–15
  clinical features, 113–14
  differential diagnosis, 116
  epidemiology and etiology, 113
  halo nevus vs., 99
  histopathology, 114
  malignant, 115
  management, 116
Spitz nevus (tumor or juvenile melanoma). *See also* Spindle- and epithelioid-cell nevus.
  malignant, 115
  pigmented variant of. *See* Spindle-cell nevus, pigmented.
Staging of melanoma, 148
Stratification of risk, 5
  ELM and, 19–21

Subungual melanoma, 187, 194–96.
  See also Melanoma, acral lentiginous.
  differential diagnosis, 188
Sunburn lentigo, 43, 44
Sunlight:
  ephelides and, 29, 31
  melanoma prevention and, 150
Sun's nevus, 72–73
Surface profile, 11
Sutton's nevus. *See* Halo nevus.
Symmetry, 10

Telemedicine, 25
Thrombosis, hemangioma, 238
Tisch nodules, 35
Topography, 11
Trigeminal nerve, nevus of Ota and, 70
Tuberous sclerosis, 35
Tyndall phenomenon, 65

Ulceration:
  acral lentiginous melanoma, 193, 196
  basal cell carcinoma, 242
  nodular melanoma, 179, 182
  pyogenic granuloma, 232
  recurrent melanoma, 217
Ultraviolet A, psoralen plus, lentigines induced by, 47

Venous lake, 238
Verruca, seborrheic. *See* Seborrheic keratosis.
Vertical growth phase (of melanoma):
  acral lentiginous, 192
  lentigo maligna, 153, 160
  superficial spreading, 166, 172–74
Vitiligo, perinevoid, 95. *See also* Halo nevus.
von Recklinghausen's disease, CALM and, 33, 34
Vulva:
  lentigines of, 57, 58
  melanoma of, 205, 208

Wart, seborrheic. *See* Seborrheic keratosis.
Watson's syndrome, 35
Westerhof's syndrome, 35
Wood's lamp, 12–13
  Mongolian spot and, 66

Xeroderma pigmentation, solar lentigines and, 47, 49

Zosteriform lentiginous nevus. *See* Nevus spilus.

ISBN 0-07-005110-0